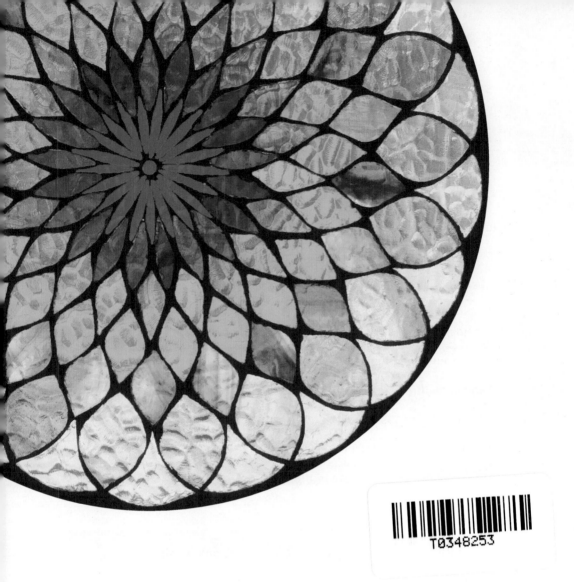

CRITICAL CONVERSATIONS FOR PATIENT SAFETY

An Essential Guide for Healthcare Students

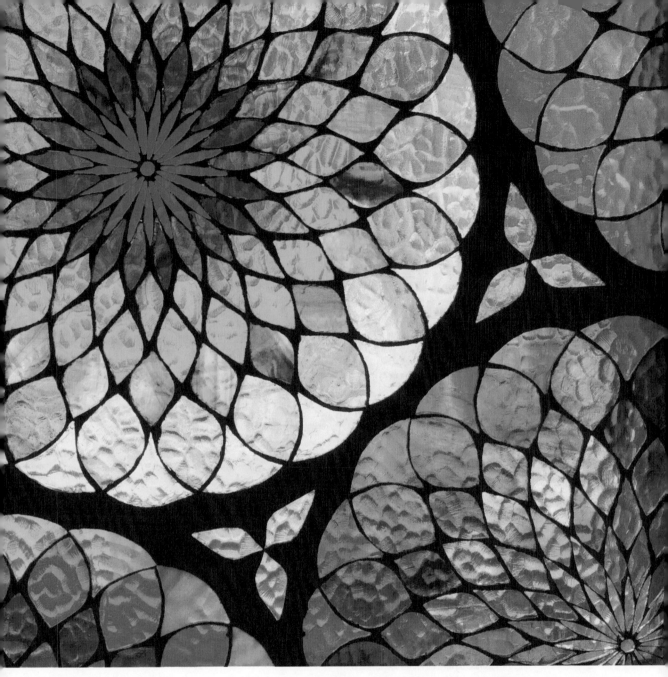

CRITICAL CONVERSATIONS
FOR PATIENT SAFETY

An Essential Guide for Healthcare Students

SECOND EDITION

Edited by **Tracy Levett-Jones**

Pearson Australia
707 Collins Street
Melbourne VIC 3008

www.pearson.com.au

Senior Portfolio Manager: Mandy Sheppard
Development Editor: Judith Bamber
Senior Project Manager: Bronwyn Smith
Production Manager: Linda Chryssavgis
External Production Manager: Rakhshinda Chishty, iEnergizer Aptara®, Ltd.
Product Manager: Erin Nixon
Content Developer: Stephen Razos
Senior Rights and Permissions Editor: Lisa Woodland
External Rights and Permissions Editors: Integra Software Services
Lead Editor/Copy Editor: Sandra Goodall
Proofreader: iEnergizer Aptara®, Ltd.
Indexer: iEnergizer Aptara®, Ltd.
Cover and internal design by Pier Vido Design
Cover artwork by Siobhan Allen
Typeset by iEnergizer Aptara®, Ltd.

Printed in Australia by the SOS Print + Media Group

ISBN 9781488623004

1 2 3 4 5 24 23 22 21 20

A catalogue record for this book is available from the National Library of Australia

Pearson Australia Group Pty Ltd   ABN 40 004 245 943

Contents

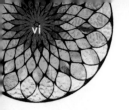

About the editor

Tracy Levett-Jones is Professor of Nursing Education at the University of Technology Sydney. Her program of research focuses on patient safety, empathy, belongingness, clinical reasoning, interprofessional education, cultural competence and simulation. Tracy has authored 10 books as well as over 200 chapters and journal articles. She has been the recipient of over three million dollars of research funding and multiple awards including an Australian Learning and Teaching Council Award for Teaching Excellence, a NSW Minister for Education and Training Quality Teaching Award, and a Pearson/Australian Nurse Teacher Society Nurse Educator of the Year Award.

Web profile: <http://www.proftlj.com/>
Twitter: @Prof_TLJ

Patient stories

Stories define:
Who we are.
Where we have come from.
Where we are going ... and
What we care about.

Stories give life!

Dana Winslow Atchley III, artist, storyteller and musician, 1941–2000

This book presents a montage of real patient stories.[3] A montage combines several contrasting and complementary stories to make a composite textual whole. Stories relate the unfolding of events, human action and feelings, and it is through stories that people make sense of their own views, values and experiences, as well as those of others. The stories included in each chapter of *Critical Conversations* are designed to bring the book to life and illustrate the key learning outcomes.

We hope you enjoy reading *Critical Conversations for Patient Safety, 2nd edition,* and that it helps you to reflect on your own performance and develop the critical conversation skills that are fundamental to safe, effective and person-centred care.

Tracy Levett-Jones and the *Critical Conversations* writing team

---

3   Throughout this book pseudonyms have been used for most of the stories except where permission has been given to use actual names.

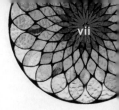

Contributors

Ms Helen Buchanan, RM RN, MFamStud. (Masters of Family Studies)
Registered Midwife, John Hunter Hospital

Dr Anne Croker, PhD, BAppSc (Physio), GradDipPubHealth
Research Fellow, The University of Newcastle Department of Rural Health

Sue Dean, RN, BA (Community Social Services), MA (Women's Health),
Grad. Dip Adult Ed, Grad. Cert Diab. Ed & Mngt.
Senior Lecturer, Faculty of Health, University of Technology Sydney

Dr Deborah Debono, PhD, BA (Psych Hons), RN, RM
Senior Lecturer, Faculty of Health, University of Technology Sydney

Dr Tania De Bortoli, BAppSc (Speech Pathology), BA (Hons) PhD
Sessional Lecturer, Charles Sturt University; Private Practitioner

Dr Lyn Ebert, PhD, RN, RM, NN, Grad Dip VET, MN, MPhil
Senior Lecturer, Deputy Head of School-Education, Head of Discipline-Midwifery
School of Nursing and Midwifery, Faculty of Health and Medicine, The University of Newcastle

Mr Wayne Farmer, B Clinical Sc, B Chiropractic Sc, Ass Dip Health Sc
Resolution Officer, NSW Health Care Complaints Commission

Dr Conor Gilligan, PhD, B.BiomedSci (Hons)
Senior Lecturer in Health Behaviour Science, School of Medicine and Public Health, The University of Newcastle

Dr Miriam Grotowski, B.Med, FRACGP, DipPsychiatryED
General Practitioner, Senior Lecturer, The University of Newcastle Department of Rural Health

Professor Colleen Hayward, DipTch B Ed B Sc Grad Cert (Cross Sector Partnerships)
Pro-Vice Chancellor (Equity and Indigenous), Edith Cowan University

Lyza Helps, RN, MN Mental Health, PhD candidate
School of Nursing and Midwifery, Flinders University

Toni Hoffman, RN, BN, RM, Master of Bioethics, Grad Cert Management
Lecturer, School of Nursing, Midwifery and Social Sciences, CQUniversity

Dr Graeme Horton, MB BS MEnvStud GDipRural FRACGP FARGP
Senior Lecturer in Medical Education and General Practice, School of Medicine and Public Health,
The University of Newcastle

Professor Ashley Kable, PhD, RN, Dip Teach Nurs Ed, Grad Dip Health Service Management
School of Nursing and Midwifery, The University of Newcastle

Professor Tracy Levett-Jones, PhD, RN, MEd & Work, BN, DipAppSc (Nursing)
Professor of Nursing Education, Faculty of Health, University of Technology Sydney

Dr Joanne Lewis, RN, MPallC, PhD
Senior Lecturer, Faculty of Health, University of Technology Sydney

Professor Elizabeth Manias, RN CertCritCare BPharm MPharm MNurs PhD FACN(DLF) MPSA MSHPA
School of Nursing and Midwifery, Deakin University

Dr Daniel McAullay, BSc, MAE & PhD
Director CRE Improving health services for Aboriginal and Torres Strait Islander children,
The University of Western Australia

Dr Rebekkah Middleton, PhD, RN, MN(Res), Grad Cert Emergency Nursing, Grad Cert Clinical Management
Senior Lecturer, Academic Program Director, School of Nursing, University of Wollongong

Professor Tracey Moroney, PhD, BN (Hons) Grad Cert Ed Studies
Head of School, School of Nursing, University of Wollongong

Dr Jonathan Mould, PhD, MSc, RSCN, RGN, RMN, Adult Cert Ed
Simulation Coordinator, Ramsay Health

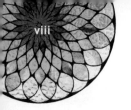

Professor Eimear Muir-Cochrane, BSc (Hons) RN, Grad Dip Adult Education MNS, PhD Credentialled MHN
Professor of Nursing (Mental Health), School of Nursing and Midwifery, Flinders University

Mrs Deb O'Kane, RN, ENB603 GradDip CN MN Grad Cert HE
Lecturer (Mental Health), School of Nursing and Midwifery, Faculty of Health Sciences, Flinders University

Associate Professor Sue Outram, PhD, RN, BA
School of Medicine and Public Health, The University of Newcastle

Ms Lorinda Palmer, MN, RN, BSc., Dip. Ed, Grad Dip (Nurs), PhD candidate
Lecturer, The School of Nursing & Midwifery, The University of Newcastle

Professor Deborah Parker, PhD, MSocSc, Grad Cert (Exec Leadership), RN
Professor of Nursing Aged Care (Dementia), Faculty of Health, University of Technology Sydney

Dr Victoria Pitt, PhD, MNur (Research), Grad Dip Nurs (Pal.care), Grad Cert Tert Teaching,
Dip ApSc (Nursing)
Lecturer, School of Nursing & Midwifery, The University of Newcastle

Professor Dimity Pond, BA Dip Ed MBBS FRACGP PhD
Professor of General Practice, School of Medicine and Public Health, The University of Newcastle

Professor Kerry Reid-Searl, RN, RM, BHlth Sc, Mclin Ed, PhD
Director of Simulation, Deputy Head of Program, School of Nursing, Midwifery and Social Sciences, CQUniversity

Associate Professor Rachel Rossiter, D.HSc, RN, MN (NP), M.Counselling, B.Counselling, B.HlthSc
School of Nursing, Midwifery & Indigenous Health, Charles Sturt University

Professor Cobie Rudd, PhD, MPH, BHlthSc(N), RN
Deputy Vice-Chancellor (Strategic Partnerships), Edith Cowan University

Dr Carla Saunders, PhD, MMedSc (Epi), BSc DipEd, Grad Cert HSM, Grad Cert Neuro, RN
Lecturer, Faculty of Health, University of Technology Sydney

Ms Robin Scott, MClinSc (MentalHNurs) RN, MACN, MACMHN, CPMHN(C)
Sessional Academic, School of Nursing, Midwifery & Indigenous Health, Charles Sturt University

Associate Professor Moira Sim, MBBS, FRACGP, FAChAM, PGDipAlcDrugAbStud
Executive Dean, School of Medical and Health Sciences, Edith Cowan University

Stephen Spencer, B Nurs (Hons), RN, PhD
Clinical Nurse Specialist, John Hunter Hospital

Dr Teresa Stone, PhD, RN, RMN, BA, M Health Management, GradCert Tertiary Teaching
Visiting Professor Faculty of Nursing, Chiang Mai University, Thailand

Dr Natalie Strobel, PhD, Postgrad Dip Clin Ex Sci, Bsc
Research Fellow, The University of Western Australia

Dr Diane Tasker, B(Phty), PhD
Private Physiotherapy Practitioner

Professor Joanne Travaglia, PhD, MEd, GradDipAdEd, BSocStuds(Hons)
Professor Health Services Management, Faculty of Health, University of Technology Sydney

Dr Anna Treloar, MA MPHC RN, PhD
Lecturer, The School of Nursing and Midwifery, The University of Newcastle, MHNIP Nurse at Integral Health, Armidale

Associate Professor Pamela van der Riet, PhD, RN, MEd, BA Dip ED (Nursing), ICU/CCU cert
School of Nursing & Midwifery, The University of Newcastle

Ms Jeannette Walsh, MHSc, BSocStud, MAASW
Faculty of Arts and Social Sciences, University of New South Wales

Dr Carla Walton, B.Sc (Psyc), D.Psyc (Clin), Grad Dip Adult Psychotherapy, MAPS
Senior Clinical Psychologist, Centre for Psychotherapy, Hunter New England Mental Health Service

Dr Karen Watson, PhD, RN, BN (Hons), BHlthRN
Lecturer, Faculty of Health, University of Technology Sydney.

The publisher would like to thank and acknowledge the valuable work of the following previous contributors to the first edition of this text:

Chapter 1 The relationship between communication and patient safety
Professor Kim Oates, *Sydney Medical School*
Associate Professor Lesley MacDonald-Wicks, *The University of Newcastle*

Chapter 2 Key attributes of patient safe communication
Associate Professor Conor Gilligan, *The University of Newcastle*
Dr Sue Outram, *The University of Newcastle*
Dr Graeme Horton, *The University of Newcastle*

Chapter 3 Why do patients complain about how health professionals communicate?
Ms Katja Beitat, *NSW Health Care Complaints Commission*

Chapter 4 An historical and cultural overview of health professionals' evolving team dynamics
Dr Kerry Hoffman, *The University of Newcastle*

Chapter 5 Interpersonal communication for interprofessional collaboration
Dr Jim Croker, *Tamworth Rural Referral Hospital, and University of New England*

Chapter 6 Clinical handover
Professor - Director Rick Iedema, *Centre for Team Based Practice & Learning in Health Care Health Schools, King's College London*

Chapter 7 Open disclosure
Professor - Director Rick Iedema, *Centre for Team Based Practice & Learning in Health Care Health Schools, King's College London*

Chapter 11 Communicating with older people
Professor Isabel Higgins, *The University of Newcastle and Hunter New England Local Health District*
Professor Jane Conway, *University of New England and University of Newcastle*
Dr Carolyn Hullick, *John Hunter Hospital*
Professor Sian Maslin-Prothero, *Edith Cowan University and Sir Charles Gairdner Hospital*
Ms Jenny Day, *The University of Newcastle*
Ms Deborah Armitage, *John Hunter Hospital*
Ms Jacqueline Hewitt, *John Hunter Hospital*

Chapter 12 Communicating with children and families
Professor Cobie Rudd, *Edith Cowan University*
Professor Anne Wilkinson, *Cancer Council WA Chair and Edith Cowan University, Perth Australia*

Chapter 20 When whistle-blowing seems like the only option
Ms Kim Elkovich, *The University of Newcastle, Self Employed Consultant—A Higher Self Pty Ltd*
Dr Penny Barrett, *Warner's Bay Private Hospital*

Chapter 21 Creating safer healthcare organisations
Professor Cobie Rudd, *Edith Cowan University*
Associate Professor Owen Carter, *Edith Cowan University*
Associate Professor Jared Dart, *The University of Queensland and NHMRC Centre for Research Excellence Quality and Safety in Integrated Primary/Secondary Care*
Emeritus Professor Cindy Gallois, *The University of Queensland*
Associate Professor David Hewett, *The University of Queensland*
Catherine Stoddart, *Department of Health WA and WA Telstra Business Woman of the Year 2012*
Adjunct professor Jill Thistlethwaite, *University of Technology Sydney*
Professor Bernadette M Watson, *The Hong Kong Polytechnic University*

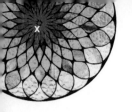

Preface

Deficiencies in healthcare communication feature in the majority of coroners' reports and quality improvement investigations and there have been repeated calls for improvement. However, over last decade studies have identified that, despite the best intentions of healthcare professionals, up to 17 per cent of patients are harmed while receiving healthcare[1] and that communication errors remain the root cause of 65 per cent of adverse outcomes.[2]

Healthcare is increasingly complex; this complexity coupled with inherent human performance limitations, even in experienced, skilled and committed healthcare professionals, means that errors will inevitably happen. However, patient-safe communication and effective teamwork can help prevent these errors from becoming consequential and harming patients. It is critically important that healthcare professionals have well-developed interprofessional communication skills, the capacity to create environments in which individuals can speak up if they have concerns, and that they share a common 'critical language' to alert team members to potentially unsafe situations. Equally important to safe healthcare is effective therapeutic communication skills, a commitment to person-centred care and the ability to recognise patients who are vulnerable and at particular risk of harm.

Critical conversations

The etymology of the word *conversation* means to share, inform and unite. It refers to the imparting or interchange of thoughts, opinions or information by speech, writing or other forms of communication. In healthcare, a 'critical conversation' is one that signals the need for immediate attention, addresses a situation that has caused (or could cause) patient (or staff) harm, or focuses attention on practices or processes that call for improvement. In essence, a 'critical conversation' is a communication interaction where important information is shared or an interchange of thoughts or opinions occurs, and that serves to unite healthcare professionals and the recipients of healthcare to achieve one common goal—improved patient safety and wellbeing.

The key aim of *Critical Conversations for Patient Safety* is the development of healthcare students' skills in safe and effective communication. Excellence in communication, including the ability to share ideas and to listen to others, is necessary to provide patients and their families with the quality healthcare that they need, deserve and expect. This requires an understanding that respect, courtesy and, above all else, empathy convert a technical interaction into a safe and caring encounter.

The stained glass images

The beautiful stained images that decorate this book are a metaphor for the collaborative approach used in its development. Just as each piece in a stained glass mosaic is beautiful in its own right, when they come together they create a magnificent work of art. In the same way, while the individual contributions, diverse disciplinary perspectives and authentic patient stories in this book each have inherent worth, together they create a rich and meaningful literary whole. And, just as viewing a scene through the different colours of stained glass transforms one's view of the world, viewing the evolving and complex nature of contemporary healthcare through a lens of patient-safe communication allows illuminative new perspectives, insights and understandings to emerge.

In writing this book, our intent was to stay true to the vision of interprofessional collaboration. In doing so, over 40 healthcare professionals and academics from different disciplines and contexts worked together to write the chapters. What became apparent is that, despite the differences in our professional roles and experiences, it was our commitment to safe and effective patient care that dominated. We shared similar views about 'what matters most' and you will see these echoing throughout the book. Person-centred care, working in partnership with patients and families, empathy, mutual respect, reflective practice, self-awareness and valuing other professions . . . these concepts resonated with each of us and are integrated throughout *Critical Conversations*. Importantly, the content of each chapter is also grounded in and informed by the authors' contemporary research in the fields of communication and patient safety.

1 Makary, M. & Daniel, M. (2016). Medical error: The third leading cause of death in the US. *British Medical Journal* (Online) 353

2 Institute for Healthcare Communication. (2018). *Impact of Communication in Healthcare*. <https://healthcarecomm.org/about-us/impact-of-communication-in-healthcare/>

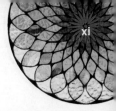

How to use this book

While there is no one way to read this book, here are some suggestions. Begin with Chapter 1—it sets the scene and will help you to understand the relationship between patient safety and communication, and how critical conversations can make a real difference to patient care. Chapter 2 provides an introduction to communication skills and Chapter 3 outlines the key attributes of patient-safe communication. With the foundation knowledge from these chapters you will be ready to explore the rest of the book. Scan the list of contents, selecting the topics that interest you most, that you are currently studying or that you have encountered in your clinical practice. Your educators may also recommend certain chapters as part of your course work.

Learning outcomes and key concepts are listed at the beginning of each chapter to provide clarity and focus. They orientate you to what you will learn and will help you to transfer your learning to new clinical situations.

Margin notes and 'Something to think about' boxes provide helpful links, hints, advice, and critical thinking questions.

Suggested readings and web resources provided at the end of each chapter will help you to extend your learning.

Critical thinking activities encourage you to maximise your learning and help you to think broadly, critically and creatively about what you have learned and, most importantly, how your learning will inform your practice.

Teaching and assessment activities provided at the end of each chapter can be used by educators in multiple ways: as stimulus materials prior to or during tutorial activities or online learning; as a guide for self-directed learning; for assignments; or for continuing professional development activities. Additionally, a number of the patient stories provide appropriate preparatory activities for simulation sessions and can be used as a framework for the development of simulation scenarios or role plays.

A glossary of terms is provided at the back of the book.

Educator resources

Digital Image Powerpoint Slides
All of the diagrams and tables from the course content are available for lecturer use.

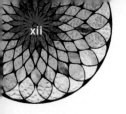

Acknowledgements

First, I would like to acknowledge and offer sincere thanks to my wonderful writing team. Their commitment to patient safety and person-centred care, along with their broad range of experiences and insights, bring every chapter to life. Their contributions have resulted in a book that I believe will inspire, motivate and engage both healthcare professionals and students.

Next, I would like to thank the expert clinicians, academics and students who reviewed the book for accuracy, authenticity and relevance. Their insights were invaluable.

Finally, thank you to the editorial and production team at Pearson, including Mandy Sheppard, Senior Portfolio Manager and Judith Bamber, Development Editor.

Reviewers

Jennifer Bassett, CQUniversity
Madeline Jones, Physiotherapist, Private Practice
Tyler Jones, Registered Nurse, Sydney Adventist Hospital
Maria Mackay, University of Wollongong
Evan Plowman, Charles Sturt University
Julie Shepherd, James Cook University
Peter Sinclair, The University of Newcastle
Cecilia Yeboah, Australian Catholic University

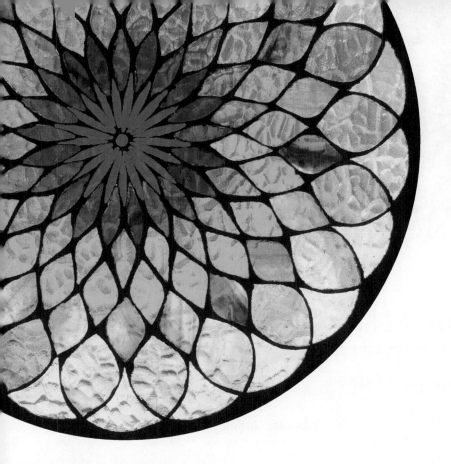

SECTION 1

Communication and patient safety

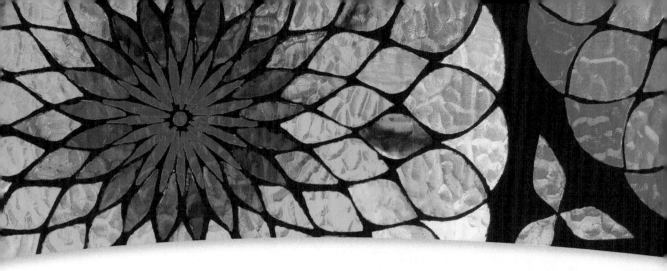

CHAPTER 1

THE RELATIONSHIP BETWEEN COMMUNICATION AND PATIENT SAFETY

Tracy Levett-Jones

LEARNING OUTCOMES

Chapter 1 will enable you to:

- discuss the relationship between communication and patient safety
- describe the impact of effective/ineffective communication on patient care
- use critical conversations to promote patient-safe communication
- reflect on your own level of communication competence and identify appropriate learning strategies for ongoing improvement.

KEY CONCEPTS

patient safety | patient-safe communication | critical conversations | communication risk factors

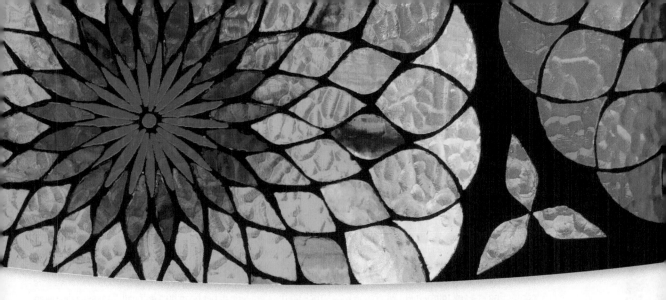

> The greatest problem with communication is the
> illusion that it has been accomplished.
>
> (George Bernard Shaw)

INTRODUCTION

When seeking healthcare, people hope and trust that their health-related problems will be appropriately managed and that their care will be safe and effective. However, despite the best intentions of healthcare professionals, healthcare errors are the third leading cause of death in developed countries. Up to 17 per cent of patients are harmed while receiving healthcare (Makary & Daniel, 2016), resulting in distress, hospital re-admissions, permanent injury, increased length of hospital stay and even death. Of these adverse events, at least 50 per cent are preventable (Bartlett et al., 2008). Although the reasons for adverse patient outcomes are diverse, research conducted between 1995 and 2005 demonstrated that ineffective communication was the root cause for nearly 66 per cent of all healthcare errors during that period (Institute for Healthcare Communication, 2018). Deficiencies in healthcare communication continue to feature in many coroners' reports and quality improvement investigations, and over the last decade there have been repeated calls for improvement.

The opportunity to improve the current situation through increased attention to the teaching of communication skills has been advocated as the most promising way forward and a pragmatic strategy for reducing healthcare errors (World Health Organization [WHO], 2011). Skilled communication is a core requirement across all healthcare disciplines (O'Keefe, Henderson & Pitt, 2011; Australian Health Practitioner Regulation Agency, 2017); this includes effective interprofessional communication (between health professionals from different disciplines), intraprofessional communication (between health professionals from the same discipline) and therapeutic communication (between healthcare professionals and patients). Despite this, many students, graduates, educators and clinicians assume that communication skills are either inherent or acquired almost serendipitously through repeated exposure to clinical practice. However, becoming a skilled and safe communicator requires active engagement in deliberate learning activities, determination and repeated practice; it also requires reflection, particularly on activities designed to improve performance. This chapter, and the ones that follow, provide the foundation

Extensive research has shown that no matter how knowledgeable a clinician might be, if he or she is not able to communicate with the patient, he or she may be of no help (Institute for Healthcare Communication, 2018).

for these types of learning activities. We illustrate the link between patient safety and communication from a wide range of disciplinary perspectives. The real-life patient stories included profile authentic and sometimes challenging situations that will cause you to re-examine many taken-for-granted assumptions as you reflect on your personal beliefs and professional understandings. Importantly, this book will enhance your communication competence and ability to practise in a way that promotes patient safety and wellbeing.

VANESSA'S STORY

Vanessa Anderson was born in 1989 and was 16 years old at the time of her death. She lived with her parents, Warren and Michelle, on Sydney's North Shore. Vanessa enjoyed good health; her only known medical conditions were asthma and migraine headaches; she did not drink or smoke. On Sunday, 6 November 2005, Vanessa was competing in a golf tournament when she was struck on the right side of her head by a golf ball. Vanessa was taken to hospital, vomiting several times en route. A CT scan was performed, and she was subsequently transferred to another, larger hospital where she was diagnosed as having a closed depressed right temporal skull fracture with temporal brain contusions. On the basis of her Glasgow Coma Score (GCS), the neurosurgical fellow classified Vanessa's head injury as mild. He then telephoned the on-call consultant neurosurgeon to advise him of Vanessa's condition, but told him that she would be transferred to the local children's hospital. He did not subsequently advise the consultant that Vanessa was not transferred but had been admitted to an adult ward instead.

On Monday, 7 November at 8:30 am, a senior medical resident, an intern on her first day in the neurosurgical unit and a nurse practitioner conducted a ward round. During the round the resident changed Vanessa's analgesic regime from Tramadol to Codeine Phosphate. The intern was responsible for making notes in Vanessa's medical records, but the notes she made were inadequate and did not include the author of the notes, the results of the physical examination and the ward-round attendees.

At approximately midday, the consultant neurosurgeon visited the ward and was told that Vanessa had been admitted under his care. He discussed the CT results and formed the view that she most likely had dural lacerations with bone fragments. He was unhappy about the poor communication, which meant that he had only just become aware of Vanessa's admission and, because of this, her surgery could not be scheduled until the following day.

Early in the afternoon of the same day, in response to Vanessa's severe pain, the resident prescribed the analgesics Panadeine Forte (2 tablets, four times a day) and Endone (5 mg, six times a day, PRN). Between 4:30 pm and 5:30 pm, an anaesthetic registrar conducted a pre-operative consultation and, in response to Vanessa's ongoing pain, she increased the dose and frequency of the Endone to 5–10 mg, three-hourly. She did not record a maximum dose. She misread the medication chart and thought that Vanessa had been prescribed Panadeine, not Panadeine Forte (Panadeine contains 8 mg of codeine and Panadeine Forte 30 mg). The anaesthetic registrar did not discuss her course of action with the nurses or the neurosurgical team.

That evening Vanessa was given two Panadeine Forte tablets at 7 pm and 12 am. She was also given 10 mg of Endone at 8 pm and 11 pm. At 1 am on the morning of Tuesday, 8 November, Vanessa buzzed for assistance. The nurse who responded observed that Vanessa could not move and sounded distressed. She lifted Vanessa's arm and it fell down limply on the bed. The nurse took some observations and noted that Vanessa's breathing was normal, that she was warm to touch and of normal colour, and that she had no shaking or stiffness. The nurse did not check Vanessa's lower limb movement or her GCS. Had she done so, Vanessa's GCS would have scored below 5, signalling that urgent medical review was necessary. However, the nurse did not believe that Vanessa was in immediate danger and, thinking that Vanessa was probably having a bad dream, did not escalate her concerns. Later, she returned to Vanessa and performed a set of neurological observations, including calling her name, asking if she was okay (to which she responded 'yes'), and requesting her to lift her arms and push her feet against the nurse's hands. Vanessa could do all these things and the nurse felt that the earlier event was not clinically significant, and that her initial view that Vanessa was simply having a bad dream was correct. The nurse did not document the events or her observations in Vanessa's chart, nor did she consult the registrar or the consultant.

At 2 am, Vanessa went to the toilet and was given a further 10 mg of Endone. The nurse later admitted that the dose of 5–10 mg Endone three-hourly struck her as unusual and that it was rare for this order to be charted in conjunction with regular Panadeine Forte. However, she felt that this was what the doctors wanted so she did not express her concerns to the anaesthetic registrar or the consultant.

Vanessa's observations were due again at 4 am; however, the nurse decided not to do these observations because Vanessa had been neurologically unchanged when she conducted the observations at around 2 am. Vanessa's father, Warren Anderson, arrived on the ward at around 3:45 am and sat in Vanessa's darkened room, then fell asleep. At around 5:30 am the nurse entered Vanessa's room and found her unresponsive. An emergency was called and CPR administered. Vanessa was pronounced dead at 6:35 am. The formal finding from a later coroner's inquest was that Vanessa died from a respiratory arrest due to the depressant effect of opiate medication.

Although Vanessa's death undoubtedly resulted from a series of system and human errors, any one of the health professionals involved may have prevented this tragic outcome had they communicated in an effective and timely manner. The NSW Deputy State Coroner, Magistrate Milovanovich, made the following statement in relation to the findings of the coronial inquest:

> The death of Vanessa Anderson at the very young age of 16 years was tragic and avoidable ... the circumstances of Vanessa's death should constantly remain in the forefront of the minds of all medical practitioners, nursing staff and hospital administrators. Vanessa's case should be used as a precedent to highlight how individual errors of judgment, failure to communicate, failure to record accurately and poor management of staff resources, cumulatively led to the worst possible outcome for Vanessa and her family.

Source: Inquest into the death of Vanessa Anderson, Coroner's Court, Westmead, Sydney, 24 January 2004. (Professor Tracy Levett-Jones was given permission by Vanessa's family to use her story in teaching students and health professionals about patient safety from the perspective of patients and their families.)

For further information about Vanessa Anderson's story, go to <http://www.ipeforqum.com.au/modules/>.

Patient safety and communication

Patient safety is defined as the prevention of errors and adverse effects to patients associated with healthcare (WHO, 2019). It is important to note that patient safety is not limited to physical safety but also includes psychological, emotional and cultural safety. Patient safety is an attribute of trustworthy healthcare systems that work to minimise the incidence and impact of, and maximise recovery from, adverse events (Emanuel et al., 2008). Patient safety is considered to be one of the most important issues facing healthcare today, and healthcare professionals need highly developed communication skills in order to manage the complexity and competing tensions that define contemporary health-care organisations. The importance of effective communication to patient safety is emphasised in the National Safety and Quality Health Service Standards (Australian Commission of Safety and Quality in Health Care, 2017), where it is specified that health professionals must facilitate structured and effective communication between health service organisations, within health service organisations, between clinicians and between clinicians and consumers.

Communication is much more than the provision of information, instructions or advice. It is a two-way process involving verbal and non-verbal skills that aims to create a shared understanding (Higgs, McAllister & Sefton, 2012). Communication is fundamental to safe healthcare. It is required for information exchange, quality decision making, creating therapeutic relationships with patients, increasing patient uptake of recommendations, enhancing patient satisfaction and improving health outcomes. Many healthcare professionals think that effective communication means giving patients clear, unambiguous information in a timely manner. This is true, but it is only part of the story. Communication involves listening as well as talking. When we listen to patients, we are less likely to jump to erroneous conclusions because we haven't seen the whole picture (this is referred to as *premature closure*).

'We think we listen, but very rarely do we listen with real understanding, or true empathy. Yet listening, of this very special kind, is one of the most potent forces for change' (Carl Rogers, 1980, p. 116).

BOX 1.1   The Australian Charter of Healthcare Rights

Safety—a right to safe and high-quality care

Respect—a right to be shown respect, dignity and consideration

Communication—a right to be informed about services, treatment, options and costs in a clear and open way

Participation—a right to be included in decisions and choices about care

Privacy—a right to privacy and confidentiality of provided information

Comment—a right to comment on care and having concerns addressed

Source: Reproduced with permission from The Australian Charter of Healthcare Rights, developed by the Australian Commission on Safety and Quality in Health Care (ACSQHC). ACSQHC: Sydney 2008.

Patients expect to be communicated with in ways that are inclusive, accurate, timely and appropriate. The Australian Charter of Healthcare Rights (Box 1.1) outlines patients' rights in regard to healthcare and emphasises that communication and working in partnership with patients underpin safe care. Indeed, communication is considered by many people to be one of the most important aspects of quality healthcare. In 2009, Australian patients and their families were surveyed in an attempt to clarify what their priorities were when undergoing healthcare (New South Wales Health, 2009). The list in Box 1.2 demonstrates the importance of communication to the survey participants' healthcare experience and illustrates the particular elements of communication that they believed were key. It is noteworthy that the only other clinical concern mentioned was in relation to pain management.

BOX 1.2   Patient survey: Top priorities for healthcare

- Healthcare professionals discussing anxieties and fears with the patient
- Patients having confidence and trust in healthcare professionals
- The ease of finding someone to talk to about concerns
- Doctors and nurses answering patients' questions understandably
- Patients receiving enough information about their condition/treatment
- Test results being explained understandably
- Patients having enough say about and being involved in care/treatment decisions
- Being given information about patient's rights and responsibilities
- Staff doing everything possible to control pain

Source: Reproduced by permission, NSW Health © 2019.

The impact of effective/ineffective communication on patient care

Effective communication impacts on patient outcomes in multiple ways. It can enhance diagnostic accuracy (Dwamena et al., 2012), improve patient satisfaction and wellbeing (Mickan & Rodger, 2005), and improve treatment adherence (such as compliance with medication and rehabilitation programs) (Zolnierek & Dimatteo, 2009) and clinical outcomes (including reduced stress and anxiety, improved pain management, self-management, mood, self-esteem, functional and psychological status) (Harms, 2007; Doyle, Lennox & Bell, 2013). Skilled communication can also enhance symptom resolution, and reduce the length of hospitalisation, healthcare costs (Mickan & Rodger, 2005) and rates of post-operative complications (Vats et al., 2010). In contrast, ineffective communication can lead to hostility, anger, confusion, misunderstandings, lack of trust, poor compliance, and greatly increased risk of error, patient harm and malpractice claims (Moore, Adler & Robertson, 2000).

Patient-safe communication is a goal-oriented activity focused on preventing adverse events and helping patients attain optimal health outcomes. It is a means by which healthcare professionals gather and share information, clarify and verify accurate interpretations of information, and establish a process for working collaboratively with both patients and other healthcare professionals to achieve common goals of safe and high-quality patient care (Schuster & Nykolyn, 2010). Every aspect of patient care depends upon how well healthcare professionals communicate with each other and the patients they care for. Clinical decisions based on incomplete or misinterpreted information are likely to be inappropriate and may cause patient harm and distress. For healthcare professionals, unsafe communication is considered to be a breach of professional standards and a leading cause of litigation (Trede, Ellis & Jones, 2012). Examples of this may include:

- inadequate or inaccurate advice on self-management
- failure to communicate in ways that the patient and their family can understand
- failure to disclose the risk of interventions and potential complications
- failure to obtain valid consent to an intervention/procedure
- failure to maintain client confidentiality
- failure to give the patient an opportunity to ask questions
- failure to respond appropriately to those questions
- failure to respect the opinion of a patient (even though the patient's opinion may be medically inaccurate, their observations are usually accurate and can be very valuable)
- failure to realise that, from the patient's point of view, there is no such thing as a 'silly question'
- failure to realise that the way we talk with patients (courteous, respectful, clear and jargon-free) can be just as important as the content of what we actually say to them
- failure to communicate with other relevant health professionals to provide a reasonable standard of care
- failure to communicate with supervisors/administrators when patient safety is in jeopardy
- failure to warn authorities, when to do so would be in the public interest (Trede et al., 2012).

Healthcare professionals should be aware that vulnerable groups of patients are at particular risk of harm from poor communication. These include older people, children, people with mental illness, people who do not speak English, people with sensory impairment (e.g. diminished hearing or limited verbal ability) and people with cognitive changes (e.g. delirium or dementia). The skills needed for patient-safe communication when caring for these groups are discussed in Chapters 11–17.

When many and varied healthcare professionals (including doctors, midwives, dentists, nurses, pharmacists, social workers, dieticians, physiotherapists, psychologists and others) are involved in patient care, ensuring exchange of accurate information in a timely manner can be difficult. Patient-safe

Patient-safe communication is a means by which healthcare professionals gather and share information, clarify and verify accurate interpretations of information, and establish a process for working collaboratively with both patients and other healthcare professionals to achieve common goals of safe and high-quality patient care (Schuster & Nykolyn, 2010).

FIGURE 1.1

Patient-safe
communication operates
within complex clinical
contexts amid myriad
potential risk factors

Source: Adapted from Schuster &
Nykolyn, 2010, p. 17.

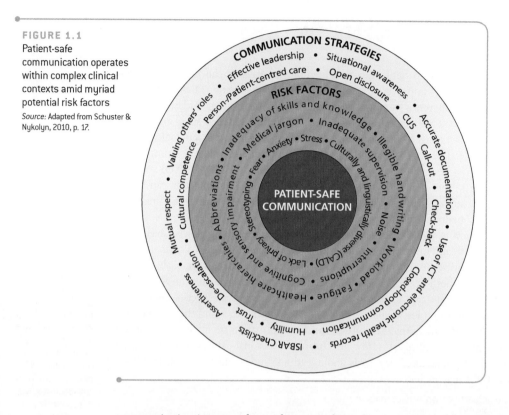

FIGURE 1.1

Patient-safe communication operates within complex clinical contexts amid myriad potential risk factors

Source: Adapted from Schuster & Nykolyn, 2010, p. 17.

communication is a complex and context-dependent process, and many human and system factors influence how effectively it transpires.

Despite healthcare professionals being well intentioned, there are numerous factors that can impact on their ability to engage in patient-safe communication. Figure 1.1 illustrates some of the risk factors for communicating safely with both patients and other health professionals. **Communication risk factors** have the potential to distort the clarity of the message being conveyed and impede the effectiveness of the process. This can lead to misinterpretation, time wasting, frustration and inaccurate decision making (Schuster & Nykolyn, 2010, p. 25). The outer circle of Figure 1.1 depicts strategies that have been identified as preventing or overcoming risk factors, improving communication and promoting patient safety. Throughout this book, these risk factors and strategies will be defined, discussed and applied to a range of clinical stories.

Using critical conversations to promote patient-safe communication

The hierarchical nature of healthcare environments presents one of the key risk factors for effective communication. Traditional cultures can make it difficult for healthcare professionals to speak up and be assertive when they are worried about patient safety. This is exacerbated by power differentials and a lack of psychological safety. The use of critical language can create clearly agreed upon communication processes that help improve communication and avoid the tendency to speak indirectly or deferentially when feeling intimidated. The ability to get everyone to stop and listen is essential for patient-safe communication. Indeed, Vanessa's story may have ended quite differently if the nurse who thought her analgesic regimen was unusual had been working in a culture where it was regarded as normal and appropriate for junior staff members to raise concerns about issues that they thought could compromise patient safety. Reflect on the patient story in Box 1.3 and consider how the use of **critical conversations** and graded assertiveness (see Box 1.4) may have given the healthcare professional involved the confidence to speak up (see Box 1.5).

BOX 1.3   Critical conversations and patient safety

In January 2004, Mr Graham Reeves was admitted to hospital for removal of a badly diseased right kidney. He had seen the surgeon a month before who documented the need for removal of the right kidney in the patient's case notes. However, possibly due to a transcription error, the hospital admission form wrongly said 'left kidney removal'. This error was transcribed to the theatre list. One of the surgeons checked the X-ray in the operating theatre, but it was the wrong way around and he misread the diseased kidney as the one on the left. The second surgeon did not look at the X-ray. Early in the operation, a medical student looked at the X-ray and said she thought it was the right kidney that should be removed. The surgeon told her she had made a mistake and continued operating, removing the left kidney (the normal kidney). Mr Reeves died of kidney failure five weeks later.

Had there been a greater culture of openness, where junior staff were encouraged to ask questions and where their concerns were taken seriously, Mr Reeves would not have died. Training in techniques such as CUSS (see Box 1.4) would have also helped the student be assertive and to escalate her concerns in a respectful way.

BOX 1.4   Examples of graded assertiveness

CUSS:

'I'm **C**oncerned

I'm **U**ncomfortable

This is not **S**afe

Stop what you are doing'.

PACE

Probe—*I don't understand why you want to do …*

Alert—*I think that will cause …*

Challenge—*Your approach will harm …*

Emergency action—*STOP what you are doing! For the safety of the patient we need to …*

Five-step advocacy

1   Attention getter—*Excuse me, Doctor.*

2   State your concern—*The patient is hypotensive.*

3   State the problem as you see it—*I think we need to get help now.*

4   State a solution—*I'll phone ICU to arrange transfer.*

5   Obtain an agreement—*Does that sound good to you?*

BOX 1.5   Learning to speak up: Primum non tacere—first do not be silent

- 'Speaking up' refers to a person in a non-dominant position expressing a concern or suggested course of action to a person in a more dominant or senior role.

- Speaking up refers to raising concerns *before* an act of commission or omission, rather than just 'hinting and hoping'.

- Healthcare professionals have a legal and ethical responsibility to advocate for patients and should never regret not having done so.

- Patients (and their loved ones) should also be encouraged to speak up.

- Speaking up requires courage and skill, but it is critical to patient safety.

- The safety and transparency of an organisational culture is demonstrated by how comfortable staff feel in speaking up when needed.

- Speaking up requires skills in graded assertiveness.

Source: Nickson (2017).

'Call-out' and 'check-back' are two other forms of critical communication that relay essential information to members of the healthcare team during emergent situations. (See Box 1.6 for examples.) The 'call-out' strategy helps team members anticipate the next steps and directs responsibility to a specific individual responsible for carrying out the task (WHO, 2011). 'Check-back' ensures that information conveyed by the sender is understood by the recipient as the sender intended. Check-back is a skill we use in our everyday lives. For example, if we give someone our telephone or credit card number over the phone, we often ask to have it read back to us so that we know it has been recorded correctly. How much more important this is when patients' lives are at risk.

While acronyms can be helpful, it is important to be aware that acronyms and abbreviations can mean different things to different professionals. For example, SB can mean 'short of breath' or 'seen by'; and PID can mean 'Pelvic Inflammatory Disease' or 'Prolapsed Intervertebral Disc'. There are many similar examples, and healthcare professionals need to be judicious when using abbreviations

---

BOX 1.6   Examples of 'call-out' and 'check-back'

Call-out

Arrest team leader: *Airway status?*

Nurse: *Airway clear.*

Arrest team leader: *Breath sounds?*

Nurse: *Breath sounds decreased on right.*

Arrest team leader: *Blood pressure?*

Nurse: *BP 96/40.*

Check-back

Doctor: *Give Adrenaline 1 milligram IV push.*

Nurse: *Adrenaline 1 milligram IV push?*

Doctor: *That's correct.*

because of the risk of misunderstanding and serious communication errors potentially leading to adverse events.

Learning to communicate in ways that promote patient safety

Although a wide body of research underpins the relationship between effective communication and positive outcomes for both patients and healthcare professionals, contemporary teaching and learning approaches do not always facilitate the development of a requisite level of communication, collaboration and teamwork skills (Woodward-Kron et al., 2013). Indeed, a review of communication skills training by Denniston et al. (2017) identified that 55 per cent of the 168 included papers focused on medical education only. Additionally, when educational opportunities are offered they tend to focus mainly on communicating with patients, and much less attention is given to communicating with other healthcare professionals. As a result, graduates and their employers consistently report that they are not well equipped to communicate and collaborate effectively as members of an interprofessional healthcare team, and consequently patient outcomes are negatively affected (Gilligan, Outram & Levett-Jones, 2014).

Both in academic settings and in clinical environments, opportunities for learning about interprofessional communication and collaboration are often overlooked. For example, in a project exploring graduates' experiences of learning about other healthcare professionals (Levett-Jones, Gilligan & Moxby, 2013), the following statement was made:

> When we were on our clinical rotations, we saw a couple of students, med students and nursing students ... but there was no interaction. We didn't actually do any study or liaising with them about patients or anything like that; it was very much segregated into 'you are a med student, you are a pharmacy student, you are a nursing student'. You don't talk to other students or learn with them; so you don't know anything about their roles.

Traditionally, communication skills have been taught primarily in academic settings and limited to one or two subjects. This is in contrast to a body of research, which suggests that attention to the development of healthcare professionals' communication skills should begin early and be continued throughout each year of study and beyond. The outcomes of an integrated approach include a more permanent understanding of the importance of communication, improvement in students' confidence and competence, reduction of clinical errors, and improved patient safety (Üstün, 2006). Additionally, research has demonstrated that applied communication skills education with strong practical and experiential components are more effective than programs that are mainly theoretical (Ahsen et al., 2010). Irrespective of the educational opportunities provided, what is very clear is that students who take the initiative by actively pursuing opportunities to learn about and practise communicating with patients and other healthcare professionals, and who seek feedback and reflect on their performance, are more likely to develop patient-safe communication skills.

Conclusion

Without doubt, effective communication leads to better outcomes for patients. It also reduces health service expenditure as there are fewer complications. Effective communication is an integral part of quality healthcare. It can take extra time but it is time saved in the long run. However, patient-safe communication can be complex and challenging, and there are many personal, contextual and organisational factors that undermine effective communication between healthcare professionals and between healthcare professionals and the people they care for. Learning to communicate in ways that promote patient safety takes personal insight, determination and an openness to change practices and habits that may have become second nature. Just as importantly, learning to communicate effectively requires active engagement in learning activities and thoughtful reflection on practice. This chapter and the ones that follow will provide students, graduates, educators and clinicians with understandings, knowledge and practical strategies that will equip them to improve their communication skills and promote patient safety.

Use of acronyms and communication tools such as CUSS, PACE, Call-out and Check-back are effective in streamlining the way healthcare professionals communicate and increasing patient safety.

'It is in the formative years of undergraduate education that attitudes are forged and skills imparted which shape the quality of engagement with patients for years to come' (Bristol Royal Infirmary Inquiry, 2001, p. 325).

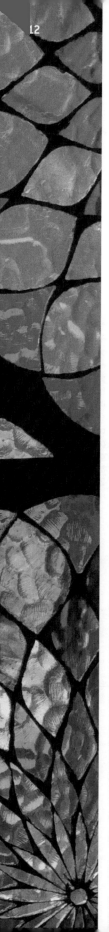

Critical thinking activities

The following excerpt is taken from a study that explored graduates' experiences of working within a healthcare team. While the scenario portrayed focuses on the interactions between a junior medical officer and a registered nurse, similar communication issues arise for all healthcare professionals irrespective of their discipline or context of work. As you read this excerpt, reflect on similar situations that you have been involved in; consider the implications for the healthcare professionals involved and the potential impact on the patients.

> *Sometimes you're fumbling your way through and you look to the nurses for a bit of a clue of what to do. I had a situation when there was a patient that I couldn't get a cannula into, he was dehydrated, but he was taking in fluids, and his diarrhoea had stopped. I tried a couple of times, went away and came back, and then decided that we were just going to go with oral fluids. And the nurse sort of made this face, but she didn't say anything. I said to her, 'You don't look very happy with that. What do you think? What's the problem?' And so she sort of exploded then and said she thought it was really a bad idea, and that 'we really have to get a line into this patient', and that 'he was going to go downhill if we don't'. So after she said that it sort of felt like quite an easy decision ... I'd been sitting on the fence and didn't really know what to do. But I wished that she'd said something, and not just sat there and made a face, because if I hadn't seen it, what would have happened to that patient?*

1   Imagine that you were the nurse in the above scenario and concerned about the junior medical officer's clinical decision. Using one of the graded assertiveness skills provided earlier in this chapter, outline how you would respond in a way that promotes both patient safety and effective interprofessional teamwork.

2   Imagine yourself as the junior medical officer in the above scenario. What would you say to the nurse to promote improved communication and collaboration in order to prevent this type of situation from occurring again?

3   Reflect on a recent clinical conversation with a patient or a colleague that did not go as well as you had expected. Identify from Figure 1.1 the contextual and interpersonal factors that may have influenced your conversation. Then consider the strategies you could use to promote patient-safe communication in the future.

Teaching and assessment activities

This activity can be used to help students gain a deeper appreciation of the roles and responsibilities of the members of the healthcare team. Begin by sharing the following quote from a graduate who participated in the previously mentioned study:

> *It's almost like a tradesman having a toolbox that they've never opened, and every now and again somebody tells them that there's a tool that could be useful, might make a certain job easier ... but if you don't know about it, you can't use it.*

Explain to students that they cannot communicate and collaborate effectively with other members of the healthcare team unless they understand, respect and value their roles.

For this activity, students should be instructed to create a table with two columns. In the left-hand column, students list the members of the healthcare team (remind students this refers to the broader team, not just the 'nursing team on ward 6' or the 'orthopaedic team', for example). In the right-hand column, students are to provide a brief description of the roles and functions of the team members, according to their current understanding.

Students should then be asked to test their knowledge about the roles and functions of the team members by seeking opportunities to observe and communicate with members of the team about their roles, what they value and how they work. The table should expand as students identify and add members of the healthcare team, and as they gain a more comprehensive understanding of their roles. It will be an invaluable resource that will help students to communicate more effectively, and work collaboratively to promote patient safety and wellbeing.

Further reading

O'Toole, G. (2011). *Core Interpersonal Skills for Health Professionals*. Chatswood, New South Wales: Churchill Livingston.

Vincent, C. (2011). *Patient Safety* (2nd edn). London: BMJ Books, Wiley Blackwell.

Web resources

Interprofessional education for quality use of medicines: This resource consists of a series of modules that have been designed to help students learn about medication safety and prepare for interprofessional practice. The modules provide a window into how health professionals communicate and work collaboratively to promote medication safety. Each module is based on an actual clinical situation; a number are re-enactments or adaptations of coronial inquests or incident reports.
<www.ipeforqum.com.au/modules/>

Patient safety resource centre: This UK website provides a range of resources related to human factors and patient safety. Of particular importance is the video titled, *Just a routine operation—patient story*.
<http://patientsafety.health.org.uk/resources/just-routine-operation-human-factors-patient-safety>

World Health Organization (2011), *Patient Safety Curriculum Guide* (multi-professional edition): This guide promotes the need for patient safety education to improve the safety of care and supports the training of all healthcare professionals on a number of priority patient safety concepts to improve learning about patient safety. <www.who.int/patientsafety/education/curriculum/ Curriculum_Tools/en/index.html>

References

Ahsen, N., Batul, S., Ahmed, A., Imam, S., Iqbal, H., Shamshair, K. & Ali, H. (2010). Developing counseling skills through pre-recorded videos and role play: A pre- and post-intervention study in a Pakistani medical school. *BMC Medical Education, 10*(1), 7.

Australian Commission on Safety and Quality in Health Care. (2017). *National Safety and Quality Health Service Standards* (2nd edn). Sydney, Australia: ACSQHC.

Australian Health Practitioner Regulation Agency. (2017). Panel decisions. Accessed June 2018 at <http://www.ahpra. gov.au/Publications/Panel-Decisions.aspx>.

Bartlett, G., Blais, R., Tamblyn, R., Clermont, R. & MacGibbon, B. (2008). Impact of patient communication problems on the risk of preventable adverse events in acute care settings. *Canadian Medical Association Journal, 178*(12), 1555–62. doi: 10.1503/cmaj.070690

Bristol Royal Infirmary Inquiry. (2001). *Learning from Bristol: The Report of the Public Inquiry into Children's Heart Surgery at the Bristol Royal Infirmary 1984–1995*. Bristol Royal Infirmary Inquiry, July 2001.

Denniston, C., Molloy, E., Nestel, D., Woodward-Kron, R. & Keating, J. (2017). Learning outcomes for communication skills across the health professions: A systematic literature review and qualitative synthesis. *BMJ Open, 7*(e014570). doi:10.1136/bmjopen-2016-014570

Doyle, C., Lennox, L. & Bell, D. (2013). A systematic review of evidence on the links between patient experience and clinical safety and effectiveness. *BMJ Open, 3*(e001570).

Dwamena, F., Holmes-Rovner, M., Gaulden, C., Jorgenson, S., Sadigh, G., Sikorskii, A. … Olomu, A. (2012). Interventions for providers to promote a patient-centred approach in clinical consultations. *Cochrane Database Syst Rev.* December 12;12:CD003267. doi: 10.1002/14651858.CD003267.pub2

Emanuel, L., Berwick, D., Conway, J., Hatlie, M., Leape, L. … Walton, M. (2008). What exactly is patient safety? In K. Henriksen, J. Battles, M. Keyes & M. Grady (Eds), *Advances in Patient Safety: New Directions and Alternative Approaches*. Rockville, MD: Agency for Healthcare Research and Quality, 19–35.

Gilligan, C., Outram, S. & Levett-Jones, T. (2014). Recommendations from recent graduates in medicine, nursing and pharmacy on improving interprofessional education in university programs: A qualitative study. *BMC Medical Education, 14*(52).

Harms, L. (2007). *Working with People*. South Melbourne, Victoria: Oxford University Press.

Higgs, J., McAllister, L. & Sefton, A. (2012). Communication in the health sciences. In J. Higgs, R. Ajjawi, L.McAllister, F. Trede, & S. Loftus (Eds), *Communicating in the Health Sciences* (3rd edn, pp. 368). South Melbourne, Victoria: Oxford University Press.

Inquest into the death of Vanessa Anderson. Westmead file No. 161/2007, Magistrate Milovanovich, NSW Deputy State Coroner. Decision handed down at Westmead Coroners Court on 24 January 2008.

Institute for Healthcare Communication. (2018). *Impact of communication in healthcare*. Accessed August 2018 at <https://healthcarecomm.org/about-us/impact-of-communication-in-healthcare/>.

Levett-Jones, T., Gilligan, C. & Moxby, A. (2013). *Interprofessional Education: Enhancing the Teaching of Medication Safety to Nursing, Pharmacy and Medical Students*. Australian Government Office for Learning and Teaching, Sydney.

Makary, M. A. & Daniel, M. (2016). Medical error—The third leading cause of death in the US. *BMJ (Online), 353*. doi: 10.1136/bmj.i2139

Mickan, S. & Rodger, S. (2005). Effective health care teams: A model of six characteristics developed from shared perceptions. *Journal of Interprofessional Care, 19*, 358–70.

Moore, P., Adler, N. & Robertson, P. (2000). Medical malpractice: The effect of doctor–patient relations on medical patient perceptions and malpractice intentions. *West J Med, 173*, 244–250.

New South Wales Health, Nursing and Midwifery Office (2009). Essentials of care project. Accessed October 2012 at <www.health.nsw.gov.au/resources/nursing/pdf/ namo_ forums/nmforum_ess_care_pres_apr08.pdf>.

Nickson, C. (2017). Speaking up. *Life in the fast lane*. Accessed August 2018 at <https://lifeinthefastlane.com/ mime/speaking-up/>.

O'Keefe, M., Henderson, A. & Pitt, R. (2011). *Health, Medicine and Veterinary Science: Learning and Teaching Academic Standards Statement*. New South Wales, Australia: Australian Government Department of Education, Employment and Workplace Relations.

Rogers, C. (1980). *A Way of Being*. Boston: Houghton Mifflin.

Schuster, P. & Nykolyn, L. (2010). *Communication for Nurses. How to Prevent Harmful Events and Promote Patient Safety*. Philadelphia: E.A. Davis.

Trede, F., Ellis, E. & Jones, S. (2012). Communication and duty of care. In J. Higgs, R. Ajjawi, L. McCallister, F. Trede & S. Loftus (Eds), *Communicating in the Health Sciences* (3rd edn). Oxford University Press, Melbourne.

Üstün, B. (2006). Educational innovation. Communication skills training as part of a problem-based learning curriculum. *Journal of Nursing Education, 45*(10), 421–4.

Vats, A., Vincent, C., Nagpal, K. & Davies, R. (2010). Practical challenges of introducing WHO surgical checklist: UK pilot experience. *British Medical Journal* (International edn), *340*(7738), 133.

Woodward-Kron, R., Flynn, E., Macqueen, S., Enright, H., & McColl, G. (2013). The state of emergency communication skills teaching in Australian medical schools: Gaps, barriers and opportunities. *Focus on Health Professional Education, 14*(3), 49–63.

World Health Organization. (2011). *World Health Organization Patient Safety Curriculum Guide* (multi-professional edition). Accessed October 2012 at <www.who. int/patientsafety/ education/curriculum/Curriculum_Tools/en/index.html>.

World Health Organization. (2019). *Health Systems: Patient Safety*. Accessed January 2019 at <http://www.euro.who. int/en/health-topics/Health-systems/patient-safety/patient-safety>.

Zolnierek, K. B. & Dimatteo, M. R. (2009). Physician communication and patient adherence to treatment: A meta-analysis. *Med Care, 47*, 826–34.

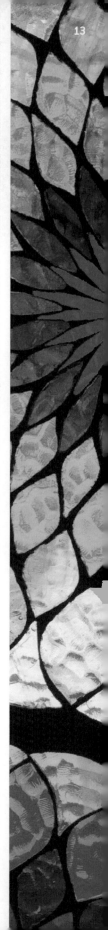

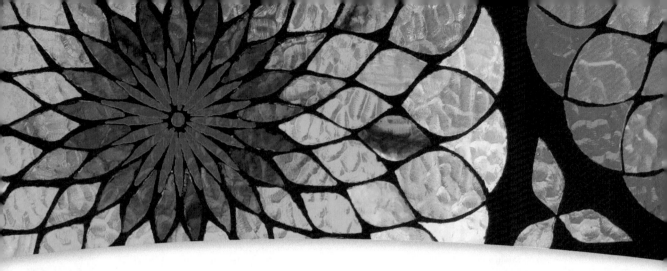

AN INTRODUCTION TO COMMUNICATION SKILLS

Sue Dean   Carla Saunders

LEARNING OUTCOMES

Chapter 2 will enable you to:

- discuss how an introduction to a patient provides the foundation for therapeutic communication
- describe the attributes and outcomes of caring communication encounters
- outline how self-awareness and intrapersonal communication influences the effectiveness of healthcare communication
- demonstrate an understanding of effective verbal and non-verbal communication skills
- outline the key attributes of effective healthcare communication
- discuss the significance of health literacy to patient safety.

KEY CONCEPTS

verbal communication | non-verbal communication | caring | self-awareness | health literacy

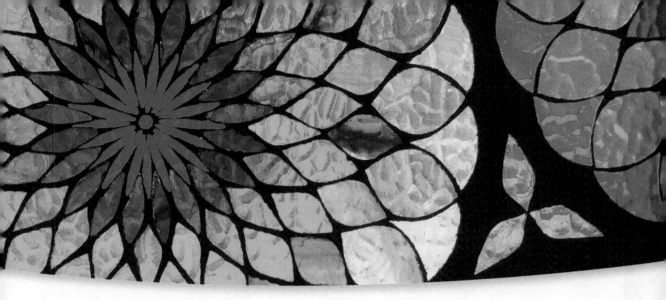

> The secret in the care of the patient lies
>
> in the care for the patient.
>
> (Francis Peabody, MD, 1880–1927. From the Harvard Medical School Graduation 1927.)

INTRODUCTION

Improvements in healthcare communication are reported to hold the greatest potential for creating healthcare environments that are safe and effective (Schiavo, 2014). This chapter will introduce you to fundamental yet critically important communication skills. Both verbal and non-verbal communication skills will be discussed and illustrated with examples and vignettes drawn from clinical practice. The relationship between caring communication encounters and patient satisfaction, safety and wellbeing will also be outlined. This chapter includes a wealth of practical examples for improving the way healthcare professionals engage with patients and for building a repertoire of strategies to promote effective communication.

KATE'S STORY

One of the most fundamental, yet often overlooked, communication skills is the ability to introduce yourself. Whilst this skill is one we don't usually think a lot about, an introduction can have a significant impact on the development of rapport with a patient and the effectiveness of the communication interaction that follows. Below is a poignant story that provides insights into the importance of this communication skill.

#hellomynameis

I am lying on a trolley in the emergency department feeling extremely unwell. My temperature is 39°C and my pulse is 150 beats per minute. It is about 36 hours since I underwent a routine extra-anatomic stent exchange, and I have developed sepsis. A young surgical doctor admits me. He does not introduce himself by name, instead plumping for 'I'm one of the doctors'. A nurse comes to administer my intravenous antibiotics. She does not introduce herself either.

Over the five days' admission I lost count of the number of times I have to ask staff members for their names. It feels awkward and wrong. Introducing yourself is the first and most basic step taught in any clinical interaction for any healthcare professional, but do we ever stop to think about how important this is? As the patient you are in an incredibly vulnerable position. The healthcare team knows so much personal information about you, yet you know next to nothing about them. This results in a very one sided power imbalance. One way to redress this imbalance is a good introduction. I believe it is the first rung on the ladder to providing truly compassionate, person-centred care. It is also vital in developing that all important rapport and trust on which to build a therapeutic relationship.

(Kate Granger, 2013)

Watch the 'Dr Kate Granger—Hello My Name Is' video to hear Dr Granger talk about why she started the #hellomynameis campaign: <www. youtube.com/watch? v=UmeQjgy4QnE>

Kate Granger was a doctor who was terminally ill with cancer. She believed that an introduction was critical to person-centred care. Her experiences led to the #hellomynameis campaign that began with this tweet in August 2013: **'I'm going to start a "Hello. My name is …" campaign. Sent Chris home to design the logo … #hellomynameis'**. By the start of 2017, #hellomynameis had made over 1.8 billion impressions with an average of six tweets an hour. Today, it is a worldwide campaign adopted by thousands of healthcare services and staff.

The first few moments of an interaction between a healthcare professional and a patient is the foundation for everything that follows. An introduction takes only seconds but it improves a patient's experience of healthcare significantly. It is the first step in discovering not only *what is the matter with the patient* but, just as importantly, *what matters to the patient.*

Source: Courtesy of Chris Pointon

Caring communication encounters

Communication makes a difference in how I feel about myself and whether I have the courage to go on. If I have a negative experience, I withdraw and close up and that's very harmful, mentally and physically.

(Thorne, Hislop, Armstrong & Oglov, 2008)

To provide person-centred care, healthcare professionals must have the ability to read the feelings and meanings associated with a person's experience, along with sensitivity to their changing emotions. A body of research demonstrates the link between caring behaviours—such as providing reassurance, touching the patient's hand and expressing support—and reduced patient anxiety, distress and depression, along with a range of other physiological and psychosocial outcomes (see Chapters 1 and 3) (Fogarty et al., 1999). Scholars have referred to these types of caring interactions as the essence of therapeutic communication (Ong et al., 2000). Caring requires well-developed intrapersonal and interpersonal communication skills, as well as the ability to create an emotional connection with patients.

A good interpersonal relationship is a prerequisite for optimal health care.

(Ong et al., 2000)

People often choose a career in healthcare because they have an empathic disposition. However, the increasingly technological nature of contemporary healthcare environments can sometimes be perceived as a barrier to empathic engagement with patients. Although there is a lot of rhetoric about caring communication interactions being neither time- nor cost-effective, these assertions are not supported by evidence. Caring encounters transcend circumstances and situational factors; they also have a positive impact on both patients and healthcare professionals (Scott, 2011). Consequently, healthcare professionals who are committed to providing person-centred care will find the time to learn, practise, refine and use their communication skills.

Communication precedes care, is integral to all of the processes that take place during care and shapes how the patient encounter unfolds and concludes. If communication is clear, accurate and attuned to the specific needs of the patient, they are more likely to be satisfied with their healthcare experience (Stewart, 1995). However, ineffective communication can result in, for example, repeat visits to healthcare providers, complaints, disputes and, sometimes, litigation. Effective communication requires a diverse skill set along with the ability to apply those skills across a wide range of healthcare settings, as well as with groups and individuals from different cultural, socioeconomic and ethnic backgrounds.

The requisite communication skills can be acquired with deliberate practice. However, students' willingness to develop their communication skills depends, to a large extent, on whether, and to what degree, they perceive they actually need to improve their skills (Dean, Zaslawski et al., 2016). In one recent study, only 18 per cent of beginning students believed that their communication skills could and should be improved. After completing a communication subject, 78 per cent of the same students came to recognise the critical importance of communication skills and that their communication skills had in fact improved (Dean, Zaslawski et al., 2016). For all healthcare students and professionals, reflection on and self-appraisal of one's communication skills is a prerequisite for learning and improvement; however, this requires a great deal of self-awareness.

Self-awareness and intrapersonal communication

Knowing and understanding yourself, and reflecting on your interactions with others, is essential to being an effective communicator. This is referred to as **intrapersonal communication** and it is premised on self-awareness. Self-awareness is being consciously aware of your thoughts, feelings, beliefs, biases, assumptions, prejudices and values, and how they might influence and/or interfere with your ability to convey or hear a message as intended, or to interpret a situation or another person's perspective. In other words, developing self-awareness requires an ongoing commitment to becoming increasingly conscious of self (Stein-Parbury, 2017). Our ability to care for patients and relate to colleagues is influenced by the extent to which we truly understand ourselves—what we think and feel, what we want and how we act. Self-awareness is also the basis of emotional intelligence, which is referred to as the ability to identify and manage the emotions of one's self and of others. One approach for improving your emotional intelligence and self-awareness, as well as gaining an understanding of how others perceive you, is by using the Johari Window (Luft, 1969) (see Figure 2.1). The four quadrants of the Johari window refer to the:

Open area—what you know about yourself and are willing to share

Blind area—what you do not know about yourself but others are aware of

Hidden area—what you are aware of about yourself but do not want others to know

Unknown area—aspects of which neither you nor anyone else are aware.

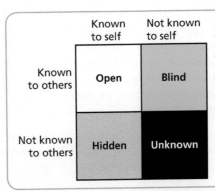

FIGURE 2.1
The Johari Window
Source: Luft, J. & Ingham, H. (1955). The Johari Window, a graphic model of interpersonal awareness. *Proceedings of the western training laboratory in group development*, Los Angeles: UCLA.

Everyone acts and behaves within all four quadrants of the *Johari Window*. We have some awareness of our skills, attitudes and perceptions, but we also hold back some of this information from others. At the same time, there are things that other people are aware of about us that we do not know—these are our blind spots. We also have 'unknown' areas—subconscious biases and experiences saved in our long-term memory that influence how we respond, react and feel.

Making a conscious decision to reflect on and learn about ourselves helps to enhance self-awareness as well as both intrapersonal and interpersonal communication skills. When communicating with a patient it is important to reflect on and self-assess ourselves, not only following the interaction but also during it. We need to be highly attuned to what is occurring, how we are feeling and why we are responding in a certain way, as this is the foundation for effective and empathic interpersonal communication. However, it is not only the verbal components of our interactions but also the non-verbal components that we must constantly notice, reflect on and examine.

Non-verbal communication skills

In reality, communication begins before you utter your first word to a patient and even before you introduce yourself. It is estimated that up to 90 per cent of our interpersonal communication is non-verbal—40 per cent through tone of voice and vocalisations and 50 per cent through posture, gestures and facial expressions (Mehrabian, 1981). Your non-verbal communication creates the patient's first impression of you. Similarly, being able to read a patient's non-verbal communication through their body language and facial expressions makes healthcare professionals more astute and insightful. Non-verbal cues often express more about a person's feelings than what they say, and, according to Christman (2015), a competent healthcare professional listens to what a patient says, but a *great* healthcare professional reads their patients' non-verbal cues in order to understand what they are really thinking and feeling. It is also important to pay particular attention to micro-expressions— the rapid, involuntary, almost imperceptible facial expressions that people might make when trying to hide their emotions. It is often these subtle cues that reveal what a person may be too embarrassed, anxious or frightened to mention (e.g. being unable to understand a diagnosis or afford prescribed medications). Seeking to understand non-verbal communication is crucial in any patient encounters, as healthcare professionals must be able to recognise and appropriately respond to people's fear, anxiety, pain or despair.

The acronym EMPATHY (Riess & Kraft-Todd, 2014) was developed to illustrate the importance of non-verbal communication to empathic encounters with patients (see Box 2.1). Similarly, SOLER is an acronym that represents an active listening approach and a way of demonstrating interest in and engagement with a patient by using effective body language (Egan, 2010) (see Box 2.2).

Cultural competence is critical to non-verbal communication, as what is acceptable in one culture may not be appropriate in another. Making eye contact is one example. In Western cultures making eye contact is considered respectful and an indication that the person we are communicating with is listening. In some cultures, though, making eye contact is considered disrespectful and rude. Touch is another example. Holding someone's hand to reassure or convey empathy can be an effective therapeutic communication skill (Dean, Lewis & Ferguson, 2016). However, in some cultures, touch may be inappropriate, particularly between different genders. Thus, it is essential to be mindful of and tailor our non-verbal (as well as verbal) communication to the individual needs of each person. Healthcare professionals also need to be able to communicate with patients who have limited or no verbal communication skills (e.g. people who are intubated or sedated in intensive care units) as this is critical to people's emotional and psychological health. See Chapter 15 for further information about communicating with people who have a verbal communication impairment.

> *Most people do not listen with the intent to understand; they listen with the intent to reply. They are either speaking or preparing to speak. They are filtering everything through their own paradigms, reading their autobiography into other people's lives.*

(Stephen Covey)

BOX 2.1   EMPATHY

Eye contact: Making eye contact facilitates patient engagement and provides the foundation for a therapeutic interaction.

Muscles of facial expression: Healthcare professionals need to be able to decode a patient's facial expressions correctly. They also need to be aware of what their own facial expressions are saying to the patient. For example, without saying a word (and without intending to) healthcare professionals can communicate disgust at the smell of malaena or a suppurating wound and, by doing so, have a negative impact on the patient and their sense of self.

Posture: Having an open posture and sitting beside a patient at eye level conveys the message that the healthcare professional is interested in the patient and willing to give them undivided attention. Conversely, standing over and looking down at a patient may be interpreted as intimidation and/or exerting power.

Affect: Making a conscious assessment of, and seeking to understand, a patient's affective or emotional state is the first step in an empathic interaction.

Tone of voice: Our tone of voice conveys as much to a patient as the actual words we speak. However, we seldom reflect on what messages we are sending with our tone of voice, nor what a patient's tone of voice might be telling us.

Hearing the whole patient: Person-centred care is a holistic approach that requires the ability to listen with our 'whole heart', and to seek to understand the patient's physical, emotional and spiritual needs.

Your response: Healthcare professionals often witness or hear about shocking and distressing events. However, we are required to respond professionally and empathically, always mindful of the impact of our response on the patients we are caring for.

Source: Riess & Kraft-Todd (2014).

BOX 2.2   SOLER—an active listening model

Square: Face the patient squarely to show that you are interested and paying attention to what they are saying.

Open: Maintain an open posture, without crossing your arms or legs to create the impression that you are open and receptive to what the patient is telling you.

Lean: Leaning forward when a person is talking to you shows that you are involved and listening to what they have to say.

Eye contact: Maintaining eye contact demonstrates that you are listening and not distracted.

Relax: It is important to avoid fidgeting, to create the impression that you are calm and completely focused on what the patient is saying.

Source: Egan (2010).

Verbal communication skills

Verbal communication is a conscious process as people typically choose their words to convey the message they want to send and the feelings they wish to express. The actual words used, as well as the way they are structured, vary between people according to their culture, socioeconomic background, age, education, role, etc. Healthcare professionals must be able to adapt their verbal communication to the individual needs and background of each patient. Later in this chapter we discuss the impact of health literacy on communication, and subsequent chapters discuss how to communicate with, for example, children, people who are angry and people from different cultural backgrounds. Review Table 2.1 for descriptors and examples of verbal and non-verbal communication techniques.

TABLE 2.1 Verbal and non-verbal communication techniques	Communication technique	Definition	Example/s
	Expressing empathy	Empathy is the ability to understand a person's feelings and perspectives, and to respond appropriately.	'The thought of having this surgery seems really frightening for you. What can I do to relieve some of your fears?' A nurse is caring for a dying patient and observes the patient's daughter, in distress, conveying that her mother is thirsty and her mouth seems very dry. The nurse positions herself at one side of the bed and gently sprays some water into the patient's mouth, simultaneously stroking her forehead and explaining what she is doing.
	Silence	Accepting pauses or silences that may extend for several seconds or minutes without interjecting. Deliberate silences are an effective communication skill as they indicate listening and allow time to collect thoughts and reflect. A quiet presence may be helpful when there are no words that can be said to make a situation better.	Sitting quietly (or walking with the patient) and waiting attentively until the patient is able to put thoughts and feelings into words. Verbal responses such as 'Take your time' can be used during periods of silence to reassure the patient that you are willing to wait until he or she is ready to respond.
	Instructing	This is similar to providing information but is usually more direct in content.	'I would like you to take a breath in and then slowly breathe out.'
	Providing information	Providing, in a simple and direct manner, specific factual information that the patient may or may not request. When information is not known, the healthcare professional states this and indicates who has it or when it will be obtained. This is different to giving advice, which is not a therapeutic communication skill. Advising increases a patient's vulnerability as it assumes they don't know what to do and that the healthcare professional knows best. It creates a sense of inadequacy in the patient.	'Your surgery is scheduled for tomorrow morning.' 'You will feel a pulling sensation when the tube is removed from your abdomen.'
	Prompting	Using short verbal statements or questions that encourage further interaction and help the patient to elaborate. It also indicates listening, much like when you are engaging in telephone communication.	'Yes.' 'Go on.' 'Mmm.' 'Uh huh.' 'Do go on.'

Communication technique	Definition	Example/s
Probing: using open-ended questions	Asking broad questions yields more information than closed-ended questions and can invite the patient to explore, elaborate, clarify, describe, compare or illustrate thoughts or feelings. Open-ended questions require more than a one-word response. It is important to consider trust when asking open-ended questions, as a patient may be reluctant to disclose personal experiences without a level of trust being established first.	'Can you fill me in a little on how you're feeling about the surgery tomorrow?' 'Describe for me what brought you to hospital today.' 'What could I do to make you feel more comfortable?'
Probing: using closed questions	Closed questions can usually be answered with a simple 'yes', 'no' or other one-word response. They limit the amount of information that is shared by the patient. They are helpful when used in a purposeful way but overuse can result in the patient feeling interrogated. Focused closed questions can be used to obtain specific information for a specific clinical situation.	'Have you been in hospital before?' 'When was the last time you had something to eat or drink?' 'Have you taken your insulin this morning?' 'Are you feeling better today?' 'Is your wife at the hospital?'
Touch	Providing *appropriate* forms of touch reinforces emotional support, encouragement, tenderness and personal attention. Because touch varies among individuals, families and cultures, the healthcare professional must be sensitive to the person's culture and personal preferences.	Placing an arm around an older person to provide a much needed and absent tactile sensory experience for someone who no longer has those experiences. Holding a person's hand when sharing some bad news. Encouraging a patient to squeeze your hand to distract them from a painful procedure. Sitting and holding a person's hand when there is nothing to be said or done to make a situation better.
Paraphrasing or restating	Actively listening for the person's basic message and then transforming those thoughts and/or feelings into similar words without losing the meaning. The paraphrased response is usually shorter and more focused than the person's statement. Paraphrasing is often used to focus and rephrase the content of what a person is saying. It also demonstrates listening and provides the person with an opportunity to confirm or deny the accuracy of the healthcare professional's interpretation of what has been said.	*Patient:* 'I couldn't manage to eat any dinner last night—the meat was tough and the vegetables tasteless.' *HCP:* 'You didn't enjoy the meal you had last night.' 'Let me just go over that; so what you are saying is …' 'In other words …'

TABLE 2.1
Verbal and non-verbal communication techniques (Continued)

(Continued)

TABLE 2.1 Verbal and non-verbal communication techniques (Continued)	Communication technique	Definition	Example/s
		Paraphrasing or restating doesn't indicate that the nurse has agreed with what the person has said—it simply implies an acceptance of their reality and indicates a desire to help.	
	Seeking clarification	A method of making the meaning of the person's message more understandable. It is used when paraphrasing is difficult (i.e. when the communication is rambling or garbled). To clarify the message, the healthcare professional requests extra input from the person, which demonstrates a desire to better understand.	Clarifying statements can begin with: 'I'm a bit confused about …' 'I'm not certain what you mean.'
	Perception checking or seeking consensual validation	A method, similar to clarifying, that verifies the meaning of specific words rather than the overall meaning of a message.	Patient: 'My husband never gives me any presents.' HCP: 'You mean he has never given you a present for your birthday or Christmas?' Patient: 'Well, not never. He does get me something for my birthday and Christmas, but he never thinks of giving me anything at any other time.'
	Offering self	Offering one's presence, interest or wish to understand the person, without making any demands or attaching conditions that the person must comply with to receive the health professional's attention.	'I'll stay with you for a while.' 'We can sit here quietly for a while; we don't need to talk unless you would like to.'
	Encouraging or acknowledging	Giving recognition, in a non-judgmental way, of a change in behaviour, an effort the person has made, or a contribution to a communication.	'You walked twice as far today with your walker.' 'You've done so well today. Yesterday you couldn't get out of bed to go to the toilet and today you have been able to use a commode.'
	Focusing	Helping the person expand on and develop a topic of importance. It is important for the healthcare professional to wait until the person finishes stating the main concerns before attempting to focus.	Patient arriving back from theatre: 'I feel terrible … sick and really wobbly.' HCP: 'Are you feeling nauseous?'
	Reflecting	Directing ideas, feelings, questions or content back to a person to enable them to explore their own ideas and feelings about a situation. Reflecting indicates listening, as it requires the skill to be able to interpret not only what is said but what is conveyed non-verbally. It also confirms the presence of emotions.	Patient: 'What can I do?' HCP: 'What do you think would be helpful?' Patient: 'Do you think I should tell my husband?' HCP: 'You seem unsure about telling your husband.'

Communication technique	Definition	Example/s
Summarising	Stating the main points of a discussion to bring into focus the relevant points. It is a brief collection of paraphrases and reflections of the person's feelings that are connected in a meaningful way. This technique may open up the discussion to different significant areas. Summarising indicates listening. It allows the healthcare professional to check their understanding and wait for feedback.	'During the past half hour we have talked about …' 'I'd just like now to sum up today's discussion …'

TABLE 2.1

Verbal and non-verbal communication techniques (Continued)

Source: Adapted from Levett-Jones, T. (2018). Communication. In A. Berman, S. Synder, T. Levett-Jones et al. (Eds), *Kozier and Erb's Fundamentals of Nursing* (4th edn). Sydney: Pearson.

NICOLE'S STORY

Nicole, a first-year nursing student, was undertaking her first clinical placement. Each day, she listened during handover as the nurses described Joyce, an older patient on the medical ward, as a 'pain', a 'nuisance', 'demanding', a 'cranky old thing', etc. When Nicole answered Joyce's call bell one morning, she took the time to talk to her. She sat beside Joyce, maintaining eye contact, giving her full attention and listening intently. Joyce told Nicole how she had been admitted to hospital as an emergency. She confided how worried she was about her cat as she hadn't been able to organise anyone to care for it while she was in hospital. Nicole asked if there was anyone she could call and Joyce gave her the phone number of one of her neighbours. Nicole immediately went and made the phone call, and organised for the neighbour to care for the cat. When she returned and explained that the cat was 'in good hands', Joyce's demeanour immediately changed. For the first time since admission she became less agitated and began to relax. Although some of the nurses had labelled Joyce as the 'demanding old girl in 217', Nicole's empathic interaction identified the real cause of Joyce's distress and agitation.

There are many environmental and interpersonal factors that can interfere with effective communication in healthcare settings—telephones, call bells, patient acuity, interruptions, time pressures, heavy workloads, stress, fatigue and negative attitudes can individually and collectively make quality communication interactions difficult. However, when healthcare professionals don't pay attention to the unique needs of each patient, and instead mislabel them as 'a pain' or 'difficult', they are making an inappropriate value judgment.

Nicole made the decision not to be unduly influenced by what she heard during handover. Instead, she took the time to develop a rapport with Joyce, establish what her concerns were, and follow up in a timely manner. The outcome from this interaction was that Joyce's distress was eased and she could focus on her recovery without worrying about her cat being left unattended.

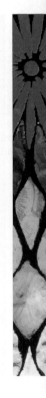

The attributes of effective healthcare communication

The Seven Cs communication model (*clear, concise, concrete, coherent, complete, courteous, compassionate*) was developed to outline the key attributes of effective written and verbal communication (Cutlip, 1952). In the section below, the Seven Cs model has been used to illustrate these attributes with reference to a range of healthcare scenarios.

Clear

No matter what type of communication (e.g. explanatory, instructive, educative), ensuring that the meaning is clear is fundamental to safe patient outcomes. When speaking to patients (or colleagues) it is important to be clear about both the purpose and the key message. If more than one message needs to be relayed, this should be stated; and the number of messages in each sentence should be minimised and described in a logical sequence. Use of jargon and unclear terms should be avoided as they can lead to confusion, uncertainty and variable interpretation (Charlton et al., 2008). The meaning of a communication interaction must be clear so that the patient can take any necessary action. Checking for patient cues that may indicate failure to understand is also critical (Uitterhoeve et al., 2009).

Example

Ineffective communication	Effective communication
'Hi John. A doctor will see you soon when blood tests are done and you have some rest.' *What is John being told exactly? The communication is vague and he is likely to request more information about timing and tests or be simply left confused as to what is going to happen to him and when.*	'Hello Mr Adams, or would you like me to call you John? My name is Sally. I am the nurse that will be taking care of you this afternoon. I am sorry that you are not feeling well. We need to take blood from your arm now to help us better understand your condition. Some of the blood test results will be available within two hours. The doctor will look at them and then speak with you about the results. Do you have any questions for me or concerns you would like to tell me about?'

Concise

In healthcare, being concise refers to keeping to the intended point of the communication. This reduces the potential for confusion that can occur when communication crosses more than one issue. An accurate and concise message is more likely to be understood and assists in keeping the person's attention. Verbose and imprecise communication can distract patients and create confusion (Adolphs, Atkins & Harvey, 2007). Examples of imprecise words include: many, soon, later and most.

Use the smallest word that does the job. (E.B. White)

Example

Ineffective communication	Effective communication
'Hi Mary. How are you feeling? Don't worry, most people with this problem recover well and don't have any real issues as a result. So, no need to worry, you should be okay soon.' *The communication with Mary is both repetitious and vague. This leaves Mary to worry about her circumstances. How many is most? How long is soon? What do they mean by 'should be okay'? Mary is not given an opportunity to voice her concerns as the healthcare professional does not wait for a response before continuing the dialogue. Communication with patients must be a two-way process that not only provides reassurance, but also leads to a better understanding of their illness.*	'Hello Mrs Lamb, how are you feeling today? It is very understandable that you are worried about your illness. What would you like to know?' 'I see, you would like to know the likely cause and progression of the illness. Is that right?' 'Research tells us that your problem was most likely caused by you having recent contact with your grandchild, who has a similar problem. It clears up in two to three weeks with a single treatment for 9 out of 10 people. It is hard to definitely know if you will need another treatment at this early stage, but your symptoms are decreasing already so that is a good sign.'

Concrete

To make communication concrete is to substantiate meaning through context—relevant clear examples, understandable facts and/or rich visuals. These approaches reduce the likelihood of the person misinterpreting the information. Healthcare professionals are predominantly trained to use verbal communication; however, visuals are the preferred communication style of many people and have been shown to help increase people's understanding of health problems and risk factors (Houts et al., 2006). Visuals can also be used to help patients rate their pain and other feelings (Scott et al., 2015).

Example

Ineffective communication	Effective communication
'To help you understand about your heart valve replacement on Tuesday I will use this textbook I found in the doctor's room. As you can see, our heart has four chambers—the right atrium, left atrium, right ventricle and left ventricle. The atria are smaller than the ventricles and have less muscular walls than the ventricles ...' *When communicating with patients with the aid of diagrams, the most effective illustrations are simple ones. For example, when explaining an aortic valve, the illustration should display a simple heart, an aorta and an aortic valve. Complex illustrations that show details not relevant to the patient's problem should be avoided. Showing inessential details can distract the patient and reduce the effectiveness of the illustration as a teaching tool.*	'It is normal for patients to ask for more information before surgery, Peter. To help you understand about your heart valve replacement on Tuesday, let's talk about what specific information you would like. From my understanding you would like to better understand what the aortic valve does and where it can be found? Is that correct? Do you think a diagram might help you to better understand?' 'Okay, I am drawing a very simple diagram of the heart with only the parts of the heart that are relevant to your operation. The aortic valve lies here between this lower left heart chamber (the left ventricle) and the main artery that delivers blood from the heart to the body (the aorta). It keeps blood flowing in the right direction as you can see by the arrow I have drawn.' 'Has this helped your understanding, Peter? Can I help you understand anything else?'

Coherent and complete

Communication is coherent if all points are connected and relevant to the message. It must also be appropriate for the receiver, and any language and terminology used needs to fit with the receiver's level of understanding.

In a complete message, all relevant information is included so the receiver is fully informed and has everything they need to take action, if applicable (Silverman, Kurtz & Draper, 2016). Complete information helps the patient make better decisions.

Example

Ineffective communication	Effective communication
'Hello Dolly. You are recovering well. You must be pleased to be going home. Don't forget what the doctor told you—pick up tablets from the pharmacy and take them BD. Give the discharge letter to your family doctor. Be sure to make an appointment later in the week. They will take over your care once you leave hospital. Leave the surgical site dressing on until you are seen—you should have no bleeding. You can go home once you have your paperwork. Best of luck.' *This communication is hurried, disconnected and confusing. It leaves a lot of unknowns and unanswered questions. Which pharmacy does he mean, the community pharmacy or the hospital pharmacy? What if the wound does bleed? Is the paperwork he refers to the same as the discharge summary he spoke about earlier? The key question to always consider when you communicate in the healthcare environment is: Are you speaking clearly and logically, and listening carefully?*	'Hello Mrs Riley, I am glad you are feeling better. Just to reinforce your doctor's instructions, when you go home you will need to see your family doctor within three days so please call as soon as possible to make an appointment. Please also see your family doctor once you have finished all the tablets or right away if you feel any worse. Your tablets can be picked up on your way out of the hospital from the pharmacy, which is at the entrance to the hospital. You need to take 2 tablets in the morning and one at night. Your wound dressing will need to stay on until your first appointment with your family doctor. If you see blood through or around the dressing, carefully remove it and replace it with the new one I have slipped in with your discharge letter.' 'Would you like me to explain any of this information again? To show me that you understand, would you mind repeating the instructions back to me?' 'I've also written these instructions on this discharge letter, along with our contact details in case you have any concerns. One copy of the discharge letter is for you to keep and the other is for your family doctor, who has also been sent an electronic copy.'

Courteous

Courteous healthcare communication is friendly, reliable and open. It is being aware of and respecting the feelings of other people, and it allows the communicator to be open to others' opinions and ideas. Courteous communication includes expressions and terms that show respect for the patient (e.g. asking a person whether they like to be called William, Bill or Mr Jackson), and it makes people feel supported and valued during interactions (Deledda et al., 2013). Courteous communication can also benefit healthcare professionals by providing a more satisfying work experience.

Example

Ineffective communication	Effective communication
'Hello dear, my name is Karen. I'll be back to help you shower and dress your wound. I will also be giving you your medications when they are due. Press the buzzer if you need anything else, but remember how busy I am today.'	'Hello Mrs James, my name is Karen and I will be your nurse today. I hope you slept well.'
This communication is business-like rather than being patient-friendly. Referring to the patient as 'dear' is discourteous. In healthcare communication, being approachable and positive, gaining eye contact and smiling are simple acts that can make a big difference to a patient's day.	'How are you feeling this morning? Can I do anything for you right now? I have five other patients to care for today so please excuse me if you don't see me as much as we would both like. Please do press your buzzer if you need me when I am out of sight and I will come as soon as I can.'
	Being courteous includes making an effort to engage in light conversation and show some interest in the patients within your care.

Compassionate

The perspective and feelings of patients should be foremost in compassionate communication. This type of communication is responsive to the feelings, perspectives and needs of patients—it implies 'walking in the shoes of others'. Compassionate communicators seek to understand the patient's views, needs, background and mindset, as well as their requirements, emotions and problems. They also modify their words, communication content and style for each person (Hawkins et al., 2008). By maintaining this focus, the patient's self-respect is maintained and a positive reaction is more likely to result.

Example

Ineffective communication	Effective communication
'Hello Mrs Crowley. You are late for your procedure so you need to quickly change into this gown and complete this paperwork so I can check your observations. After this, I will prepare you for your procedure. You will need to have an IV inserted in your hand before the procedure begins. Your family will need to go outside now.'	'Hello Mrs Crowley, my name is Andrew and I am the nurse that will be taking care of you this morning. We were expecting you earlier, is everything alright?'
This rushed one-way communication is inconsiderate of the patient and their circumstances. It risks the patient losing a sense of control. The communication does not allow for an understanding of the current patient circumstances, nor their broader context. These include the reason for their delay, an understanding of the patient's need for family members to be present, whether they understand what the nurse has told them, and their individual needs; yet these factors could have a direct bearing on the outcomes of the procedure. An assumption of 'one size fits all' in terms of patient understanding and context is adopted, yet every patient is different.	'Okay, good. I'm glad everything is alright. I want to first let you know the steps we take with you before your procedure. Please stop me if I am speaking too fast or you need to clarify anything.'
	'First, I will ask you to change into this gown. It opens to your back and you do not have to remove your underpants. Next, I will ask you to complete some forms and I will be here to help you in case you do not understand what is required. I will then check your temperature, blood pressure and heart rate so we can detect any changes during and after the procedure. After this, I will prepare you for your procedure by inserting a tube in your hand for IV fluids. This allows the anaesthetist to give you fluid and medications during the procedure. You should be taken to theatre on a trolley within the next half an hour. Your family are welcome to stay while you wait. Do you have any questions or concerns at this stage?'

Read Box 2.3 and reflect on some of your own experiences with communication.

BOX 2.3   What can job interviews tell us about healthcare communication encounters?

Job interviews can be highly stressful events even for the most experienced people. They are intellectually and emotionally demanding as they have the potential to significantly influence a person's future career aspirations. A job interview requires a person to hand over control of personal power and it creates a feeling of being exposed. Amid this stressful situation the person can find it difficult to hear, understand and respond to the questions being asked by members of the interview panel. Differences in education and power levels between interviewers and interviewees can result in different communication styles that can further complicate the process. Alternatively, job interviews can be helpful and even pleasant experiences, depending on the attitudes and communication skills of those conducting the interview.

The patient experience can be similar to the interview process, but with the feelings much more magnified, especially when the health problem is serious. Effective communication can make a significant difference to the patient's healthcare experience. If the healthcare professional is difficult to understand, distracted or disinterested, the patient may sense that their concerns are not a priority and feel reluctant to ask questions. Alternatively, communication that is clear, concise, concrete, coherent, complete, compassionate and courteous helps to facilitate a rapport between the healthcare professional and the patient, and they are more likely to express their concerns and ask questions.

Health literacy

Health literacy refers to how people understand information about health and healthcare, and how they use that information to make decisions. An important factor in achieving optimal health outcomes is for patients to understand and appropriately act on healthcare advice. When people have this ability, they are said to be health literate. Almost 60 per cent of Australian adults have a low level of health literacy (Australian Commission on Safety and Quality in Health Care [ACSQHC], 2014), and it is estimated that these people are 1.5–3 times more likely to experience a serious adverse health outcome (ACSQHC, 2014).

While health information is now freely and widely available from the internet, and many people use this information to try to gain a better understanding of their own or their loved one's health concerns, research has shown that most online health information is written at a level that the average person cannot accurately understand (Cheng & Dunn, 2015). Healthcare professionals therefore have a key role in assessing patients' health literacy skills and providing patient education that is aligned with these assessment results (Brach et al., 2012). Failing to take into account a person's health literacy level can result in ineffective communication, use of language that is unfamiliar to patients, or provision of instructions that are not clear (Cafiero, 2013). Educating patients is a key healthcare professional role and integral to safe patient care. Fundamental to education is determining how well a patient or their family comprehends and recalls information they have been given. The example below highlights how healthcare professionals may not only cause confusion if patient understanding of healthcare information is not adequately assessed but also potentially cause significant harm.

MR SCHRODER'S STORY

Mr Carl Schroder, an 81-year-old man, was diagnosed with emphysema 10 years ago and his condition has recently worsened. He is attending an appointment with the practice nurse to receive education on how to better manage his emphysema at home with the use of oxygen as required. The nurse has brought several pages of

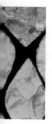

printed instructional information for Mr Schroder about when and how to use the oxygen safely. After the nurse explains the instructions, she gives him the printed information and states that he can read it at home where he will have more time. The nurse opens the door of the consulting room and wishes Mr Schroder well. At his next appointment with his family doctor, Mr Schroder is found to be very unwell. He responds to the doctor's question about how many hours a day he is using oxygen by saying, 'I have tried to use it a few times but it doesn't seem to work. I have never been very good at understanding written instructions.'

Each healthcare professional has a responsibility to identify patients who require communication support so that even the most vulnerable patients gain every possible benefit from their healthcare (Cho et al., 2008). Health literacy assessment provides important information about the patient and allows healthcare professionals to appropriately modify their communication when needed. A large variety of tools are available to assess people's health literacy. These include those that evaluate general health literacy or an understanding of specific illnesses and others that assess health literacy for different patient languages or healthcare environments.

One evidence-based approach for confirming a person's understanding of what is being explained to them is the teach-back method (Dinh et al., 2016). This method is premised on the belief that, if a patient (and/or family member) understands the information that has been provided, they will be able to 'teach it back' accurately. If the patient cannot translate the information accurately, the healthcare professional should clarify or modify the information provided and reassess the patient's understanding. While this method benefits the patient, it also assists healthcare professionals to better understand the effectiveness of their communication skills, as it confirms (or refutes) whether they have explained the information in a way that the patient understands. Experts recommend that healthcare professionals check every patient's understanding of the information provided about their health problem, treatment plan, medications, self-management and other important areas by using this quick teach-back method (Brega et al., 2015) and documenting in the patient's healthcare record.

The teach-back method

1	2	3	4	5
Important information needs to be relayed to the patient	The healthcare professional communicates the information to the patient	The healthcare professional asks the patient to explain the information that has just been provided	The healthcare professional recognises that the patient is unable to teach-back correctly	The healthcare professional asks the patient to explain the information that has just been provided
Information about the patient's health problem, treatment, self-management, medications and other important aspects of healthcare.	Care is taken to plan patient communication using plain language and explaining any technical terms.	The patient is respectfully asked to teach the information back to the healthcare professional in their own words and to identify anything they do not understand or any further information that is required. The healthcare professional emphasises the reason why this is important, i.e. to ensure they have provided information in a way that meets the patient's needs.	The patient is provided the information again with further clarification, tailored to the identified needs of the patient.	The patient is respectfully asked to teach the information back in their own words and to again identify anything they do not understand. This step is repeated as required using different approaches to ensure understanding. Key information can also be written to help patient's to remember the instructions when they get home.

Conclusion

The ability to be a 'good' communicator is sometimes viewed as an inherent skill or trait. In reality, safe and effective patient communication is a practical skill that can be learnt and improved through deliberate practice. As healthcare professionals, your ability to communicate is a crucial clinical skill. Focused attention to and reflection on your current level of verbal and non-verbal communication skills, together with a commitment to ongoing improvement, will impact on your relationships with both patients and colleagues. This chapter has provided a plethora of ideas and strategies for examining and improving your communication skills, and adding to your repertoire of professional capabilities.

Critical thinking activities

1   Healthcare professionals often need to share complex information with patients. These types of explanations require you to break down information into manageable chunks and to structure the way you communicate this information to enhance comprehension.
    • Imagine trying to give someone only verbal instructions on how to draw the string of shapes in Figure 2.2. What would be challenging about doing this?

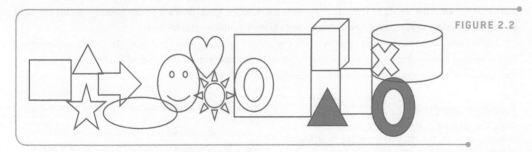

FIGURE 2.2

    • Then consider other complex instructions that you may need to provide to patients (e.g. self-catheterisation, blood glucose monitoring, administration of a subcutaneous injection) and the most effective way of doing so.
2   Have you ever tried to have a conversation with someone who was clearly distracted—scrolling through Facebook posts, thinking about something else, not maintaining eye contact or interrupting you. How did this make you feel?
    • Then think about experiences that you have had when seeking treatment from a healthcare professional. Did they make you feel valued, respected, listened to and understood? If so, how did they do this?
    • Did they engage with you in an empathic manner, taking into consideration your feelings, perspectives and needs? If so, how did they do this?
    • What have you learnt from these types of encounters that you can apply in your own practice?

Teaching and assessment activities

Activity 1

Developing self-awareness through mindfulness meditation

If we are serious about increasing our self-awareness, we need to stop thinking and doing and learn to listen to our inner selves. Mindfulness meditation is the perfect practice to help students focus and gain a sense of equanimity. Access this link for one example of a 10-minute loving kindness meditation: <https://www.virtualempathymuseum.com.au/wp-content/uploads/2018/10/Kindness-Visualisation-first_mix.mp3>.

Activity 2

Listening exercise

In pairs, select one student to be the listener and one student to be the speaker. The speaker speaks for about 5 minutes, retelling a story of a situation that was a comfortable one (e.g. attending an event, participating in a ceremony, receiving an award). The listener may only make three statements during the interaction, yet must somehow get the

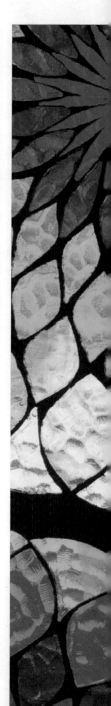

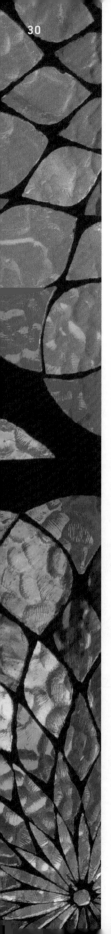

speaker to continue speaking for the allotted time. Switch roles and repeat the exercise. When finished, discuss your answers to these questions:

1 How did it feel to be the speaker when the person listened yet didn't exchange much information?
2 Were any non-verbal communication signals encouraged by the listener?
3 How uncomfortable was the silence?
4 How did it feel to just listen without the pressure to contribute to the communication?
5 How did the speaker feel about having the freedom to say whatever he/she wanted?

Activity 3

Reading people's feelings

This activity is very useful in demonstrating how important it is to correctly identify feelings and how it is very easy to incorrectly identify them. It also demonstrates the uniqueness of 'feelings'—a feeling experienced by one person in a particular situation may not seem feasible to another person. So it is for our patients. It is important to correctly identify how a patient is feeling in order for us to respond appropriately and empathically.

Print out a list of feeling words on individual cards: happy, scared, bored, angry, anxious, sad, surprised, worried, excited, confused, frustrated, embarrassed, joyful, disgusted, jealous, grieving, dread, horrified, confident, uneasy, confident, hopeful, optimistic, shy, nervous, vulnerable, neglected, ashamed—there are many more you can add to the list.

In groups, put the cards in the middle of the table. Ask a student to pick up a card (without looking at it), show it to the others at the table and get the others to non-verbally act out that feeling, one-by-one. The person holding the card must work out what the feeling is. The activity continues around the group until the person holding the card correctly identifies the feeling. Repeat, using different cards and students, until allocated time runs out.

Another exercise, using the same cards, is to ask one student to hold up a card and for students who see the feeling card to verbally communicate a situation or time that they might experience that feeling. All students in the group can take turns in retelling a story or situation until the feeling is correctly identified.

Further reading

Brega, A. G., Barnard, J., Mabachi, N. M., Weiss, B. D., DeWalt, D. A., Brach, C. … West, D. R. (2015). *AHRQ Health Literacy Universal Precautions Toolkit* (2nd edn). (Prepared by Colorado Health Outcomes Program, University of Colorado Anschutz Medical Campus under Contract No. HHSA290200710008, TO#10.) AHRQ publication no. 15-0023-EF. Rockville, MD: Agency for Healthcare Research and Quality. Access December 2018 at <https://www.ahrq.gov/sites/default/files/publications/files/healthlittoolkit2_3.pdf>

World Health Organization. (2013). *Health literacy: The solid facts*. Copenhagen: WHO Regional Office for Europe.

Accessed December 2018 at <http://www.euro.who.int/_data/assets/pdf_file/0008/190655/e96854.pdf>

Web resources

Explore the healthcare experiences of patients at the following sites:

Patient Opinion Aust:
<https://www.patientopinion.org.au/>

Care Opinion: What's your story:
<https://www.careopinion.org.uk/>

MTD Training Academy: Basic communication skills:
<http://www.mtdacademy.com>

Pfizer clear health communication initiative: Health literacy:
<https://www.pfizer.com/health/literacy>

The *Always Use Teach-back!* training toolkit: This resource provides a very useful range of tools and videos to support an assessment of patient understanding.
<http://www.teachbacktraining.org/>

Video: US Institute of Healthcare Innovation. *What Is Teach-Back?*
<https://www.youtube.com/watch?v=bzpJJYF_tKY>

Video: North Western Melbourne Primary Health Network. *Teach back—a technique for clear communication.*
<https://www.youtube.com/watch?v=d7O2HIZfVWs>

References

Adolphs, S., Atkins, S. & Harvey, K. (2007). Caught between professional requirements and interpersonal needs: Vague language in healthcare contexts. In *Vague Language Explored* (pp. 62–78). London: Palgrave Macmillan.

Australian Commission on Safety and Quality in Health Care. (2014). *Health Literacy: Taking Action to Improve Safety and Quality*. Sydney: ACSQHC.

Brega, A. G., Barnard, J., Mabachi, N. M., Weiss, B. D., DeWalt, D.A., Brach, C. & West, D. R. (2015). *AHRQ Health Literacy Universal Precautions Toolkit*. Rockville, MD: Agency for Healthcare Research and Quality.

Brach, C., Keller, D., Hernandez, L.M., Baur, C., Dreyer, B. … Schillinger, D. (2012). *Ten Attributes of Health Literate Health Care Organizations*. Washington, DC: Institute of Medicine of the National Academies.

Cafiero, M. (2013). Nurse practitioners' knowledge, experience, and intention to use health literacy strategies in clinical practice. *Journal of Health Communication*, *18*(1), 70–81.

Charlton, C. R., Dearing, K. S., Berry, J. A. & Johnson, M. J. (2008). Nurse practitioners' communication styles and their impact on patient outcomes: an integrated literature review. *Journal of the American Association of Nurse Practitioners*, *20*(7), 382–8.

Cheng, C. & Dunn, M. (2015). Health literacy and the Internet: A study on the readability of Australian online health information. *Australian and New Zealand Journal of Public Health*, *39*(4), 309–14.

Cho, Y. I., Lee, S. Y., Arozullah, A. M., Crittenden, K. S. (2008). Effects of health literacy on health status and health service utilization amongst the elderly. *Social Science & Medicine*, *66*, 1809–16.

Christman, C. (2015). *How to Read Minds & Influence People: The Science of Nonverbal Communication and Everyday Persuasion* (2nd edn). USA: Createspace Independent Publishing Platform.

Cutlip, S. M. (1952). *Effective Public Relations: Pathways to Public Favor*. New York: Prentice Hall.

Deledda, G., Moretti, F., Rimondini, M. & Zimmermann, C. (2013). How patients want their doctor to communicate. A literature review on primary care patients' perspective. *Patient Education and Counseling*, *90*(3), 297–306.

Dean, S., Lewis, J. & Ferguson, C. (2016). Is technology responsible for nurses losing touch? *Journal of Clinical Nursing*. doi: 10.1111/jocn.13470

Dean, S., Zaslawski, C., Roche, M. & Adams, J. (2016). 'Talk to them': Teaching communication skills to students of traditional Chinese medicine. *Journal of Nursing Education and Practice*, *6*(12), pp 49–56.

Dinh, T. T. H., Bonner, A., Clark, R., Ramsbotham, J. & Hines, S. (2016). The effectiveness of the teach-back method on adherence and self-management in health education for people with chronic disease: A systematic review. *JBI Database of Systematic Reviews and Implementation Reports*, *14*(1), 210–47.

Egan, G. (2010). *The Skilled Helper* (9th edn, p. 136). Belmont, California: Brooks/Cole Publishing Company.

Fogarty, L., Curbow, B. Wingard, J., McDonnell, K. & Somerfield, M. (1999). Can 40 seconds of compassion reduce patient anxiety? *Journal of Clinical Oncology*. *17*(1), 371.

Hawkins, R. P., Kreuter, M., Resnicow, K., Fishbein, M. & Dijkstra, A. (2008). Understanding tailoring in communicating about health. *Health Education Research*, *23*(3), 454–66.

Houts, P. S., Doak, C. C., Doak, L. G. & Loscalzo, M. J. (2006). The role of pictures in improving health communication: A review of research on attention, comprehension, recall, and adherence. *Patient Education and Counseling*, *61*(2), 173–90.

Granger, K. (2013). Healthcare staff must properly introduce themselves to patients. *BMJ*, *347*: f5833. doi: 10.1136/bm

Levett-Jones, T. (2018). Communication. In A. Berman, S. Synder, T. Levett-Jones, et al. (Eds), *Kozier and Erb's Fundamentals of Nursing* (4th edn). Sydney: Pearson.

Luft, J. (1969). *Of Human Interaction: The Johari Model*. Palo Alto, CA: Mayfield.

Mehrabian, A. (1981). *Silent Messages: Implicit Communication of Emotions and Attitudes*. Belmont, CA: Wadsworth.

Ong, L., Visser, M., Lammes, F., De Haes, J. (2000). Doctor–patient communication and cancer patients' quality of life and satisfaction. *Patient Education and Counseling*, *41*(2), 145–56.

Riess, H. & Kraft-Todd, G. (2014). E.M.P.A.T.H.Y.: A tool to enhance nonverbal communication between clinicians and their patients. *Academic medicine*, *89*(8), 1108–12. doi: 10.1097IACM.0000000000000287

Schiavo, R. (2014). *Health Communication: From Theory to Practice* (2nd edn) . San Francisco: Jossey-Bass Public Health.

Scott, H. (2011). *Empathy in Healthcare Settings*. University of London, UK: Goldsmiths Research Online.

Scott, S. E., Birt, L., Cavers, D., Shah, N., Campbell, C. & Walter, F. M. (2015). Patient drawings of their melanoma: A novel approach to understanding symptom perception and appraisal prior to health care. *Psychology & Health*, *30*(9), 1035–48.

Silverman, J., Kurtz, S. & Draper, J. (2016). *Skills for Communicating with Patients* (3rd edn). London: CRC Press.

Stein-Parbury, J. (2017). *Patient & Person* (7th edn). Chatswood, Australia: Elsevier.

Stewart, M. A. (1995). Effective physician-patient communication and health outcomes: A review. *CMAJ: Canadian Medical Association Journal*, *152*(9), 1423.

Thorne, S., Hislop, T., Armstrong, E. & Oglov, V. (2008). Cancer care communication: The power to harm and the power to heal? *Patient Education and Counseling*. *71*(1), 34–40.

Uitterhoeve, R., Bensing, J., Dilven, E., Donders, R., demulder, P. & van Achterberg, T. (2009). Nurse–patient communication in cancer care: Does responding to patient's cues predict patient satisfaction with communication. *Psycho-Oncology*, *18*(10), 1060–68.

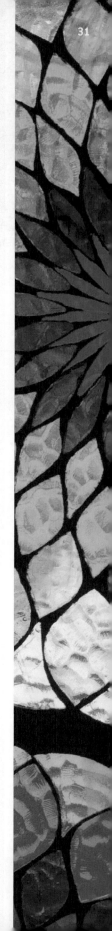

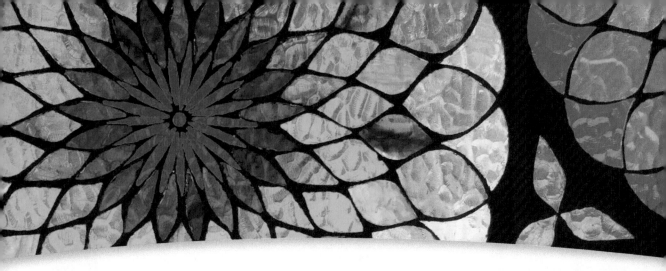

CHAPTER 3

KEY ATTRIBUTES OF PATIENT-SAFE COMMUNICATION

Tracy Levett-Jones

LEARNING OUTCOMES

Chapter 3 will enable you to:

- describe the principles, practices and outcomes of person-centred care[1]

- explore the relationship between person-centred care and patient-safe communication

- describe the attributes and attitudes that promote patient-safe communication

- discuss the impact of interprofessional and team-based communication on patient safety

- reflect on your personal attributes and consider how they have the potential to enhance or detract from your ability to be person-centred and clinically safe.

KEY CONCEPTS

patient-safe communication | person-centred care | interprofessional communication | teamwork

---

1 The terms 'person-centred' and 'patient-centred' care are often used interchangeably. In this book we use the term 'person-centred care' as this is the term commonly used in healthcare literature. We acknowledge that for some disciplines the term patient-centred care is preferred. Both terms are conceptually similar, and emphasise the central roles of patients, families and carers in aspects of care, as well as in the broader approach to improving health service planning and delivery.

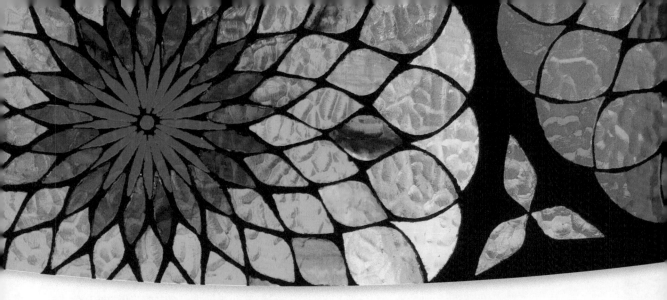

> We are guests in our patients' lives; and we are their hosts
> when they come to us. Why should they, or we, expect
> anything less than the graciousness expected by guests
> and from hosts at their very best. Service is quality.
>
> (Berwick, 1999, p. 9)

INTRODUCTION

In Chapter 1, patient-safe communication was defined as a goal-oriented activity focused on pre-venting clinical errors and helping patients attain optimal health outcomes. Patient-safe communi-cation was described as an essential foundation for working collaboratively with both patients and other healthcare professionals to ensure safe care (Schuster & Nykolyn, 2010). Person-centred care is the most important attribute of patient-safe communication, and we begin Chapter 3 by discussing the benefits of this approach to patients, healthcare professionals and healthcare organisations. We then outline the importance of interprofessional communication and teamwork to patient safety. In the chapters that follow, these issues are discussed in greater depth with specific clinical examples provided.

MRS GRUZENSKI'S STORY

Professor Donald Berwick, an internationally recognised leading authority on quality and safety in health-care, gave a graduation address at Yale Medical School on 24 May 2010. The following story is an excerpt from that address, and it begins by recounting an email that Professor Berwick received from Mrs Jocelyn Gruzenski in 2009:

> 'My husband was Dr William Gruzenski, a psychiatrist for 39 years. He was admitted to hospital after developing a cerebral bleed with a hypertensive crisis. I was denied access to my husband except for very strict visiting, four times a day for 30 minutes; my husband was hospitalised behind a locked door. He wanted me present in the ICU, and he challenged the ICU nurses and doctors saying, "She is not a visitor, she is my wife". But, it made no difference. My husband was in the ICU for eight days out of his last 16 days alive, and there were a lot of missed opportunities for us. His care was not individualised to meet his needs; he wanted me there more than I was allowed. I feel it was a very cruel thing that was done to us. My husband and I loved each other very deeply and we wanted to share our last days and moments together. We both knew the gravity of his illness, and my husband wanted quality of life, not quantity.'

'What might a husband and wife, aware of the short time left together, wish to talk about in their last days? Someone stole all of that from Dr and Mrs Gruzenski. A nameless someone. I suspect an unknowing someone with "rational" words such as "It's our policy", "It's against the rules", "It's in your own best interest". This is the voice of power; and power can be, to borrow Mrs Gruzenski's word, "cruel".'

Donald Berwick continued his address to the graduating students:

'Today you take a big step into power. With your anatomy lessons and your stethoscope, you enter today a life of new and vast privilege. You will not always feel powerful or privileged—not when you are filling out endless forms and struggling through hard days of too many tasks. But this will be true: In return for your years of learn-ing and your dedication, society will allow you to hear secrets from frightened human beings that they are too scared to tell anyone else. Society will permit you to use drugs and instruments that can do great harm as well as great good. Society will let you make rules. And in that role, with that power, you will meet Dr and Mrs Gruzenski over and over again. You will meet them every day—every hour. They will be disguised as a new mother afraid to touch her premature baby. Disguised as a construction worker too embarrassed to admit that he didn't under-stand a word you said after "It might be cancer". Disguised as the alcoholic who was the handsome champion of his soccer team and dreamed of being an architect someday. Disguised as the child or the 90-year-old grand-mother over whom you tower. Disguised as the professor in the MRI machine who has been told to lie still, but who desperately needs to urinate and is ashamed. Disguised as the man who wants you to call him "Bill", and as the man who prefers to be called "Dr Gruzenski". Mrs Gruzenski wrote, "My husband was a very caring physician and administrator for many years, but during his hospitalisation, he was not even afforded the respect of being called 'Doctor'." Dr Gruzenski wanted to be called, "Dr Gruzenski". But, they did not do so. You can. That choice is not in the hands of nameless power. It is your choice; your power.

'What is at stake here may seem a small thing in the face of the enormous healthcare world you have joined. But that small thing is what matters. I will tell you: it is *all* that matters. All that matters is the person. The per-son. The individual. The patient. The poet. The lover. The adventurer. The frightened soul. The wondering mind. The learned mind. The Husband. The Wife. The Son. The Daughter. It is all about choice. You have a magical opportunity. Yes, you can hide behind the protocols and policies. You can lock the door and say, "Sorry, Mrs Gruzenski, your 30 minutes are up." But, you can also *unlock* the door. You can ask, "Shall I call you 'Dr Gruzenski'?" "Would you like to be alone?" "Is this a convenient time?" "Is there something else I can do for you?"'

Source: Reproduced with permission: Jocelyn Anne Gruzenski and Dr Donald Berwick.

Person-centred care

Recognition that person-centred care is arguably the most important attribute of patient-safe commu-nication is changing the landscape of contemporary healthcare education. The traditional view of patients as passive recipients of care has given way to one where patients are seen as active participants and integral members of the healthcare team. Patients (and their families) are now seen to have a vested interest and valuable perspective in ensuring safe care.

There are various definitions of the term 'person-centred care', with each underpinned by principles such as *empathy*, *dignity*, *autonomy*, *respect*, *choice*, *transparency*, and a desire to help individuals lead *the life they want*. Person-centred care is built on the understanding that patients bring their own experiences, skills and knowledge about their condition and illness. It is a *holistic* approach to the planning, delivery and evaluation of healthcare that is grounded in *mutually beneficial partnerships* between healthcare professionals, patients and families.

> *[Person-centredness] is an approach to practice established through the formation and fostering of healthful relationships between all care providers, service users [consumers] and others significant to them in their lives. It is underpinned by the values of respect for persons, individual rights to self-determination, mutual respect and understanding.*
>
> (McCormack & McCance, 2017, p. 60)

Healthcare professionals who practise person-centred care are *ethical*, *open-minded*, *self-aware* and have a profound sense of *personal responsibility* for actions (*moral agency*). They place the 'person' at the centre of healthcare and consider their needs and wishes as paramount (McCormack & McCance, 2017). Person-centred clinicians:

- appreciate that people have a unique life history that influences their healthcare experience
- seek to understand the patient's perspective
- inform and involve patients in their care
- promote active involvement of family and friends
- elicit patient preferences
- check and confirm information with patients
- share treatment decisions
- respect patients' culture, values and personal beliefs
- provide physical and emotional comfort and support
- maintain patients' dignity
- design care processes to suit patients' needs, not the provider's needs
- ensure coordination and continuity of care
- are transparent and provide access to health information
- are sensitive to non-medical and spiritual dimensions of care
- guide patients to appropriate sources of information on health and healthcare
- educate patients on how to protect their health and prevent occurrence or recurrence of a disease
- provide support for self-care and self-management
- communicate information on risk and probability.

Source: Australian Commission on Safety and Quality in Health Care (ACSQHC), 2011; Institute for Patient- and Family-Centered Care, 2013; Shaller, 2007.

Person-centred care in practice

What we say, how we speak and the words we use have a significant impact on our patients. The right words can calm, comfort and reassure. The wrong words can produce anxiety and create confusion, anger or frustration in situations that are often fraught and stressful. When communicating in a person-centred way, showing respect and gaining trust is essential for enhancing patient cooperation and improving clinical outcomes.

Person-centred care is an ongoing process that requires professional competence, sound interpersonal skills, self-awareness, commitment to patient care and strong professional values (Australian College of Nursing, 2014). The Australian Commission on Safety and Quality in Health Care (ACSQHC, 2017) advocates that person-centred care may help address some of the health inequalities experienced by vulnerable or disadvantaged populations, such as the young, elderly, disabled or mentally ill; those from culturally and linguistically diverse backgrounds, or rural and remote areas; and Aboriginal and Torres Strait Islander peoples.

Evidence indicates that exposure to and reflection on authentic patient stories is an effective learning strategy, and one that can cause attitudinal shifts and behavioural change (Shapiro, 2011). Reflect on Mr Teddle's story in Box 3.1 and consider how the use of a person-centred approach may have influenced how the scenario unfolded.

BOX 3.1   Mr Treddle's story

Mr Treddle, 82 years old, was being discharged from hospital following admission for a TIA (transient ischaemic attack). His doctor gave him a written referral to his GP (general practitioner) and a prescription for his discharge medications. The pharmacist dispensed the prescribed medications. The dietitian provided a written dietary plan, as Mr Treddle had not been eating a diet appropriate for his type 2 diabetes. The registered nurse gave Mr Treddle a written discharge summary and reminded him to make an appointment to see his GP later that week. The ward clerk organised for him to go home in one of the hospital cars driven by a volunteer. While driving him home, the volunteer discovered that:

- Mr Treddle had no close family and lived alone in a caravan park
- the caravan park was 12 kilometres from his GP and the closest shops; he did not drive and there was no public transport
- Mr Treddle had macular degeneration and could not read the instructions written on the discharge summary or on his medication containers
- Mr Treddle had attempted suicide on two occasions.

Mr Treddle had been in hospital for a week and had interacted with numerous healthcare professionals, but during his hospitalisation Mr Treddle had not shared any of the information that he had discussed with the volunteer driver during the 40-minute car ride.

- *Why do you think this might have been?*
- *How could the healthcare professionals have interacted with Mr Treddle in a person-centred way that allowed him to feel comfortable in sharing his personal situation with them?*
- *How might the lack of person-centred care evident in this situation have impacted on Mr Treddle's safety and wellbeing post discharge?*

Person-centred care and patient safety

The literature increasingly demonstrates that there are many benefits to person-centred care (for patients, healthcare professionals and healthcare organisations). Foremost among these is improved communication and patient safety. Studies show that when healthcare professionals, patients and families work in partnership, the quality and safety of healthcare rises, costs decrease, and provider and patient satisfaction increase (Institute for Patient- and Family-Centered Care, 2013).

Organisations in which person-centred care is practised in a consistent way have reduced numbers of clinical errors, decreased readmission rates, lower infection rates (Institute for Patient- and Family-Centered Care, 2013), fewer medication errors (Bolster & Manias, 2010), decreased mortality rates and a shorter average length of stay (Institute for Patient- and Family-Centered Care, 2013; Meterko et al., 2010). In the care of patients with chronic conditions, studies indicate that person-centred care can improve disease management, reduce anxiety and improve quality of life (Bauman, Fardy & Harris, 2003; Stewart et al., 2000).

Person-centred language includes verbal and nonverbal communication. Asking patients how they prefer to be addressed establishes the foundation for a therapeutic relationship. By contrast, referring to a patient as 'a bowel resection' or 'the one with dementia' deprives them of the respect to which they are entitled. The use of acronyms such as AIDET (Acknowledge, Introduce, Duration, Explanation, Thank you)—see Box 3.2—can help healthcare professionals communicate in a person-centred way.

'Person-centred care should be a component of undergraduate and postgraduate education for all healthcare professionals' (ACSQHC, 2011).

BOX 3.2 **Using AIDET to improve communication and promote person-centred care**

1 **Acknowledge the patient.** Smile and make eye contact. Call the patient by his or her name. Consider the patient's prior experiences of healthcare.

2 **Introduce yourself.** Your name and role, and what you're planning to do.

3 **Duration of process/procedure.** Provide the patient with the length of time expected for processes, procedures, waiting, etc.

4 **Explanation.** Discuss what you're doing and why, what is next, and what procedures or tools you are using. Clarify whether the patient understands your explanation and has any questions. (Remember: explore—explain—explore.)

5 **Thank you.** Thank the patient for their time, information and cooperation.

Attitudes that promote patient-safe communication

If you were asked to list the specific attributes that healthcare professionals need in order to ensure patient-safe communication, you might reflect on the clinical experiences you have had and identify specific behaviours that you believe influenced patient outcomes. Patient-safe communication behaviours (both with patients and with other healthcare professionals) were also the focus of Chapters 1 and 2. What is perhaps more challenging is to identify the attitudes, beliefs and personal values that underpin healthcare professionals' behaviours and communication style. In the following section, we make the implicit explicit by discussing how attitudes influence patient care and why *self-awareness* is pivotal to effective communication. It is important to remember that each episode of communication will make a difference; whether it is a positive difference will depend on the attitudes and behaviours of the healthcare professionals involved.

A body of research has examined the influence of attitudes on healthcare professionals' behaviours. One recent study (Lapkin, Levett-Jones & Gilligan, 2012) identified that a student's attitude is the most significant predictor of their intention to practise in a way that enhances patient safety. This finding is supported by a meta-analysis of 87 studies that concluded there is significant evidence that attitudes and intentions can be used to predict actual behaviour (Sheppard, Hartwick & Warshaw, 1988). Although behavioural changes can occur as a result of social pressure and expectations, such changes are often short-lived if not accompanied by attitudinal changes. Attitudes are malleable and evolve over time, often in response to experiences and education.

As healthcare professionals, it is important that we are aware of our own attitudes, values and beliefs, as preconceptions, assumptions and biases can negatively influence our ability to be person-centred and to engage in patient-safe communication. Healthcare professionals' personal philosophies influence how we communicate with patients, particularly those who are vulnerable (e.g. have cognitive changes, have a mental illness, are from culturally and linguistically diverse backgrounds, or are socioeconomically disadvantaged). Failure to reflect on and question our assumptions and prejudices may negatively affect our communication competence. Table 3.1 illustrates three cognitive errors that can result from flawed assumptions and beliefs.

Ability is what you're capable of doing.

Motivation determines what you do.

Attitude determines how well you do it.

(Raymond Chandler)

Error	Definition
Ascertainment bias	When a health professional's thinking is shaped by prior assumptions and preconceptions (e.g. ageism).
Fundamental attribution error	The tendency to be judgmental and blame patients for their illnesses (dispositional causes) rather than examine the circumstances (situational factors) that may have been responsible. People from marginalised groups tend to be at particular risk of this error.
Overconfidence bias	A tendency to believe we know more than we do. Overconfidence reflects a tendency to act on incomplete information, intuition or hunches. Too much faith is placed on opinion instead of carefully collected cues.

TABLE 3.1
Examples of cognitive errors resulting from flawed assumptions and beliefs

Source: Adapted from P. Croskerry (2003). The importance of cognitive errors in diagnosis and strategies to minimise them. *Academic Medicine, 78*(8), 1–6.

Interprofessional and team-based communication

It would be naive to bring together a highly diverse group of people, no matter how talented, and expect that, by calling them a team, they will in fact behave as a team. Professional football teams can spend 40 hours a week practicing their teamwork skills in preparation for the weekend game when their teamwork really counts. Yet healthcare teams rarely spend an hour a week practicing teamwork skills, even though their ability to function as a team counts every day of every week.

(Wise, Beckhard, Rubin & Kyte, 1974)

Although most educational opportunities tend to focus on communication with patients, interprofessional and team-based communication is also critical to patient safety. Even the isolated general practitioner in a solo rural medical practice will routinely need to communicate with others in his/her daily work, for example a pathology laboratory (to order a test or receive results), a specialist ('The result indicates a malignancy; can you give an opinion?') or a nurse practitioner ('Can I have your advice on this patient's wound management?'). The more complex the working environment, the greater the potential for errors and the greater the need for effective communication between health professionals.

In order to communicate effectively with either patients or colleagues, healthcare professionals need to be *confident* and *knowledgeable*. This includes having a breadth and depth of domain-specific knowledge that is grounded in a solid evidence base. Just as importantly, healthcare professionals need to know the limits of their professional knowledge and skills, when to refer to other members of the team, the most appropriate person to consult, and how to access the help and advice they require. This requires *humility* about one's own limitations, recognition that they are a member of a team, *mutual respect*, confidence in their fellow team members and recognition of potential communication barriers. The transfer of appropriate information between team members, whether by written or electronic means, needs to be as seamless as possible. Communication barriers, such as the uneven uptake of technology among the team, need to be anticipated and overcome (Pierce & Fraser, 2009).

At times, raising concerns about patients and accessing help can be challenging. This is when health professionals need skills in *patient advocacy* and the ability to be *assertive* without being confrontational, judgmental or aggressive. This includes the ability to question 'up or down' the hierarchy where appropriate. Table 3.2 provides examples of behaviours that promote patient-safe communication between members of the healthcare team. Chapter 6 describes these behaviours in further detail.

In healthcare, the notion of the 'team' is sometimes more rhetoric than reality. A team is not just a group of people who are co-located or caring for the same group of patients. A team is a group of people who do collective work and are *mutually committed* to a *common purpose* (Hill & Lineback, 2012). Effective team communication skills are as important to patient safety as technical skills or expert knowledge (Katzenbach & Smith, 2004). A landmark report 'To Err Is Human' (Institute of Medicine, 1999) concluded that patient safety was a function of how well healthcare professionals perform effectively in teams. A 2006 World Health Organization report titled 'Working Together for Health' recognised that healthcare professionals are able to carry out their responsibilities more efficiently if they are members of effective teams that have well-developed interprofessional communication processes. Further, the report stated that it is not enough merely to have experience in working in a healthcare team; healthcare professionals must understand and adopt the values that underlie teamwork.

Conclusion

This chapter introduced the concept of person-centred care and discussed how it is essential to patient-safe communication. It then discussed the attributes that promote effective communication with both patients and other members of the healthcare team. This is just the beginning, however. In the chapters that follow these concepts will be expanded and applied to a wide range of different situations and patient groups. The diverse views of many different healthcare professionals will provide insights that are both illuminative and thought provoking.

Domains	Patient-safe communication behaviours
Person-centred care	Including patient/family in discussion
	Seeking and considering patient's social and medical history
	Equipping patients with the skills to identify problems and to play an active role in their management
Communication and interaction	Maintaining eye contact (if appropriate)
	Demonstrating open body language
	Being polite and friendly
	Active listening
	Discussing together
	Asking questions
	Coordinating actions
	Expressing concerns freely
	Speaking up when unsure
	Communicating openly
Teamwork and cooperation	Awareness of and respecting the roles of team members
	Supporting others
	Understanding the needs of the team
	Recognising when a team member needs help
	Managing conflict
	Asking for help
	Valuing others' contribution
	Sharing accountability and responsibility
Problem solving and decision making	Collaborative problem solving
	Shared option generation
	Shared risk assessment
	Shared decision making
	Reviewing outcomes
Leadership and management	Taking the initiative
	Maintaining clinical standards
	Delegating
	Demonstrating gradated assertiveness
	Creating a 'no-blame' culture
Situational awareness	Noticing and anticipating—identifying future problems and discussing contingencies
	Recognising the capabilities of others, cross-checking, and contacting outside sources when necessary
Adherence to guidelines	Being familiar with and adhering to relevant guidelines, policies and evidence-based resources
Documentation	Documenting clearly, accurately, contemporaneously and concisely
	Accessing and clarifying medical records
	Using electronic communication processes

TABLE 3.2
Teamwork and communication behaviours that promote patient safety

Source: IPE for QUM Facilitator guide, Copyright © 2012 School of Nursing and Midwifery Faculty of Health, University of Newcastle.

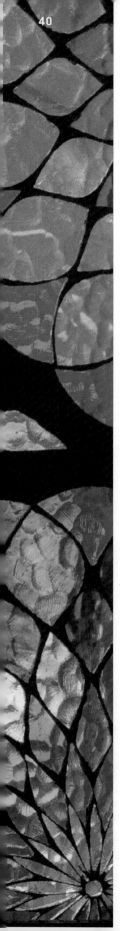

Critical thinking activities

Charmel and Frampton (2008) suggest that person-centred care is not merely philosophical, it is sound business practice. Consider this statement as you reflect on the story below.

> *We arrived in the ward—a very frightened, confused and depressed woman and her worried husband—and were kept waiting for a long time without explanation.*
>
> *In due course the psychiatrist appeared. He addressed my wife directly. I was ignored, but I tagged along. The family unit of a man and his wife had become a patient and an appendage. We entered the room. Then ominous silence for a while. No introductions; the doctor without a name. No introductions or explanation [as to] who might have been the unknown young observer sitting in on the consultation. The patient had become an item on a conveyor belt. The doctor faced the desk and had his back to us. At no time did he turn round to face us. I entered the discussion only when I felt that my comments were needed since my wife, because of her mental state, could not answer all the questions. I felt that my presence was not welcome.*

Source: Reproduced with permission from Patient Centred Care: Improving Quality and Safety through Partnerships with Patients and Consumers, developed by the Australian Commission on safety and Quality in Health Care(ACSQHC), ACSQHC: Sydney 2011.

1   How do you think patient safety could have potentially been affected by the communication that occurred in this scenario?
2   If you could turn back the clock and 're-script' this scenario, how would you change the interaction so that person-centred and patient-safe communication was evident?
3   If person-centred care is 'sound business practice', how might the type of interaction described in this story affect the 'business' of a healthcare organisation?

According to a systematic review conducted in 2009, the most effective way to promote patient safety using a person-centred approach is through communication training for healthcare professionals (Zolnierek & DiMatteo).

4   Reflect on your educational experiences and identify whether, and to what extent, your learning has enhanced your ability to communicate effectively and practise in a patient-safe manner. Then consider the learning opportunities that you have independently negotiated, or could negotiate, to ensure that your communication skills are patient-safe and person-centred.
5   Reflect on your attitudes and consider how they have the potential to enhance or detract from your ability to be person-centred and clinically safe.

Teaching and assessment activity

Too often, healthcare professionals think that person-centred care is synonymous with being kind and caring. While it does include these attributes, person-centred care also includes specific clinical behaviours that have a direct impact on patient safety. The following activity can be a classroom-based discussion, individual reflection or written assessment item. If it is undertaken in the classroom, students should work in small groups.

Using *evidence-based resources*, describe specific behaviours and attitudes that would help to facilitate person-centred care that is designed to improve:

- medication safety
- infection control
- clinical reasoning
- care of a confused older person
- care of a person with persistent pain
- care of a person from a non-English-speaking background
- care of a person who is angry or aggressive.

Further reading

Australian Commission on Safety and Quality in Health Care. (2011). *Patient-Centred Care: Improving Quality and Safety through Partnerships with Patients and Consumers.* Sydney: ACSQHC. Accessed September 2018 at <https://www.safetyandquality.gov.au/wp-content/uploads/2012/03/PCC_Paper_August.pdf>.

Web resources

Come into My World—How to Interact with a Person Who Has Dementia: This educational resource focuses on person-centred care. It includes a workbook and series of communication interactions that are both positive and negative, and demonstrates how organisations and healthcare professionals can promote the use of a person-centred approach. <nursing.flinders.edu.au/comeintomyworld/media/video.php?video>

Institute for Patient- and Family-Centered Care: This US website provides numerous practical resources, including assessment tools, publications and multimedia resources, produced by the institute and other leading patient-centred care organisations.
<www.ipfcc.org>

World Health Organization—Patients for Patient Safety: This website is designed to ensure that the perspective of patients and families is a central reference point in education and in designing systemic quality and safety improvements.
<http://www.who.int/patientsafety/patients_for_patient/regional_champions/en>

References

Australian College of Nursing. (2014). *Person-Centred Care Position Statement.* Accessed September 2018 at <https://www.acn.edu.au/sites/default/files/advocacy/submissions/PS_Person-centered_Care_C2.pdf>.

Australian Commission on Safety and Quality in Health Care. (2017). *National Safety and Quality Health Service Standards* (2nd edn). Sydney: ACSQHC.

Australian Commission on Safety and Quality in Health Care. (2011). *Patient-Centred Care: Improving Quality and Safety through Partnerships with Patients and Consumers.* Sydney: ACSQHC. Accessed July 2018 at <www.safetyandquality.gov.au/wp-content/uploads/2012/03/PCC_Paper_August.pdf>.

Bauman, A., Fardy, H. & Harris, P. (2003). Getting it right: Why bother with patient-centred care? *Medical Journal of Australia, 179,* 253–6.

Berwick, D. (1999). *The Permanente Journal, 3*(1), 1–91. Accessed October 2012 at <xnet.kp.org/permanentejournal/winter99pj/insides.pdf>.

Bolster, D. & Manias, E. (2010). Person-centred interactions between nurses and patients during medication activities in an acute hospital setting: Qualitative observation and interview study. *International Journal of Nursing Studies, 47*(2), 154–65.

Charmel, P. & Frampton, S. (2008). Building the business case for patient-centred care. *Healthcare Financial Management, 62*(3), 80–5.

Hill, L. & Lineback, K. (2012). *Good Managers Lead through a Team.* Accessed at <blogs.hbr.org/hill-lineback/2012/04/good-managers-lead-through-a-t.html>.

Institute of Medicine. (1999). *To Err Is Human: Building a Safer Health System.* Accessed at <www.nap.edu/openbook.php?isbn=0309068371>.

Institute for Patient- and Family-Centered Care. (2013). *Partnering with Patients and Families to Enhance Safety and Quality: A Mini Toolkit.* Institute for Patient- and

Family-Centered Care, Bethesda. Accessed September 2018 at <http://www.ipfcc.org/resources/Patient-Safety-Toolkit-04.pdf>.

Katzenbach, J. & Smith, D. (2004). *Harvard Business Review on Teams That Succeed.* Cambridge, USA: Harvard Business School Press.

Lapkin, S., Levett-Jones, T. & Gilligan, C. (2012). A cross-sectional survey examining the extent to which interprofessional education is used to teach nursing, pharmacy and medical students in Australian and New Zealand Universities. *Journal of Interprofessional Care, 26*(5), 390–6.

McCormack, B. & McCance, T. (2017). *Person-Centred Practice in Nursing and Health Care: Theory and practice.* Oxford: Wiley-Blackwell.

Meterko, M., Wright, S., Lin, H., Lowy, E. & Cleary, P. (2010). Mortality among patients with acute myocardial infarction: The influences of patient-centered care and evidence-based medicine. *Health Services Research, 45*(5, Pt 1), 1188–204.

Pierce, D. & Fraser, G. (2009). An investigation of medication information transfer and application in aged care facilities in an Australian rural setting. *Rural & Remote Health, 9*(3), 1090.

Schuster, P. & Nykolyn, L. (2010). *Communication for Nurses. How to Prevent Harmful Events and Promote Patient Safety.* Philadelphia: E.A. Davis.

Shaller, D. (2007). *Patient-Centered Care: What Does It Take?* United States: Picker Institute and The Commonwealth Fund.

Shapiro, J. (2011). Illness narratives: Reliability, authenticity and the empathic witness. *Medical Humanities, 37,* 68–72.

Sheppard, B., Hartwick, J. & Warshaw, P. (1988). The theory of reasoned action: A meta-analysis of past research with recommendations for modifications and future research. *Journal of Consumer Research, 15,* 325–43.

Stewart, M., Brown, J., Donner, A., McWhinney, I., Oates, J., Weston, W. & Jordan, J. (2000). The impact of patient-centered care on outcomes. *Journal of Family Practice, 49*(9), 796–804.

Wise, H., Beckhard, R., Rubin, I. &, Kyte, A. (1974). *Making Health Teams Work.* Cambridge, MA: Ballinger.

World Health Organization. (2006). *Working Together for Health. The World Health Report.* Geneva: WHO.

Zolnierek, H. & DiMatteo, M. (2009). Physician communication and patient adherence to treatment: A meta-analysis. *Medical Care, 47,* 826–34.

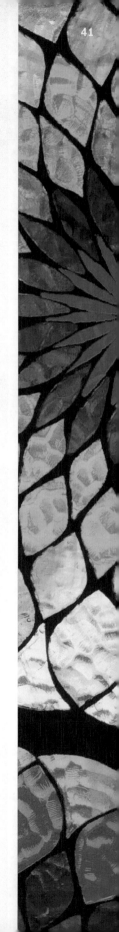

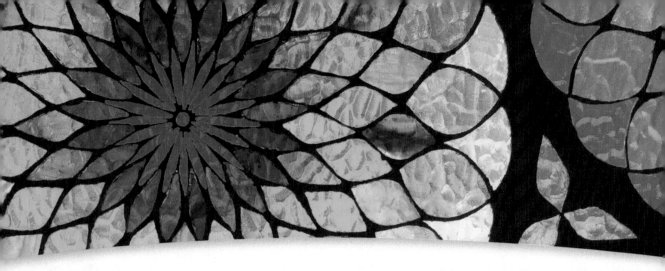

WHY DO PATIENTS COMPLAIN ABOUT HOW HEALTHCARE PROFESSIONALS COMMUNICATE?

Ashley Kable   Wayne Farmer

LEARNING OUTCOMES

Chapter 4 will enable you to:

- discuss the increasing incidence of patient complaints associated with communication issues
- identify the factors that motivate patients or family members to make a complaint about healthcare professionals' communication
- outline strategies that healthcare professionals can use to prevent and manage complaints about communication.

KEY CONCEPTS

healthcare complaints | listening | responding | prevention of complaints

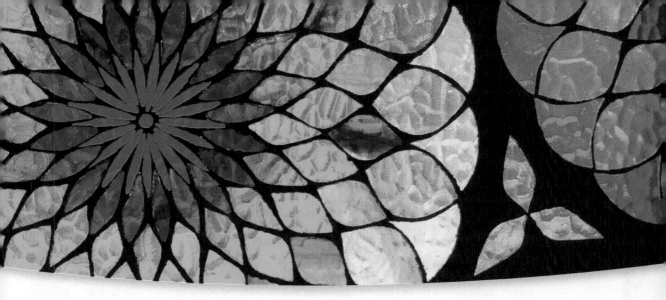

'I'd like a second opinion—I couldn't understand the first.'

(Pugh, 2012)

INTRODUCTION

When a person is concerned or dissatisfied with aspects of their healthcare experience they may decide to complain, and when they do, they have a range of potential options for raising their concerns. A patient may complain directly, or a complaint may be lodged by family, friends or other people on the patient's behalf. Complaints can be made to the healthcare professional/s concerned (who may be able to resolve them quickly), or their managers, members of parliament, the ombudsman, the Australian Health Practitioner Regulation Agency (AHPRA) or the media. Additionally, independent complaints commissions exist in many states and territories. For example, in New South Wales, people can submit a complaint to the NSW Government Health Care Complaints Commission (HCCC), an independent body that deals with complaints about healthcare professionals and healthcare services.

The manner in which healthcare professionals communicate with each other, and with the patients they care for or their families, often contributes to complaints. Communication issues are one of the most common reasons for healthcare complaints in Australia. Complainants may be dissatisfied with the healthcare professional's manner, the type of information provided, the inadequacy of responses, and a perceived failure to recognise and respond to factors that are unique to a patient's circumstances. Importantly, healthcare professionals could prevent many complaints through better communication, and those that do eventuate, if addressed in a timely and appropriate way, do not need to escalate.

This chapter explores the reasons that people complain about communication interactions related to healthcare and discusses how healthcare professionals can prevent or reduce the number of complaints that occur.

GEORGE'S STORY

George attended the emergency department (ED) of a tertiary hospital with his wife, Norma, and daughter, Lucy. George was 82 years old and had an existing cardiac condition. Two weeks previously he had been rushed to the same hospital by ambulance and had required emergency treatment. On this occasion, George, Norma and Lucy were concerned because he had been experiencing episodes of dizziness and breathlessness over the past five hours and his symptoms were not improving.

On arrival at the hospital, George was able to walk slowly with some assistance from Norma. He was able to speak but had some difficulty because of his breathlessness. Norma explained to the receptionist that George had been at the ED two weeks previously, as he had a problem with his heart, and that he was again feeling dizzy and breathless. Norma asked whether he needed a medication to be put under his tongue, as had occurred during his previous presentation. She suggested that the receptionist might be able to access the details of his last presentation on her computer. The receptionist told her that the hospital did not keep patient records in the ED and that George, Norma and Lucy should take a seat and wait for the triage nurse to call them.

Ten minutes later the triage nurse called them and Norma explained that George had a cardiac condition, that he had been admitted to the ED just two weeks earlier in relation to this, and that they were concerned about his dizziness and difficulty breathing. The nurse took George's blood pressure, told them it was fine, and told them that they should wait to be called again. She advised that they could expect to wait up to five hours.

As the evening unfolded, George's condition deteriorated. Two hours after the initial triage, George's dizziness had increased and was more constant, he was feeling tight in the chest and he was finding it even more difficult to breathe. Norma and Lucy approached the triage nurse once again and raised their concerns about his deteriorating condition. They asked that he be seen by a doctor as soon as possible or that staff, at least, put a medication under his tongue as they had done on the previous occasion. They were told to return to their seat and wait. Norma and Lucy felt that the triage nurse was very dismissive in response to their concerns and was treating them as if they were a nuisance. The staff did not speak with George and they did not carry out any further assessment.

Two hours passed and George deteriorated further. He was now unable to sit upright and was slumping over in his chair. He also had chest pain, numbness in his neck and arm and could barely speak. Norma and Lucy were now very distressed and frustrated. They believed that George was likely to die if treatment was delayed further. Norma approached the triage nurse once again and, although she could see that the nurse was busy with another patient, she voiced her concerns about George's continuing deterioration and asked that a doctor attend to George straightaway. The triage nurse turned in Norma's direction and, in an angry and dismissive tone, stated that she was busy with a patient and that Norma would have to wait her turn. On this occasion, Norma did not return to her seat. She felt very angry and frustrated and stated in a loud voice, 'So it's okay that my husband has a heart attack while I wait my turn? Is that what you want?' The triage nurse replied angrily, 'I don't have to take your abuse. Sit down or I will call security.' The nurse then turned her back on Norma and ignored her while attending to the other patient.

Norma and Lucy had expected the triage nurse to speak to George and make some effort to reassess him. When this did not occur, their frustration and anger escalated further. They voiced their concerns to the triage nurse again and security officers were asked to intervene. Norma and Lucy were escorted out of the ED waiting room and a conversation ensued with the security officers.

While Norma and Lucy were speaking with the security officers, George was assessed by a medical officer in the ED. It was established that he was acutely unwell. He was experiencing a ventricular tachycardia (VT) storm and he required emergency medical treatment to restore his normal heart rhythm.

As a result of this experience, George's family made a complaint to the New South Wales HCCC. George, Norma and Lucy, with the assistance of one of the Commission's resolution officers, met with the hospital representatives to discuss their concerns. The hospital acknowledged that the four-hour wait was not ideal. They explained that the assessment had been delayed due to the excessive workload being experienced in

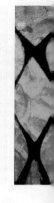

the ED on the night George presented. The hospital agreed that there were quite a number of shortcomings, both with respect to the manner in which the triage nurse and other staff had communicated with the family and with the standard of clinical care. The hospital agreed that the ED staff should have monitored George more closely while he was waiting to see the medical officer and that the triage nurse had failed to act on important information provided by Norma and Lucy. It was also acknowledged that the triage nurse should have done more to respond to the family's concerns, given that they were, quite understandably, in a distressed and anxious state. Rather than de-escalating the situation, the manner in which the triage nurse had communicated with the family had contributed quite significantly to the increased tensions between the staff and the family.

Source: NSW Government Health Care Complaints Commission. Used with permission. Names changed to maintain confidentiality.

- Do you feel that George's family was justified in making a complaint?
- How could the triage nurse have managed the situation better?
- What strategies could have been used to de-escalate the situation?
- How do external factors, such as time and resource pressure, impact on communication with patients?

Refer to Chapter 19 for more information about the prevention and management of anger and aggression.

SOMETHING TO THINK ABOUT

The increasing incidence of patient complaints

In Australia and internationally, complaints about healthcare professionals have increased. In the United Kingdom (UK) in 2017, 7577 complaints were made regarding doctors (General Medical Council [GMC], 2017, p. 31). This equates to approximately one in ten doctors being the subject of a complaint. In Germany, complaints about physician–patient relationships increased by 9.3 per cent over a four-year period (Schnitzer et al., 2012) and in Australia, complaints about all registered healthcare professional groups are also increasing (AHPRA, 2017). In NSW, communication issues are the second most common type of complaint made to the HCCC. There were 6319 complaints made to the HCCC in the year 2016–17, which represents a growth of 53 per cent over the past five years and 132 per cent over the last decade (HCCC, 2017, p. 4).

Two of the most frequently reported concerns involve the quality of communication and issues about interactions between patients and healthcare professionals. In the latest UK report, complaints about communication increased by 69 per cent and lack of respect by 45 per cent (GMC, 2017). A content analysis of eight studies that examined the nature of patient complaints identified that 19 per cent resulted from unprofessional conduct (during interactions with patients) and 17 per cent identified poor health professional–patient communication (Montini, Noble & Stelfox, 2008). Another study conducted at a major hospital in Australia reported that, of 1308 complaints, 71 per cent were related to poor communication (Anderson, Allan & Finucane, 2001). These studies indicate that poor communication is a common issue and of significant concern to patients and their families.

This is further illustrated by an analysis of the types of complaints to the New South Wales HCCC. Of the complaints received by the HCCC from 2012 to 2013 and from 2016 to 2017, 40 per cent related to the treatment provided, including concerns about inadequate treatment, diagnosis, unexpected treatment outcomes and complications, or delay in treatment (HCCC, 2017). The second most common type of complaint (17%) related to the communication between healthcare professionals and patients and their families. For complaints about communication, 56 per cent of these concerned the attitude and manner of health professionals, 27 per cent concerned inadequate information having been provided, and 16 per cent concerned incorrect or misleading information. A smaller number of communication issues related to special needs not being accommodated; this included people from

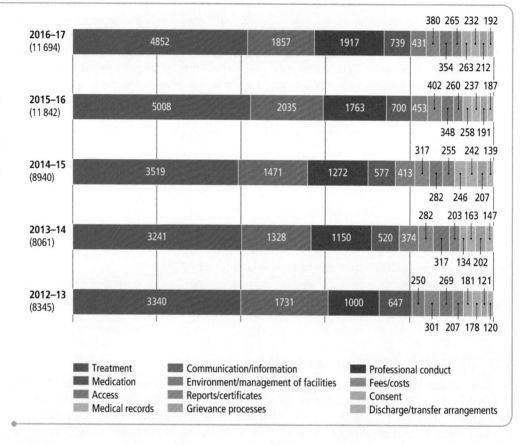

FIGURE 4.1
Issues raised in complaints to the New South Wales HCCC, 2012/13 to 2016/17

Source: NSW Government Health Care Complaints Commission. (2017). *Annual Report 2016/17*, Chart 12, p. 19. Used with permission. Accessed December 2018 at: <www.hccc.nsw.gov.au/Publications/Annual-Reports/default.aspx>

culturally and linguistically diverse backgrounds not being offered an interpreter, or the lack of support for people with a disability or requiring special assistance. Figure 4.1 illustrates the types of complaints the HCCC received between the periods of 2012/13 and 2016/17.

The high number of complaints related to healthcare professionals' attitudes suggests that we need to consider, not only the facts provided to patients, but also the way that information is delivered. 'Attitude' can relate to the patient perceiving that the healthcare professional is rude, discourteous, negative, unsympathetic, patronising or overbearing (see Box 4.1). In addition, information can be inadequate if the patients or their families cannot be understood it because the healthcare professional uses medical jargon or conveys only selective information (e.g. when test results are not placed into the context of what the information actually means for the patient and the possible treatment options). Sometimes, information provided to the patient is incorrect or misleading. When healthcare professionals fail to check that patients understand the information provided, they miss an opportunity to clarify and correct misunderstandings.

Often complaints are made about multiple issues, with communication being one part of a larger complaint. For example, when a patient complains about inadequate treatment, he or she may also be concerned about the attitude and manner of the healthcare professional who provided the care. Also, when several issues are raised in a complaint, they do not necessarily occur at the same time. For example, when a patient experiences an unexpected complication, the healthcare provider may not explain why this occurred and what the implications are for further treatment and care. Additionally, patients and family members often make complaints in order to obtain information and explanations they are unable to get directly from the healthcare professionals involved (HCCC, 2017).

BOX 4.1 Summary of issues raised in complaints to the New South Wales Health Care Complaints Commission

- Healthcare professionals' attitudes or manners that are rude, discourteous, negative, lacking in sympathy, patronising (e.g. elderspeak) or overbearing.

- Provision of incorrect or misleading information, or conflicting information from different healthcare professionals.

- Provision of incomplete or inadequate information, including incomprehensible verbal or written advice, jargon, other communication barriers (e.g. accents, environmental noise), or failure to provide information to patients and carers.

- Special needs not accommodated, such as provision of interpreters, sign language, disability support, print size in documents, literacy problems.

- Interprofessional communication failures (Nagpal et al., 2012), including workplace bullying.

Complaints where communication is a key issue are usually referred to the HCCC Resolution Service. The aim is to provide a forum for the relevant parties to have their experiences acknowledged and questions answered, and for their concerns to be resolved (see Melissa's story). When people have experienced a negative outcome, explanations (and, where appropriate, an apology) may contribute to resolving the complaint and achieving closure for both the patient and the healthcare professionals involved.

MELISSA'S STORY

Melissa complained to the HCCC about a consultation in a GP practice that had been interrupted several times, without apparent reason. Melissa felt that the doctor had behaved in a rude and unprofessional manner.

The doctor provided a response to the complaint. He explained that he had interrupted the consultation to attend to an emergency in the practice rooms as no other staff had been available. He acknowledged that he had not explained this to Melissa when he left or returned to the consultation. He apologised to her, acknowledging that the consultation did not meet his usual standards and that he understood why the complaint had been lodged. Melissa accepted the doctor's apology. She understood that the doctor had needed to attend to the emergency, and she said she would not have made the complaint if the doctor had explained the situation to her at the time.

Although this was an emergency situation, and the doctor probably had no time to explain why he suddenly had to leave during the consultation, it would have been simple to address the reason for his departure when he returned to the consultation room. A brief explanation could have prevented this patient from feeling that she had not received adequate attention, which left her feeling offended, disregarded and disrespected. It could also have prevented the lodgement of the complaint. Once the doctor provided an explanation, Melissa understood the urgency of the situation and the unavoidable demands placed on him during the consultation.

Source: New South Wales Health Care Complaints Commission. Used with permission. Names changed to maintain confidentiality.

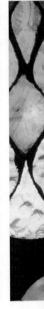

What motivates people to make a complaint?

In a survey of 1007 complaints, the primary motivation for complaining was to prevent other patients experiencing the same adverse event in the future (Bark et al., 1994; Cave & Dacre, 2008). Approximately 72 per cent of these complaints involved insensitivity by healthcare professionals

(Bark et al., 1994; Cave & Dacre, 2008; Friele & Sluijs, 2006); and 78 per cent related to communication breakdown between healthcare professionals and patients (and their families) (Donaldson & Cavanagh, 1992).

Some complainants are seeking an apology for distress they have experienced. Others are looking for a healthcare practitioner or organisation to be blamed, punished or held accountable when there has been an adverse event or outcome. Complainants may also have tried to raise their complaint with the healthcare professional in the first instance but have not felt heard, or have received an inadequate or inappropriate response. As mentioned earlier, people who make a complaint to an external body may view this as an avenue to get the information and explanation they need in order to make sense of what has happened. Some complainants consider the healthcare professional has betrayed them; some simply feel overpowered by the healthcare professional and lack the confidence to raise their concerns directly. Occasionally, the complainant may have a personal grievance against a healthcare professional.

It is worth noting that very few people complain simply to make trouble for a healthcare professional and, in contrast to what many people think, financial compensation is not usually a primary motivation for complaints. In fact, some reports suggest that less than 7 per cent of patients complain because they want financial compensation (Cave & Dacre, 2008; Friele & Sluijs, 2006). In a study of 1047 patients (Andrews et al., 1997), it was identified that this figure may actually be as low as 1.2 per cent.

It is also worth noting that, after something has gone wrong, a timely and appropriate apology from the healthcare professional or facility, along with appropriate action, may prevent or resolve a complaint. However, an incomplete, inappropriate or insincere apology can actually have the opposite result and fuel a complaint (Iedema et al., 2007) rather than resolve it, and may be the actual reason that people complain to an external body. (See Chapter 8 for more information about open disclosure.)

Preventing patient complaints about communication

Chapter 3 introduced the concept of person-centred care. Many of the strategies described below are consistent with a person-centred approach and illustrate how you can prevent complaints or manage them effectively.

Answering questions promptly and providing complete and understandable explanations

When you answer questions and provide explanations, you should be particularly careful to give accurate information in a user-friendly format. Check that the information is correctly understood by the person receiving it by asking simple questions to confirm that the message has been interpreted accurately. For example: 'When you are discharged, what medications will you take?'; 'How often will you take them?'; 'Will you take them with food?'; 'Will you need to get a prescription for them?'; 'Do you have written instructions for your medications?'. See Chapter 2 for information about the heath literacy of patients, the need for healthcare professionals to be aware of this when providing information or instructions, and how to use the teach-back method to confirm people's understanding of what is being explained to them.

Conveying respect towards and about others

Using a person-centred approach and professional manner with patients and colleagues (as described in Chapters 3 and 11) will convey respect to the listener, as well as respect about others who are mentioned in the conversation or described in documentation. This approach can also help to defuse or de-escalate a difficult situation and alleviate patient anxiety (e.g. 'I can understand why you would feel distressed about this. Would you like to tell me a bit more about it?'). Using the approach with colleagues will maintain open lines of communication between healthcare professionals and ensure effective working relationships.

CHAPTER 4 WHY DO PATIENTS COMPLAIN ABOUT HOW HEALTHCARE PROFESSIONALS COMMUNICATE?

49

Listening and clarifying

When you talk you are only repeating what you already know. But if you listen you may learn something new.

(Anon.)

The clinical examples provided in this chapter consistently demonstrate the importance of listening *and* clarifying. Asking simple questions about information provided by a patient can help you to clarify and confirm the important elements contained in what they have attempted to communicate. When people are questioned about the information they provide, they are more likely to feel like they have been listened to. Simple questions can be a very useful way of clarifying the intended message. For example: 'What makes you think that?'; 'What works for you?'; 'Does anyone else know about this?'; 'What are you most concerned about?'.

Responding to concerns

It is important to respond to the information provided. If a carer or patient advises a healthcare professional that the patient feels worse, it is reasonable for him or her to expect that the healthcare professional will respond by assessing the patient or referring them for further attention. If a colleague expresses concern about a patient, responding to and following up information that can prevent deterioration in a patient's status manifests professional trust and respect. For example: 'Is your pain worse?'; 'I'm going to check your blood pressure again'; 'Can I have a look at your wound?'; 'Is your pain constant?'; 'I will ask the doctor to come and check on you'.

Healthcare professional accountability and communication

The clinical examples provided earlier in this chapter identified the issues of professional accountability and communication. Patients and their families are vulnerable and depend on healthcare professionals communicating with them effectively. Professional accountability extends into responsible clinical engagement with patients and their families, including shared decision making and respecting individuals' beliefs and preferences. Professional accountability also involves recognising that when patients (or their family) bring something to your attention it should not be dismissed; rather, it should be considered carefully, as the information is likely to be clinically significant, and listening and responding appropriately may prevent a patient from deteriorating further.

Appropriate apologies

The New South Wales Ombudsman (NSW Ombudsman, 2009) has developed a practical guide for apologies, with the aim of assisting individuals and organisations to respond appropriately and effectively to situations where the actions of healthcare professionals have caused harm. The principles of and skills for effective apologies must become part of the repertoire of clinical skills for all health professionals (Cave & Dacre, 2008). (See Chapter 8 for more information about apologies and open disclosure.)

Responding to complaints

Wherever possible, it is more desirable to implement local systems and processes that allow complaints to be identified and resolved quickly so escalation of formal complaints can be prevented, rather than the complaints being managed by an external authority or commission.

Documentation and effective communication

Investigations of adverse events frequently find that documentation has been missing, been inadequate or not been available at the time it was needed (Wilson et al., 1995). As a result, there have been some system changes that have the potential to improve the availability and quality of documentation, such as electronic medical records (Nagpal et al., 2012). Documentation provided to patients should use language that they can understand and be in a format that is user-friendly, such as large print for visually impaired people and unambiguous instructions.

Regulatory organisations

Internationally, heathcare professional regulatory authorities have begun to implement a range of strategies designed to prevent or reduce the number of complaints. These strategies include appointing employer liaison officers, launching confidential helplines for doctors, piloting a national induction program for doctors, and reforming fitness-to-practise procedures (GMC, 2017). Similar strategies are becoming evident in Australia to regulate the registration of healthcare professionals and respond to complaints and notifications (AHPRA, 2012).

Communication skills training for health professionals

Taking advantage of opportunities to learn and practise communication skills is essential for healthcare professionals in order to become skilled in managing challenging conversations, such as those that concern complaints or end-of-life decision making (see Chapter 20), those with angry or aggressive patients (see Chapter 19), those with people from culturally and linguistically diverse backgrounds (see Chapter 17), and those with vulnerable people generally (Levin et al., 2010). Simulations with actors or standardised patients create a safe learning environment where skills can be learnt and mistakes do not affect real patients. Seeking constructive feedback following these types of learning opportunities allows learners to reflect on and improve their performance. In addition, there are a number of resources available to assist healthcare professionals to improve their communication skills and the way they respond to complaints, including resources from the National Health and Medical Research Council (2004) and the NSW Ombudsman (2009).

Patient advocates

For more information about patient advocates access: <http://www. patientadvocates. com.au/what-is-a-patient-advocate. html>

Some patients and their families may feel overwhelmed about attempting to engage with healthcare professionals if they are concerned about their situation, and may not understand the processes and interactions that occur around them. In these circumstances, it is possible for them to access a patient advocate to act on their behalf. Patient advocates accompany patients to medical appointments in order to ask questions, and explain disease concepts and treatment options. Patient advocates provide a valuable service for people (or their carers) who are ill, confused (about negotiating the healthcare system) and vulnerable, and who need someone to provide practical and emotional support.

Conclusion

Patients frequently complain about negative experiences encountered when interacting with healthcare professionals. They may have received information that is confusing, incomplete, inadequate or delivered in a manner that conveys a lack of respect and empathy. This can alienate them from the healthcare system, diminish the quality and effectiveness of therapeutic interactions, and result in inadequate support and clinical management for the patients. Patients and their families may ultimately submit a formal complaint because they feel that their concerns have not been heard, and frequently because they wish to ascertain whether their experience can be prevented from occurring again and affecting other patients.

There are many strategies that healthcare professionals can use to prevent complaints, improve the quality of communication with their patients and improve the experience that patients have when engaging with healthcare services. Additionally, if complaints are effectively managed at a local level with an apology and/or open disclosure, the need for escalation is often prevented, along with the associated emotional and psychological distress for all concerned.

Critical thinking activities

Mary underwent elective surgery to repair an incisional hernia at a stoma reversal site. Post-operatively, she developed abdominal pain, nausea and vomiting. The surgical registrar advised Mary and her husband, Theo, that it was not unusual to develop these symptoms after surgery, and that the plan was to continue to monitor her and to discharge her once the symptoms resolved.

By day two, Mary was feeling quite unwell. Her abdominal pain was now severe and her analgesic regime was not providing effective relief. The nausea and vomiting had not settled and she was not passing urine. Mary told the attending nurse about the severity of her pain. The attending nurse was quite concerned about the irregularity of a post hernia repair patient experiencing unresolved and severe pain. She mentioned this to Mary and Theo, and voiced her concerns to a junior medical officer and the surgical registrar.

When Mary was reviewed by the surgical team, Theo explained that Mary was in considerable pain. Mary, however, was reluctant to disclose the full extent of her pain and how unwell she was feeling, as she did not want to appear ungrateful for the care she was receiving. The surgical team did not press Mary on this issue. They advised that they would continue to monitor her and they were hopeful her symptoms would resolve soon. Mary and Theo felt somewhat reassured by this, although they were still a little concerned and confused as the attending nurse continued to voice her concerns to them about Mary's condition.

Later that afternoon, Mary was reviewed by a nephrology visiting medical officer (VMO). The nephrology VMO was concerned that Mary may have been suffering from an acute abdomen and asked the attending nurse to contact the surgical registrar for discussion. The nurse discussed her concerns with the surgical registrar over the telephone and passed on the message from the nephrology VMO. The registrar replied that he felt that Mary was stable from a surgical point of view and that she required management for the suspected renal dysfunction only. He ended the call and he did not speak with the nephrology VMO.

Mary deteriorated further during the evening of day two and the next day. The nephrology VMO reviewed her again just before midday on day three and, suspecting intra-abdominal sepsis caused from the surgery, contacted the surgical VMO who, prior to that point, had not been informed of Mary's deterioration.

Mary was taken back to theatre on the afternoon of day three. She was found to have a bowel perforation with an abscess cavity, and a necrotic omentum and segment of small bowel. Following surgery, Mary remained in a critical condition and required cardiac support due to ongoing sepsis and renal failure. Mary continued to deteriorate and she passed away on day five. The family made a complaint to the New South Wales HCCC.

Source: New South Wales Health Care Complaints Commission. Used with permission. Names changed to maintain confidentiality.

1   Why do you think Mary's family decided to lodge a complaint with the Health Care Complaints Commission?
2   Did the healthcare professionals caring for Mary engage in patient-safe communication?
3   In what areas do you feel the communication could have been improved?
4   When the media reports stories from people about adverse outcomes or medical errors they have experienced, what do you think has motivated people to tell their story?

Teaching and assessment activities

The following letter of complaint submitted to the NSW HCCC can be used as a stimulus for classroom discussion or as an assessment item.

I was admitted to Hospital A on 13/3/16 for gynecology issues and pain. (I have Polycystic Ovary Syndrome [PCOS] diagnosed 2013.) During my 3-day admission I was seen by 7 different doctors. One doctor listened to me and wanted to help. The other 6 doctors did not want to listen to me or know what it has been like for me the past 2½ years with PCOS and pain, nor did they want to listen to what I have been through and the medications I have tried. I felt that I was being bullied into what they wanted as they came around in teams of two. I wanted to put an end to my pain and PCOS but they blamed my weight, my age (being only 31 they thought I may want more children). I made it clear that I do not want any more children; I have two, an 11 year old (who is on the autism spectrum with an intellectual disability) and a six year old. They told me my pain was in my head and that I was depressed (as I broke down explaining about the pain and the effect it is having on my life and family). I wanted for it all to be taken out. I no longer wanted this condition to control my life. They wanted to do a hysteroscopy and either an ablation or insertion of a mirena. I told them straight out that I did not want the mirena. They basically told

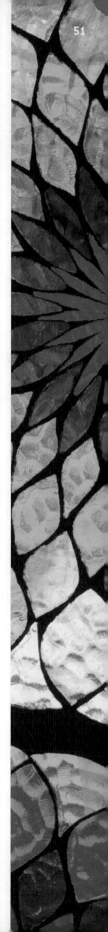

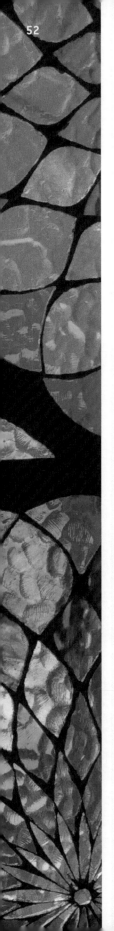

me I had no choice. I also told them that I have been to four different IVF and hormone specialists and even my own GP has stated that the mirena won't work as it can cause more cysts and more pain and discomfort and they still did not want to listen. My GP had placed on the referral to them that surgical intervention is now needed. I have been in and out of hospital since 2013 with the same issue. I was also insulted by one of the nurses. She stated that the clothes I was wearing was [sic] inappropriate as there were children and men around. I was wearing track pants and a singlet top. She brought me down a gown to wear but I did not wear it as I was feeling hot, uncomfortable and did not want to move. Later on that night the same nurse brought me my next round of pain medication (endone). I told her I did not want it as I was feeling sick (as I was nil by mouth and was given endone every 4 hours). She ignored me. At 9 pm when my partner arrived I started to vomit. I had scans and more blood tests done on the 14th and on the morning of 15th, as the nurses were doing handover around my bed, [they] discussed the cancer that was revealed by the ultrasound. I was upset as none of the six doctors had come around to discuss anything. When two doctors finally showed up they didn't mention anything about the cancer, only that they were going to put the mirena in and do a biopsy, and left it at that. As they were walking out they stated that something showed up in the ultrasound and it was maybe a fibroid or an adenomyosis, and before I could ask any questions or ask about the cancer they were gone. I was discharged still in pain and still having my issues, with more questions than answers and was told the procedure will be done in the next 90 days. I now have to go to my GP with my questions and ask for another referral to see someone else as I am not confident in the ability of the doctors at Hospital A, nor do I want them to do any procedures.

Source: New South Wales Health Care Complaints Commission. Used with permission. Names have been changed to protect confidentiality.

1   What aspects of the communication outlined in this letter concern you?

2   What aspects of the healthcare professionals' communication do you think could be improved?

3   Construct three questions that could have been asked by the healthcare professionals to more effectively engage with the patient and other healthcare professions, and elicit relevant information in this situation.

4   What strategies do you think could be used to assist healthcare professionals to engage and communicate with patients and their families more effectively?

Further reading

Aubusson, K. (2018, March 10). When a patient advocate becomes the patient in desperate need of help. *The Sydney Morning Herald*. Accessed December 2018 at: <https://www.smh.com.au/national/when-a-patient-advocate-becomes-the-patient-in-desperate-need-of-help-20180304-p4z2rb.html>.

Australian Broadcasting Commission. *PM: Woman Dies of Drug Overdose after Hospital Blunder*. Accessed December 2018 at: <www.abc.net.au/pm/content/2012/s3609775.htm>.

Australian Health Practitioner Regulation Agency. (2017). *Annual Report 2016/17: AHPRA and National Boards*. Accessed December 2018 at: <www.ahpra.gov.au/Legislation-and-Publications/AHPRA-Publications.aspx>.

Bartholomew, K. (2004). *Speak Your Truth: Proven Strategies for Effective Nurse–Physician Communication*. MA, USA: HCPro, Inc. ISBN 1-57839-556-9.

General Medical Council. (2018). *The State of Medical Education and Practice in the UK: Our Findings in 2018*. Accessed December 2018 at: <https://www.gmc-uk.org/about/what-we-do-and-why/data-and-research/the-state-of-medical-education-and-practice-in-the-uk>.

Web resources

NSW Government Health Care Complaints Commission. What if a complaint is made about me?
<www.hccc.nsw.gov.au/Complaints/What-if-a-complaint-is-made-about-me-/default.aspx>

NSW Government Health Care Complaints Commission. Responding to a complaint lodged with the Commission.
<http://www.hccc.nsw.gov.au/Information/Information-For-Health-Providers/Responding-/default.aspx>

NSW Government Health Care Complaints Commission. Dealing with complaints—A guide for health service providers.
<http://www.hccc.nsw.gov.au/Information/Information-for-health-providers/Dealing>

NSW Government Health Care Complaints Commission. Case studies.
<www.hccc.nsw.gov.au/Publications/Case-Studies/default.aspx>

CEC REACH Program Toolkit.
<http://www.cec.health.nsw.gov.au/quality-improvement/people-and-culture/reach>

Australian Health Practitioner Regulation Agency.
<https://www.ahpra.gov.au/>

References

Australian Health Practitioner Regulation Agency. (2012). *Annual Report 2011/12: AHPRA and National Boards*.

Australian Health Practitioner Regulation Agency. (2017). *Annual Report 2016/17: AHPRA and National Boards*.

Anderson, K., Allan, D. & Finucane P. (2001). A 30-month study of patient complaints at a major Australian hospital. *Journal Quality in Clinical Practice*, 21(4), 109–11.

Andrews, L., Stocking, C., Krizek, T., Gottlieb, L., Krizek, C., Vargish, T. & Siegler, M. (1997). An alternative strategy for studying adverse events in medical care. *The Lancet*, *349*, 309–13.

Bark, P., Vincent, C., Jones, A. & Savoy, J. (1994). Clinical complaints: A means of improving quality of care. *Quality in Health Care*, *3*, 123–32.

Cave, J. & Dacre, J. (2008). Dealing with complaints. *British Medical Journal*, *336*, 326–8.

Donaldson, L. & Cavanagh, J. (1992). Clinical complaints and their handling: A time for change? *Quality in Health Care*, *1*(1), 21–5.

Friele, R. & Sluijs, E. (2006). Patient expectations of fair complaint handling in hosptials: Empirical data. *BMC Health Services Research*, *6*, 106.

General Medical Council. (2017). *The State of Medical Education and Practice in the UK 2017*. Accessed January 2019 at <https://www.gmc-uk.org/-/media/about/somep-2017/somep-2017-final-full.pdf?la=en&hash=B6AD13C9D672F7FCD927498A3F50BB0A2A4286F2>.

Iedema, R., Mallock, N., Sorensen, R., Manias, E., Tuckett, A., Williams, A., et al. (2007). *Final Report: Evaluation of the Pilot of the National Open Disclosure Standard*. Sydney: University of Technology, Sydney.

Levin, T., Horner, J., Bylund, C. & Kissane, D. (2010). Averting adverse events in communication skills training: A case series. *Patient Education and Counseling*, *81*, 126–30.

Montini, T., Noble, A. A. & Stelfox, H. T. (2008). Content analysis of patient complaints. *International Journal for Quality in Health Care*, *20*(6), 412–20.

Nagpal, K., Arora, S., Vats, A., Wong, H. W., Sevdalis, N., Vincent, C. & Moorthy, K. (2012). Failures in communication and information transfer across the surgical care pathway: interview study. *BMJ Quality and Safety*, *21*, 843–9.

National Health and Medical Research Council. (2004). *Communicating with Patients. Advice for Medical Practitioners*.

NSW Government Health Care Complaints Commission. (2017). *Annual Report 2016/17*.

NSW Ombudsman. (2009). *Apologies. A Practical Guide*. (2nd edn). Sydney: NSW Ombudsman.

Pugh. (2012). *Cartoon: Complaints against GPs Have Hit a Record High*. London: Mail Online.

Schnitzer, S., Kuhlmey, A., Adolph, H., Holzhausen, J. & Schenk, L. (2012). Complaints as indicators of health care shortcomings: Which groups of patients are affected? *International Journal for Quality in Health Care*, *24*(5), 476–82.

Wilson, R., Runciman, W., Gibberd, R., Harrison, B., Newby, L. & Hamilton, J. (1995). The Quality in Australian Health Care Study. *The Medical Journal of Australia*, *163*(9), 458–71.

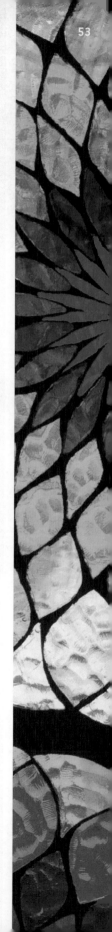

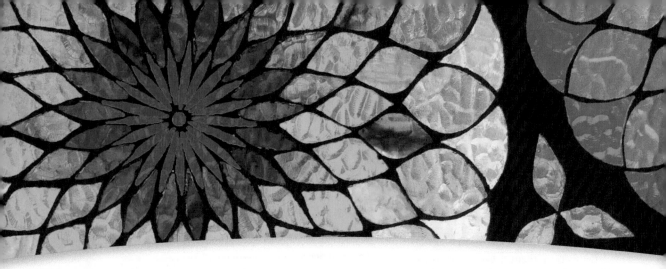

CHAPTER 5

AN HISTORICAL AND CULTURAL OVERVIEW OF HEALTHCARE PROFESSIONALS' EVOLVING TEAM DYNAMICS

Lyn Ebert

LEARNING OUTCOMES

Chapter 5 will enable you to:

- identify how traditional hierarchical and power structures influence the way healthcare professionals work together in contemporary healthcare settings
- describe how healthcare teamwork has evolved over the last century
- discuss current challenges to working effectively in healthcare teams
- outline strategies for demonstrating respect for and valuing of the roles of other team members
- describe the relationship between person-centred care, teamwork and patient safety
- outline potential strategies for learning to work more effectively in healthcare teams.

KEY CONCEPTS

culture | history | teamwork | tradition | hierarchy | professional identity

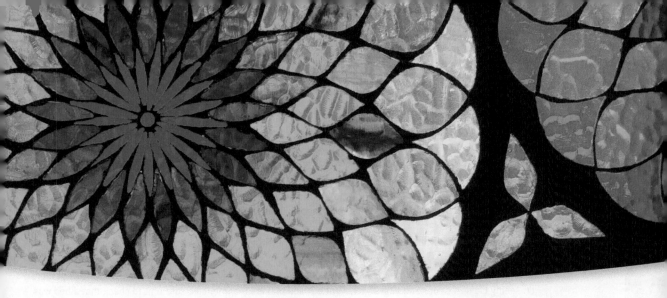

We cannot accomplish all that we need

to do without working together.

(Richardson, n.d.)

INTRODUCTION

An examination of critical patient incidents has shown that patient outcomes are adversely affected by poor teamwork and communication failures. Conversely, effective collaboration between healthcare professionals results in reduced mortality and morbidity, decreased length of stay in hospital, and reduced healthcare costs (Weller, Boyd & Cumin, 2014). However, in contemporary healthcare environments, effective teamwork, collaboration and communication can be challenging (Dunn et al., 2018). This chapter explores how evolving cultural, historical, educational and social processes have influenced relationships between healthcare professionals in contemporary healthcare contexts. We also discuss how tradition influences healthcare hierarchies and the impact this has on patient safety. The chapter concludes with suggestions for a way forward and emphasises the importance of understanding and valuing the roles of 'others' in order to work effectively as a team.

ELAINE'S STORY

Elaine Bromiley was married and a mother of two young children, Victoria and Adam, at the time of her death. She enjoyed good health apart from sinus problems. In 2005, she was admitted to hospital for routine sinus surgery. At the commencement of the surgical procedure the anaesthetist and his assistant were unable to intubate or ventilate her. After 5 minutes, they were joined by an anaesthetist from an adjoining theatre and the surgeon. Three nurses also answered a call for help. The three experienced and well-regarded consultants continued with the attempts to intubate Elaine, using a variety of techniques and equipment, for approximately 10 minutes. Elaine remained cyanotic during this period of time, with oxygen levels at 40 per cent or lower.

The nurses, meanwhile, recognised the gravity of the situation early on and knew what needed to be done. Using their own initiative they brought a tracheostomy set into the operating theatre. The senior nurse announced to the consultants that the tracheostomy set was available, but there was no response. One of the other nurses, on seeing Elaine's colour and vital signs, went out and phoned the intensive care unit to check that a bed was available. She came back to the operating theatre and told the consultants that a bed was available. However, she was ignored by the consultants and got the impression that they felt she was overreacting; consequently, she cancelled the ICU bed.

For a further 15 minutes, the three consultants continued with their attempts to intubate Elaine to the exclusion of any other option. At the end of 25 minutes, Elaine's oxygen level was 90 per cent but only for a short period of time before dropping again to 40 per cent for another 10 minutes. The decision was made to cancel the surgery and to allow Elaine to wake up naturally. She was taken to recovery but did not wake up; she died in the intensive care unit 13 days later.

At the inquest into Elaine's death, it was identified that there was a loss of control among the medical team as well as a breakdown in leadership, communication, situational awareness, prioritisation and decision making. It was identified that, although the nurses knew what was happening and what should be done, they did not know how to make themselves heard, how to be assertive and how to escalate their concerns.

Source: Used with permission from Martin Bromiley.

Elaine Bromiley's full story, titled *Just a routine operation*, is available at <https://www.youtube.com/watch?v=JzlvgtPlof4>

Tradition, power and hierarchy

The way in which healthcare professionals have worked together throughout history has been influenced by economic, professional and political forces, which have reflected corresponding societal changes (McKay & Narasimhan, 2012). Historically, power and control within healthcare contexts were exerted by physicians; the roles and scope of practice of other healthcare members were largely dismissed in relation to patient care, planning and decision making (Dunn et al., 2018). In the middle ages, law, medicine and the ministry were professions dominated by upper-class men who were able to pay for their education (Jefferson, Bloor & Maynard, 2015). In 1512, a British act of parliament secured licensing for physicians and surgeons, giving them control over the practice of medicine (Colson & Ralley, 2015). During this time and for centuries afterwards, doctors were trained and rewarded for having the attributes of leadership, daring, independence, autonomy, self-sufficiency, innovation, delegation and risk taking. Notably, the capacity to collaborate, communicate and work effectively in teams was only recently recognised as integral to competence, and of equal importance to highly developed knowledge and clinical skills.

Other healthcare professions, such as pharmacy (originally part of the apothecaries and Grocers' Mercantile), have been in existence since the 1600s (Colson & Ralley, 2015). In 1617, English apothecaries obtained a special charter that gave them a monopoly and prevented grocers from selling medicines. Physicians objected, fearing that this would mean apothecaries would become competitors in the practice of medicine. However, by the end of the 17th century, physicians' long and costly education, along with the limited numbers of graduates, led to shortfalls in medical care. Apothecaries sometimes helped to fill the gap by practising medicine without a licence; however, those who did were prosecuted by the Royal College of Physicians (Colson & Ralley, 2015). The physician's licence allowed only physicians to diagnose disease, choose remedies and order their application. Apothecaries were only allowed to advise patients and to give medical aid. Clarity about the roles gradually emerged and led to the apothecaries and physicians working together from then on in a somewhat uneasy relationship (Colson & Ralley, 2015). Ongoing tensions continued, with some physicians viewing pharmacists as retailers as well as healthcare providers, since pharmacy is the only healthcare profession reimbursed for its sale of a product rather than a service (Rigby, 2010). Even today, physicians often oppose pharmacists as the first point of call for minor ailments, as typically occurs in community pharmacies. This has, at times, led to adversarial relationships between physicians and pharmacists (Rigby, 2010).

Historically, nursing was arduous and ill-paid, with patients cared for by female members of family, religious orders, the poor (Jefferson et al., 2015), or people considered unfit for other work, such as criminals, vagrants and immoral women, all of whom had little training (McKay & Narasimhan, 2012). The National Archives Education Service (n.d.) reports that, during the Crimean War, Florence Nightingale persuaded army physicians in male-dominated hospitals that trained nurses could be helpful to them. However, the nurses worked at the physician's discretion, and their worthiness was equated to their degree of helpfulness to doctors (Open Learn, 2016).

The first nursing schools set up by Nightingale were run like the army, with an emphasis on hierarchy, discipline, authority, punishment and adherence to rigid procedures and rules (Karimi & Masoudi Alavi, 2015). Integral to the Nightingale system was a formalised instructional program for the training of nurses. In this system, students were carefully selected by the matron on the basis of both their educational and moral standards. The qualities of a 'good nurse', as described by Nightingale, included the ability to carry out orders in a humble and deferential way (Nightingale, 1881, cited by Open Learn, 2016). Nurses were socialised to obey and respect authority, and their membership of the healthcare team depended on their acceptance of their subordinate role. Nurse training was carried out as an apprenticeship, with nurses taught the skills required to assist doctors.

This form of nurse education was transported to Australia when Lucy Osborn and five other nurses, who were prepared in the Nightingale system, arrived in Sydney on 5 March 1868 to manage and staff the Sydney Infirmary (now called Sydney Hospital), and to establish and supervise a local training school for nurses. Lucy Osborn and her staff faced a long and difficult fight against prejudice and ignorance in their efforts to reform the Sydney Infirmary as they were thwarted at every turn by suspicion and jealousy, especially among the hospital's doctors.

In Australia, the Nightingale system became so fundamental to nursing education that it remained essentially unchanged and unchallenged for almost a century. However, in the latter half of the 20th century this system came under increasing pressure to change. Essentially, the Nightingale system placed an emphasis on learning nursing procedures to prepare nurses as quickly as possible for ward duties, without providing the necessary theoretical instruction. This resulted in the production of nurses who were limited in their ability to challenge practices, cope confidently with scientific and technological advances in healthcare, and evolve with social changes occurring in the community.

The 1970s ushered in changes, along with the growing feminist movement. Nursing became increasingly professionalised in Australia as nursing education began to move to universities in the 1980s, with all nurses entering the profession through higher education pathways by 1993 (Department of Health, 2013). This resulted in nurses having greater control over their own education and knowledge base. Gender roles were also changing, with growing numbers of female doctors and male nurses (Jefferson et al., 2015). The hierarchical nature of healthcare was changing as well, and relationships were becoming more complex. However, there were still differences in power, perspective, education, pay and status between medicine and nursing (McKay & Narasimhan, 2012).

A nurse must begin her work with the idea firmly implanted in her mind that she is only the instrument by whom the doctor gets his instructions carried out; she occupies no independent position in the treatment of the sick person (McGregor Robertson, 1902, cited in Fagin & Garelick, 2004).

The object of the game is as follows: the nurse is to be bold, have initiative and be responsible for making significant recommendations while, at the same time, she must appear passive. This must be done in such a manner as to make her recommendations appear to be initiated by the physician (Stein, 1967).

Poor collaboration and communication can lead to adverse patient outcomes. 'Most nurses are afraid to call Dr X when they need to and frequently won't call. Their patient's safety is always in jeopardy because of this' (Sirota, 2007).

Allied health professionals are qualified tertiary-educated health practitioners who include social workers, physiotherapists, occupational therapists, podiatrists, speech pathologists and a range of other professions.

Tensions between doctors and nurses have existed throughout history. In 1967, Stein described the 'doctor–nurse game', a manipulative relationship designed to manage these tensions. The object of the game was to avoid open disagreement at all costs by carefully managing relationships to ensure that the existing hierarchy was not openly challenged. Both the doctor and nurse were said to gain from the game: doctors from nurses' knowledge and nurses in self-esteem. In the 1990s, Stein revisited the 'doctor–nurse game' and found that nurses had begun to demand respect, and they were more likely to challenge doctors and offer advice. Conversely, Holyoake (2011) suggests the game still remains, with nurses more dependent on the medical profession than ever.

In some quarters, tension between the medical and nursing professions has not abated. This is particularly evident in the resistance of the medical profession to nurse practitioners, who were, for a long time, viewed as being in competition with doctors. Interestingly, since 2000, when nurse practitioners were first endorsed in Australia, the negative attitudes of doctors towards nurse practitioners have abated somewhat; yet at the same time some senior nurses have become increasingly resistant to the advanced role (Maclellan, Higgins & Levett-Jones, 2015). In the United States, collaborative interprofessional relationships between doctors and nurses are perceived differently by the professional groups. Doctors perceive the relationships more positively than nurses, with nurses voicing greater dissatisfaction with interprofessional communication and collaboration (Siedlecki & Hixson, 2015).

Allied health professions are relatively young, with most developing over the last century, although some are able to trace their beginnings back much further. The 20th century saw a proliferation of these professions, and the relationships between allied health professionals and other members of the healthcare team are variable. Physiotherapists support individuals and populations to develop, maintain and restore functional ability and movement, maximising quality of life through habilitation and rehabilitation, and facilitating physical, social and emotional wellbeing (World Confederation for Physical Therapy London, 2016). The origins of physiotherapy can be traced to Sweden, where Per Henrik Ling commenced the Royal Central Institute of Gymnastics (RCIG) in 1813 (Dahl-Michelsen, 2015).

The demand for physiotherapists grew globally when physical rehabilitation was required for wounded soldiers during the First World War, with the first school of physiotherapy being established in Washington D.C. (Washington University School of Medicine, 2009). However, as physiotherapists increased their scope of practice (working with those who had limitations of movement), the medical profession became concerned with the potential for professional boundary crossing, and in 1934, they exerted their influence to change the educational requirements for physiotherapists. Physiotherapy education became harder for males to enter, redirecting the profession towards a female dominated profession and making it more subservient to the medical profession (Dahl-Michelsen, 2015). Regardless of professional obstacles, the physiotherapy profession has continued to grow, with their scope of practice now encompassing the knowledge and skills to diagnose and implement interventions to prevent impairments and restrictions related to movement, function and health (World Confederation for Physical Therapy London, 2016). While physiotherapy has been legitimised as a profession, there is sometimes a struggle for professional recognition in the workplace (Jaros, 2015).

Occupational therapy, similar to physiotherapy, has faced challenges in developing a professional identity (Binyamin, 2017). It was first recognised as a health profession through the work of the National Society for the Promotion of Occupational Therapy (now called the American Occupational Therapy Association [AOTA]) during the early 1900s. The profession expanded during the Second World War, as a greater number of practitioners were required to support the recovery of returning soldiers' (O'Brien, 2013). As a profession, occupational therapy has continued to develop its own body of discrete knowledge, which has helped with differentiation from other healthcare professions (Hocking & Wright-St Clair, 2011). However, occupational therapists also report some conflict and tensions with other healthcare professionals due to 'turf wars' and perceived role overlap (Chung et al., 2012).

A further overlap of professional roles that can lead to turf wars occurs between social workers and nurses, especially when case management is involved (Schneiderman, Waugaman & Flynn, 2008). The overlapping of professional boundaries is occurring more often as healthcare moves away from professionally defined structures and silos towards 'flatter' organisations, requiring new roles and greater collaboration (Davies, Goodman & Cripacc, 2008). The proliferation of other allied health roles such as naturopaths, osteopaths, chiropractors and physician assistants has also added to the turf wars, with doctors in particular.

The evolution of teamwork

Societal change and a political emphasis on quality healthcare as a right for all citizens, along with a greater emphasis on person-centred care and increasing consumer involvement in stakeholder groups, have led to significant changes to healthcare delivery (Delaney, 2018). A gradual move away from healthcare characterised mainly by unpredictable, acute, simple diseases towards the care of patients with multiple, chronic diseases has also shifted the focus from discrete hospital admissions to ongoing community care and primary health approach. Hospital systems have been changing as well, with a growing emphasis on ambulatory and managed care, and integration of services (Schneiderman et al., 2008). Coupled with growing evidence that working together collaboratively enhances patient safety, there has been an increasing emphasis on the effectiveness of relationships between healthcare professionals (Weller, Boyd & Cumin, 2014).

While there has been a growing understanding of the need for improved teamwork for healthcare professionals, attempts to improve collaboration have been in existence for many years. In England in the 1920s, the Dawson Report advocated a 'team approach'. This team approach, however, was based on a military model of frontline primary care and was basically a triage system (Baldwin, 2007). In this context, nursing and allied health professionals, according to Baldwin, perceived the developing concept of teamwork as a means of achieving professional acceptance, and so were willing to adopt it.

During the Second World War, interprofessional collaboration between medical and nursing teams who were working together to treat injured soldiers began to demonstrate how effective collaboration in teams could be. Following the war, in 1948, a hospital outreach service in the United States employed teams of physicians, nurses and social workers, and was an early attempt at teamwork in primary healthcare (Baldwin, 2007).

The notion of working together to achieve a shared goal is not new. More than 30 years ago, Weiss and Davis (1985) argued for collaborative practice as the way to improve patient safety and defined it as 'the interactions between nurse and physician that enable the knowledge and skills of both professions to synergistically influence the patient care provided' (p. 299). It is increasingly recognised within the healthcare environment that poor interprofessional communication results in ineffective teamwork, increases healthcare costs and adversely affects health outcomes for the recipient of care (Weller, Boyd & Cumin, 2014). Healthcare environments that lack supportive leadership, and where leaders make decisions in isolation, are demonstrated to have poorer outcomes and to be less efficient than those teams where input and inquiry from all team members is equally valued, respected and promoted (Murray, Sundin & Cope, 2017). However, while the importance of teamwork and collaboration has been increasingly emphasised, a number of factors continue to undermine collaborative practice (Sirota, 2007); these include:

■ disruptive physician behaviour and lack of interprofessional respect

■ passive-aggressive behaviours by healthcare professionals who consider themselves to be disempowered

■ feelings of being 'taken for granted', with work and roles not understood or valued by other team members

■ different focus and orientation for different professions; for example, 'care' as opposed to 'cure'

■ gender differences and power differentials; for example, the mainly female nursing and allied health professions

■ nurses (and others) unwilling to 'rock the boat' by challenging authority

■ the 'doctor–nurse game' still being played

■ differing education levels

■ turf wars when roles overlap

■ the diverse and ever increasing array of healthcare professions, specialties and subcultures, each with its own terminology and norms

■ different professions training separately, leading to misunderstandings and miscommunication.

Contemporary challenges of working in healthcare teams

While many of the factors that have been found to impact negatively on healthcare professionals' ability to work collaboratively remain current, the complexity of today's healthcare environment creates additional challenges. These include the constantly shifting boundaries in professional roles and responsibilities, as well as changing team compositions, stressful working conditions, and increasing patient co-morbidities, needs and expectations. Furthermore, team members can have differing views on their role in providing care, and a limited understanding of the roles and responsibilities of others (Nancarrow et al., 2013).

Healthcare professionals often work as separate entities within the same environment and, although a common goal to achieve the best possible health outcomes for the client is often espoused, decisions made in isolation, and a lack of effective communication between members of the team, can result in failure to achieve that goal. The inability to work effectively in teams can be attributed to differing views on professional status as well as differing, and at times overlapping, professional boundaries (Lancaster et al., 2015). The individual healthcare professional's way of being within the healthcare environment is shaped by their personal beliefs and values, and their developing professional identity, which in turn impacts on their collaborative capacity. Frenk and colleagues (2010) propose that professional separateness or 'tribalism', resulting from the enculturation and socialisation of members within a discipline, maintains hierarchical structures and power imbalances within healthcare settings. Professional tribalism fosters competition within and between healthcare professions, which in turn reduces cooperation and collaboration, resulting in poorer healthcare for the client. Despite the increasing push for interprofessional education within health disciplines, professional silos continue to exist in the healthcare context with often devastating outcomes resulting for the healthcare consumer (Weller, Boyd & Cumin, 2014).

Valuing and respecting the roles of other team members

For collaborative communication and teamwork to work, they need to be valued and respected by all members of the team, including senior healthcare professionals. When senior team members value their own group over other groups, it can lead to poor team relationships by all team members. Junior members of the team learn and replicate the behaviours and attitudes of their senior colleagues. Conversely, role modelling collaborative communication and the attributes of effective teamwork by senior members of the team has the potential to increase collaborative communication behaviours by all team members. Effective healthcare teams are characterised by interprofessional communication that is non-hierarchical in nature, by a sense of collective agency, and by a culture of shared mental models (Weller, Boyd & Cumin, 2014). It has been demonstrated that interprofessional collaborative teams in which there is mutual respect and goal sharing deliver, not only better patient outcomes, but also increased job satisfaction (McKinley & Perino, 2013). According to Frenk and colleagues (2010), such teams minimise 'tribalism', which allows healthcare professionals to work with, and learn from and about each other. These findings are supported by McKeon and colleagues (2006) who report that observing how others work enhances understanding and valuing of roles, which fosters mutual respect and supports interprofessional collaboration. Dunn et al. (2018) argue that collaborative relationships cannot exist when members of the team do not value or respect the differing professional perspectives of all members of the decision-making team. Feeling professionally valued within the healthcare environment can be defined as being highly regarded and considered with respect or importance through the valuing of one's actions and reactions within the healthcare encounter (Ebert, 2012). The challenge facing healthcare educators and managers today is to create the conditions that foster the valuing and respect of different professionals and their role/s within the healthcare team. For more information about interprofessional collaboration refer to Chapter 6; for the characteristics of effective teams, see Box 5.1.

BOX 5.1   Characteristics that define effective healthcare teams

- Good communication
- Respecting/understanding roles
- Appropriate skill mix
- Commitment to quality process and outcomes of care
- Appropriate team processes and resources
- Shared vision
- Flexibility (of team and individuals within)
- Effective leadership and management
- Supportive team relationships
- Shared training and development opportunities
- Positive personal attributes of individuals
- Professional rewards and development opportunities

Source: Nancarrow et al. (2013).

Person-centred care and teamwork

While the differences between and within the health professions are evident and too often divisive, there is nevertheless a degree of irony, as the different professions share one common, unifying and eminently important goal—the delivery of person-centred care. Although the terms may vary (e.g. 'patient-centred', 'client-centred', 'family-centred' or 'woman-centred'), the intent remains the same, and each profession is committed to the importance of partnership between the care provider and the care recipient as fundamental to effective healthcare and optimal health outcomes.

A way forward: Strategies for learning to work more effectively in healthcare teams

Students enter their respective degrees with an individual identity shaped by the wider socio-political context. They often have preconceived ideas about their role within the healthcare

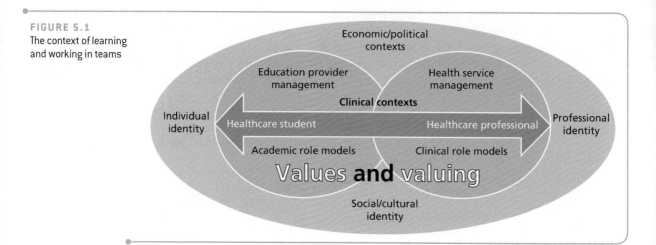

FIGURE 5.1
The context of learning and working in teams

environment, their professional identity and the roles of other professional groups. However, in order to promote teamwork, and thus improve patient outcomes, it is important to foster a joint identity among healthcare professionals as person-centred healthcare experts—rising above their professional identities as doctors, nurses, physiotherapists and so forth. This 'joint identity' as members of an interconnected team is facilitated when healthcare professionals are provided with both formal and opportunistic experiences to learn with, from and about each other, to enable effective collaboration and improve health outcomes (Canadian Interprofessional Health Collaborative, 2010). These experiences need to be premised on an underlying philosophy of mutual respect (see Figure 5.1).

Interprofessional education (IPE) enhances learners' ability to communicate effectively and work as part of an interprofessional team (Reeves, 2016). IPE has the greatest impact when those learning together have equal status, experience a cooperative atmosphere, have institutional support, are aware of group similarities and differences, and perceive the members of different professional groups positively (Reeves, 2016). In the absence of a sense of equality, valuing and respect, IPE will do little to improve attitudes in the classroom or the healthcare environment. Only when people learn or work together *with a shared common goal* will their attitudes change (Allport, 1954). Furthermore, cross-disciplinary socialisation, with healthcare professionals spending time together throughout all learning contexts (including clinical practice), facilitates respect for differences and understanding of role differentials (Richter et al., 2006). Education, therefore, is one phase of a multifaceted and ongoing approach in the development and maintenance of effective healthcare teams.

Conclusion

This chapter described the impact of culture, history, education and social processes on teamwork and collaboration between healthcare professionals. It then discussed how patient safety is influenced by traditional and hierarchical approaches. It is evident that social, political and gender-based organisational structures, both past and present, continue to impact on the current contexts in which healthcare teams function. The challenges of working together collaboratively are multifaceted, but they include competitiveness and 'turf wars' as well as a lack of role awareness and failing to understand and value the roles of other team members. Role modelling and IPE are viewed as strategies for developing collegial healthcare relationships, but both require organisational and professionally endorsed support. Working as part of an effective healthcare team, where members understand, value and respect each other can improve patient safety as well as other healthcare outcomes.

Critical thinking activities

The following excerpt is taken from a study that explored graduates' experiences of working within a healthcare team. While the scenario portrayed focuses on the interactions between a junior medical officer and a registered nurse, similar communication issues arise for all healthcare professionals, irrespective of their discipline or context of work.

Communicating with nurses is hard; there's always a lot of tension there. Although you hear about it before you start working, you don't really figure it out until you experience it. I'm in the ED and when I ask the nurses to do things, they often go to the bottom of the list, even if it's something that from the patient's point of view needs to be done soon. A patient that came in with a stroke didn't get aspirin for three hours, and I had to ask the nurse again and again and again. But I feel like it was because I was an intern ... if someone more senior asked her she would've done it.

1   What social, historical or cultural factors do you believe may have influenced the interprofessional interactions in this scenario?
2   Reflect on similar situations that you have been involved in and consider the implications for the healthcare professionals involved as well as the potential impact on the patient.
3   What insights have you gained from this chapter that you can use when exposed to these types of situations?
4   How well have your educational experiences prepared you to work as part of an effective interprofessional team?
5   What personal and professional attributes do you possess that either help or hinder your ability to work in teams?

Teaching and assessment activities

Communication scenarios

Instructions for educators:

1   Divide students into groups of three, giving each group a role-play scenario from the list below. One student is healthcare professional 1; one student is healthcare professional 2; and the third student is the observer/healthcare consumer (taking into consideration the communication principles and strategies used in the interaction, and providing feedback).
2   The observing student (healthcare consumer) should use the observation prompts below to provide feedback.
3   Healthcare professionals 1 and 2 are to provide feedback on how they felt during the interaction.

Role play 1: Providing evidence-based care using a person-centred approach

Healthcare professional 1: Registered midwife, Sarah
Healthcare professional 2: Medical resident, Christine (first week doing obstetric rotation)

Situation

Sarah is caring for Rebel, a 30-year-old woman who is in a relationship with her partner, Jessie. Rebel is 28 weeks pregnant; this is her first pregnancy and she is well. She is a fitness instructor and has a BMI of 22. Her ultrasound shows her baby is of average weight and size for gestational age. There is no history of diabetes in Rebel's family. Jessie's baby was born at home with a private midwife. Rebel and Jessie have moved to the area recently for Jessie's new job.

Christine advises Rebel that she should have a glucose tolerance test (GTT) in order to screen for gestational diabetes and, therefore, reduce the risk to the baby of sustaining a birth trauma and/or becoming a diabetic in later life.

Activity

Sarah (healthcare professional 1) is to approach the resident, Christine (healthcare professional 2) to discuss evidence-based midwifery care and how a woman-centred approach could be employed to meet Rebel's needs.

Clinical guidelines

All women between 24 and 28 weeks gestation should be offered testing for diabetes. Appropriate tests when a woman has risk factors for hyperglycaemia in the first trimester are glycated haemoglobin (HbA1c), or fasting blood glucose.

Level of evidence

Consensus-based recommendation—that is, a recommendation formulated in the absence of quality evidence (where a systematic review of the evidence was conducted as part of the search strategy).

Source:

Department of Health. (2018). *Clinical Practice Guidelines: Pregnancy Care*. Canberra: Australian Government Department of Health.

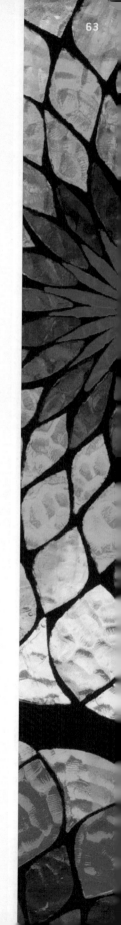

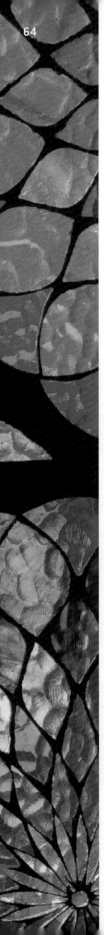

Role play 2: Hand hygiene

Healthcare professional 1: New graduate nurse, Jason

Healthcare professional 2: Registered nurse, Carolyn

Situation

Jason is working with four patients on a busy medical ward. One patient (Joe) has dementia and requires help eating his lunch. While Jason is assisting Joe with his lunch another nurse, Carolyn, enters the room to undertake a set of observations on a newly admitted patient. Jason notices that Carolyn does not observe hand hygiene.

Activity

Jason (healthcare professional 1) is to approach Carolyn (healthcare professional 2) to discuss healthcare-associated infections (HAIs) and the relationship between HAI and hand hygiene.

Clinical guidelines

In Australia, there are approximately 200 000 HAIs in acute healthcare facilities annually. Prevention of HAIs is everybody's responsibility. Hand hygiene is a standard precaution shown to reduce HAIs, and should be undertaken before and after every episode of patient contact.

Sources:

- Australian Guidelines for the Prevention and Control of Infection in Healthcare (2010). Available at: <https://www.nhmrc.gov.au/guidelines-publications/cd33>.
- Hand Hygiene Australia (2018). Available at: <http://www.hha.org.au>.

Role play 3: Unprofessional behaviour

Healthcare professional 1: ED nurse, Sara

Healthcare professional 2: Social worker, Gillian

Situation

Sara has admitted a woman (Kylie) who presented as a sexual assault victim to the ED. Sara requested the social worker (Gillian) to see Kylie for support. After the social worker briefly introduced herself to Kylie she excused herself to step outside. Sara and Kylie both overhear a personal conversation, with Gillian saying (on her mobile), 'I'll be late home as a sexual assault has just turned up'.

Gillian is near the end of her shift, there is no one covering the evening shift, and she wants to go home as she has people coming for dinner. She stepped outside the door to make a personal phone call, not realising her conversation could be overheard.

Activity

Sara (healthcare professional 1) needs to address with Gillian (healthcare professional 2) the personal communication episode overheard by the woman, and how the content of her conversation was unprofessional and disrespectful to the woman.

Clinical guidelines

The Australian Association of Social Workers' Practice Standards (2013) outline the practice expectations required of all social workers. Social Worker Standard 2.1 requires a social worker to 'Represent the social work profession with integrity and professionalism' (p. 10).

The Registered Nurse Standards for Practice (Nursing and Midwifery Board of Australia, 2016) should be evident in current practice. Registered Nurse Standard 2.1 requires registered nurses to 'Advocate on behalf of people in a manner that respects the person's autonomy and legal capacity'; and Standard 2.7 requires registered nurses to 'Actively foster a culture of safety and learning that includes engaging with healthcare professionals and others, to share knowledge and practice that supports person-centred care' (p. 3).

Sources:

- Australian Association of Social Workers. (2013). *Practice Standards*. Available at: <https://www.aasw.asn.au>.
- Nursing and Midwifery Board of Australia. (2016). *Registered Nurse Standards for Practice*. Available at: <http://www.nursingmidwiferyboard.gov.au>.

Student observation prompts

As you observe the interaction between the two healthcare professionals, take into consideration the following communication principles and strategies. Your role is to observe and provide feedback to your colleagues.

Were any/all of the steps in AIDET utilised by healthcare professional 1?

(Tick)   **Yes**   **No**

Acknowledge the person

Introduce yourself

Duration of process or procedure

Explanation

Thank you

Using the ISBAR mnemonic, what did you observe in healthcare professional 1?

Identifying themselves

Explaining the **Situation**

Providing a **Background** to the problem

Summarising your **Assessment**

Providing a **Recommendation** regarding future interactions

Did you notice any of the SOLER principles?

Squarely facing the person

Open posture

Leaning towards the speaker

Eye contact maintained

Relaxed while attending

At the end of the feedback session provide general observations about how the role play unfolded.

Further reading

Chen, A. H., Kiersma, M.E., Keib, C. N. & Cailor, S. (2015). Fostering interdisciplinary communication between pharmacy and nursing students. *American Journal of Pharmaceutical Education*, *79*(6), 1–10.

Garon, M. (2012). Speaking up, being heard: Registered nurses' perceptions of workplace communication. *Journal of Nursing Management, 20*, 361–71.

Lauren B. (2017). Communicating between healthcare disciplines: An educator's perspective. *JOJ Nurse Health Care, 2*(3): 555589.

Shlafer, R. J., McRee, A., Gower, A. L. & Bearinger, L. H. (2016). Better communication for better public health: Perspectives from an interdisciplinary training program. *Health Promotion Practice*, *17*(2), 165–8. doi:10.1177/1524839915627453

Shoham, D. A., Harris, J.K., Mundt, M. & McGaghie, W. (2016). A network model of communication in an interprofessional team of healthcare professionals: A cross-sectional study of a burn unit. *Journal of Interprofessional Care, 30*(5), 661–7. doi:10.1080/13561820.2016.1203296

Web resources

Australian Commission on Safety and Quality in Health Care. Clinical Communications.
<https://www.safetyandquality.gov.au/our-work/clinical-communications/>

Australian Commission on Safety and Quality in Health Care. Inter-professional communication and team climate in complex clinical handover situations (in the Post Anaesthesia Care Unit).
<https://www.safetyandquality.gov.au/our-work/clinical-communications/clinical-handover/national-clinical-handover-initiative-pilot-program/inter-professional-communication-and-team-climate-in-complex-clinical-handover-situations-in-the-post-anaesthesia-care-unit/>

World Health Organization. Being an effective team player.
<http://www.who.int/patientsafety/education/curriculum/who_mc_topic-4.pdf>

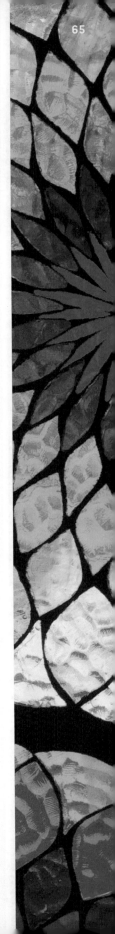

References

Allport, G. (1954). *The Nature of Prejudice*. Cambridge, MA: Addison-Wesley.

Baldwin, D. (2007). Some historical notes on interdisciplinary and interprofessional education and practice in health care in the USA. *Journal of Interprofessional Care, 21*(S1), 23–7.

Binyamin G. (2017). Growing from dilemmas: Developing a professional identity through collaborative reflections on relational dilemmas with role partners. *Israeli Journal of Occupational Therapy, 26*(1), H9–H27.

Canadian Interprofessional Health Collaborative. (2010). *A National Interprofessional Competency Framework*. Accessed May 2018 at: <https://www.cihc.ca/files/CIHC_IPCompetencies_Feb1210.pdf>.

Chung, C. L. R., Manga, J., McGregor, M., Michailidis, C., Stavros, D. & Woodhouse, L. J. (2012). Interprofessional collaboration and turf wars how prevalent are hidden attitudes? *The Journal of Chiropractic Education, 26*(1), 32–9.

Colson, J. & Ralley, R. (2015). Medical practice, urban politics and patronage: The London 'commonalty' of physicians and surgeons of the 1420s. *The English Historical Review, 130*(546), 1102–31. doi: 10.1093/ehr/cev261

Dahl-Michelsen, T. (2015). Curing and caring competencies in the skills training of physiotherapy students. *Physiotherapy Theory & Practice, 31*(1), 8–16.

Davies, S., & Goodman Cripacc, C. (2008). Supporting quality improvement in care homes for older people: The contribution of primary care nurses. *Journal of Nursing Management, 16*, 115–20.

Delaney, L. J. (2018). Patient-centred care as an approach to improving health care in Australia. *Collegian, 25*(1), 119–23.

Department of Health. (2013). Review of Australian Government Health Workforce Programs: 7.1 Nursing and Midwifery Education. Australian Government. Accessed May 2018 at: <http://www.health.gov.au/internet/publications/publishing.nsf/Content/work-review-australian-government-health-workforce-programs-toc~chapter-7-nursing-midwifery-workforce–education-retention-sustainability~chapter-7-nursing-midwifery-education>.

Dunn, S. I., Cragg, B., Graham, I. D., Medves, J. & Gaboury, I. (2018): Roles, processes, and outcomes of interprofessional shared decision-making in a neonatal intensive care unit: A qualitative study. *Journal of Interprofessional Care*. doi: 10.1080/13561820.2018.1428186

Ebert, L. (2012). Woman-centred care and the socially disadvantaged woman: An interpretative phenomenological analysis (unpublished doctoral dissertation). University of Newcastle, NSW, Australia.

Fagin, I. & Garelick, A. (2004). The doctor–nurse relationship. *Advances in Psychiatric Treatment, 10*, 277–86.

Frenk, J., Chen, L., Bhutta, Z., Cohen, J., Crips, N., Evans, T., … Zurayk, H. (2010). Health professionals for a new century: Transforming education to strengthen health systems in an interdependent world. *The Lancet, 376*, 1923–58.

Hocking, C. & Wright-St Clair, V. (2011). Occupational science: Adding value to occupational therapy. *Journal of Occupational Therapy, 58*(1), 29–35.

Holyoake, D. (2011). Is the doctor–nurse game still being played? *Nursing Times, 107*, 12–14. Accessed May 2018 at: <https://search-proquest-com.ezproxy.newcastle.edu.au/docview/1038954864?accountid=10499>.

Jaros, A. A. (2015). The course of the professional development and the level of job satisfaction among physiotherapists. *Medical Studies, 31*(1), 26–34.

Jefferson, L., Bloor, K. & Maynard, A. (2015). Women in medicine: Historical perspectives and recent trends. *British Medical Bulletin, 114*(1), 5–15. doi: 10.1093/bmb/ldv007

Karimi, H., & Masoudi Alavi, N. (2015). Florence Nightingale: The Mother of Nursing. *Nursing and Midwifery Studies, 4*(2), e29475. doi: 10.17795/nmsjournal29475

Lancaster, G., Kolakowsky-Hayner, S., Kovacich, J. & Greer-Williams, N. (2015). Interdisciplinary communication and collaboration among physicians, nurses, and unlicensed assistive personnel. *Journal of Nursing Scholarship: An Official Publication of Sigma Theta Tau International Honor Society, 47*(3), 275–84.

McKay, K. & Narasimhan, S. (2012). Bridging the gap between doctors and nurses. *Journal of Nursing Education and Practice, 2*(4), 52–5.

McKeon, L. M., Oswaks, J. D. & Cunningham, P. D. (2006). Safeguarding patients: Complexity science, high reliability organizations, and implications for team training in healthcare. (quiz 305-6) *Clinical Nurse Specialist, 20*, 298–304.

McKinley, C. J. & Perino, C. (2013). Examining communication competence as a contributing factor in health care workers' job satisfaction and tendency to report errors. *Journal of Communication in Healthcare, 6*(3), 158–65. doi: 10.1179/1753807613Y.0000000039

Maclellan, L., Higgins, I. & Levett-Jones, T. (2015). Medical acceptance of the nurse practitioner role in Australia: A decade on. *Journal Of The American Association Of Nurse Practitioners, 27*(3), 152–9. doi:10.1002/2327-6924.12141

Murray, M., Sundin, D. & Cope, V. (2017). The nexus of nursing leadership and a culture of safer patient care. *Journal of Clinical Nursing, 27*(5–6), 1287–93.

Nancarrow, S. A., Booth, A., Ariss, S., Smith, T., Enderby, P. & Roots, A. (2013). Ten principles of good interdisciplinary team work. *Human Resources for Health, 11*(19). doi: 10.1186/1478-4491-11-19

O'Brien, J. C. (2013). *Introduction to Occupational Therapy*. E-Book. St Louis, Missouri: Elsevier. Accessed May 2018 at: <https://books.google.com.au/books?isbn=0323266398>.

OpenLearn. (2016). *Florence Nightingale on What Makes a Good Nurse*. UK: The Open University. Accessed May 2018 at: <http://www.open.edu/openlearn/health-sports-psychology/health/health-studies/florence-nightingale-on-what-makes-good-nurse>.

Reeves, S. (2016). Why we need interprofessional education to improve the delivery of safe and effective care. *Interface: Comunicação, Saúde, Educação, 20*(56), 185–97. doi: 10.1590/1807-57622014.0092

Richardson, B. (n.d.). BrainyQuote.com.

Richter, A., West, M., Van Dick, R. & Dawson, J. (2006). Boundary spanners' identification, intergroup contact, and effective intergroup relations. *Academy of Management Journal, 49*, 1252–69.

Rigby, D. (2010). Collaboration between doctors and pharmacists in the community. *Australian Prescriber, 33*, 191–3.

Schneiderman, J., Waugaman, W. & Flynn, M. (2008). Nurse social work practitioner: A new professional for health care settings. *Health and Social Work, 33*, 149–54.

Siedlecki, S.L. & Hixson, E.D. (2015). Relationships Between Nurses and Physicians Matter. *OJIN: The Online Journal of Issues in Nursing, 20*(3). doi: 10.3912/OJIN.Vol20No03PPT03

Sirota, T. (2007). Nurse/physician relationships: Improving or not? *Nursing, 37*(1), 52–5.

Stein, L. (1967). The doctor–nurse game. *Archives of General Psychiatry, 16*(6), 699–703.

The National Archives Education Service. (n.d.). *Florence Nightingale—Why Do We Remember Her?* Report upon the state of the hospitals of the British Army in the Crimea and Scutari. Accessed May 2018 at: <https://nationalarchives.gov.uk/documents/education/florence.pdf>.

Weiss, S. & Davis, H. (1985). Validity and reliability of the Collaborative Practice Scales. *Nursing Research, 34*(5), 299–305.

Weller, J., Boyd, M. & Cumin, D. (2014). Teams, tribes and patient safety: Overcoming barriers to effective teamwork in healthcare. *Postgrad Medical Journal, 90*(1061), 149–54.

Washington University School of Medicine. (2009). *Women in Health Sciences Health Professions Development of the Field of Physical Therapy*. St Louis, Missouri: Bernard Becker Medical Library. Accessed May 2018 at: <http://beckerexhibits.wustl.edu/mowihsp/health/PTdevel.htm>.

World Confederation for Physical Therapy London. (2016). *Policy Statement: Description of Physical Therapy*. Accessed May 2018 at: <http://www.wcpt.org/policy/ps-descriptionPT>.

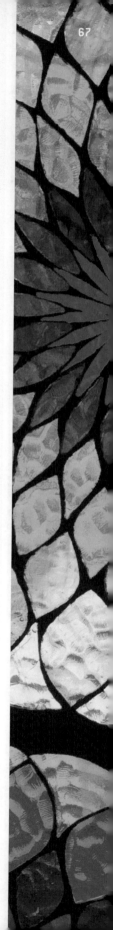

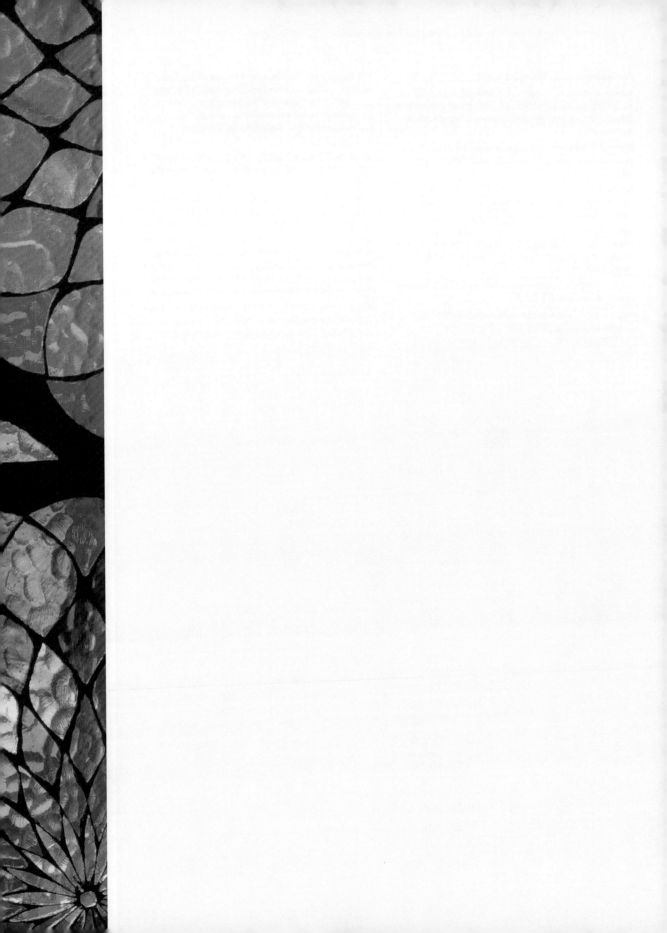

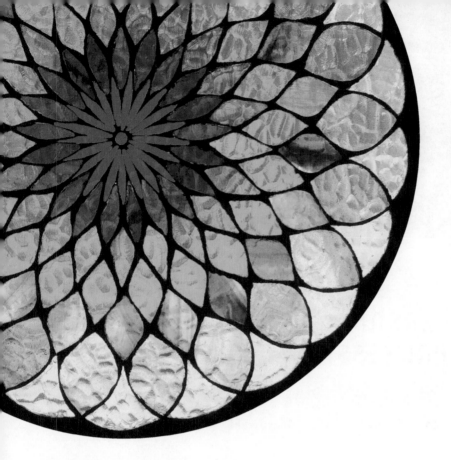

SECTION 2

Improving interprofessional communication to promote patient safety and wellbeing

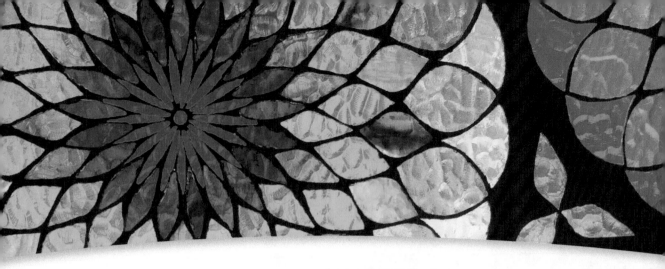

CHAPTER 6

INTERPERSONAL COMMUNICATION FOR INTERPROFESSIONAL COLLABORATION

Anne Croker   Miriam Grotowski   Diane Tasker

LEARNING OUTCOMES

Chapter 6 will enable you to:

- identify key differences and potential contributions brought to collaborative situations by healthcare professionals
- discuss person-centred care as an impetus for working collaboratively with others to ensure patient safety
- explain the role of respect in interpersonal communication for interprofessional collaboration
- outline key issues to consider when communicating with other healthcare professionals
- describe key capabilities that enhance interprofessional collaboration.

KEY CONCEPTS

interpersonal communication | interprofessional collaboration | person-centred care | respect | shared purpose

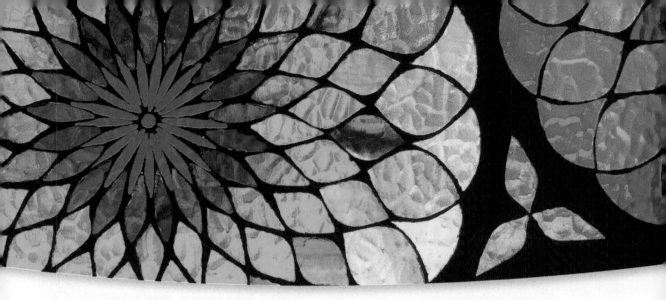

Working together with indifference?

Our aspiration is to be working together within difference!

(Croker, 2011, p. 324)

INTRODUCTION

Although we talk so easily and so often about *interprofessional collaboration*, it is important to remember that it is people as *individuals* who collaborate, rather than *professions*. And, as individuals, we are all different. The nature of interpersonal communication for interprofessional collaboration is shaped by the way we deal with the differences encountered in our practice as individual healthcare professionals.

This chapter explores interpersonal communication as a core component of interprofessional collaboration. In highlighting the interpersonal nature of communication, we emphasise the importance of individuals and their relationships in the ongoing process of sharing knowledge, information, thoughts and perspectives. This emphasis on individuals and relationships also underpins our conceptualisation of interprofessional collaboration as the intentional practice of people representing different professions working together through their communication, decision making and actions to achieve a common purpose (Croker, Higgs & Trede, 2016).

The chapter begins by discussing some of the differences that are brought into collaborative situations. Following a discussion of the notions of respect and person-centred care, the key components of communicating with others in clinical settings are explored. The chapter concludes by reflecting on the value of being aware of self, others and the situation when we collaborate with individuals from other healthcare professions.

Bringing differences together

You know [we, as healthcare professionals] are just so completely different. We're not different with regards to ideals (for patient care) … But in terms of our personalities, the way we get jobs done, agendas, all different. And I think that's fantastic.

(Croker, 2011, p. 330)

As healthcare professionals we need to respond to our patients' varied health issues, personalities and situations, and in doing so, we need to engage with our colleagues' differences. These differences can relate to history, disciplinary perspectives, personal characteristics, experiences and the contexts in which we collaborate. We also bring the professional roles that we acquire as part of our healthcare professional education and socialisation. At the same time, we bring our different ways of seeing the world, our varied ways of interacting with others, our range of personal and professional experiences, and our particular situations at the time of communicating. Understanding others' particular situations, while embracing their professional and personal differences, can bring a rich range of skills, capabilities, perspectives and values to collaborative situations. Although patient safety is a complex notion, experienced clinicians are aware of the value of multiple different perspectives for minimising oversights and preventing errors.

However, the degree to which differences are valued and the ease with which they are embraced can vary. Some healthcare professionals work together closely, valuing their colleagues' differences and caring about each other—that is, they are together within their differences. Other healthcare professionals may find their work colleagues more distant and, while their colleagues are notionally part of the team, their working style is not necessarily integrated or inclusive—that is, they are together, but with indifferent attitudes towards each other. These different experiences are described in the following story.

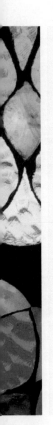

BEING TOGETHER: WITH INDIFFERENCE AND WITHIN DIFFERENCE

Staff at a general practice recently heard about the death of a 50-year-old man, a long-term and well-known patient at their practice. He left behind him a wife and two teenage sons, also patients at the practice. The practice doctors, nurses and reception staff worked with each other and with the family during the man's long-term illness. One of his sons now has an appointment with the doctor. It is a difficult consultation; on the surface it is unrelated to his father's recent death, yet it is unsettlingly accompanied by an undercurrent of deep loss.

Working together with indifference

At the end of the consultation, the doctor takes a brief break in the tea room to look out the window and mentally prepare for the next consultation. The chat between the nurse and the practice manager is welcomed as a background distraction, but it does not address the emotion of the consultation. Then voices from the waiting room provide the impetus for 'Next patient, please'.

While staff in this situation worked cooperatively during the father's illness, there was insufficient understanding of each other's roles or sense of 'caring togetherness' to carry over to related situations.

Now imagine the same scenario, but with a different outcome.

Working together within difference

At the end of the consultation, the practice nurse spontaneously (but 'knowingly') meets the doctor in the tea room. Her acknowledgment of the challenging nature of the consultation is appreciated. They 'touch base' about the implications for the family of the death of a father, and the sadness the practice staff feel when a long-term patient dies. The practice manager (also aware of the situation) drops in to say that the reception staff have

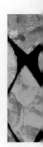

arranged a new baby check as the next consultation, because 'new life and a joyful focus' might be welcome after the sadness inherent in the last consultation. Following a short, shared silence and nod of agreement, the nurse and doctor smile at each other and begin discussing the details of the next consultation.

Although not physically present during the son's consultation, staff members are 'tuned in' to their colleague's work. In supporting each other to provide quality patient care, they draw on their shared experiences with this particular family, the numerous other occasions they have worked collaboratively and the respect they have for each other's roles and contributions.

In aspiring to work *together within our differences,* we need to appreciate the value and challenges of working with others who have been socialised into their particular professional roles and who bring their individual contexts to the collaborative situations. We also need to be aware of the influence of different team structures on collaboration. Understanding and grappling with issues related to education, socialisation, individual contexts and team structures provides a strong foundation for valuing differences that are brought to clinical situations.

Socialisation of professional roles is the process through which students learn the roles, common values, problem-solving approaches and language of their profession. The resulting rich diverse roles and understandings underpin the need for and importance of collaboration. Viewing these differences positively enables us to engage constructively with other healthcare professionals. A healthcare professional explains this as follows:

From our backgrounds we have different ways of approaching, getting information or dealing with the information that [patients and carers] are giving us. It's so nice to watch someone else at work.

(Croker, 2011, p. 229)

Interprofessional education provides opportunities for students and healthcare professionals to learn with, from and about each other, and to collaborate more effectively as members of an interprofessional team (World Health Organization, 2010). Interprofessional education allows us to recognise, respect and value the differences between people and professions.

Integral to engaging constructively with professional diversity is both being open to others' clinical reasoning and being able to explain our own. 'Clinical reasoning' is a 'broad term denoting the thinking, judgements and decision-making involved in clinical practice', recognising that healthcare professionals '... often need to make decisions based on their professional knowledge and judgment in situations where there are no right answers, and where textbook and research is insufficient, or needs to be adapted to the particular client' (Ajjawi, Higgs & McAllister, 2012, pp. 206–7). Encouraging others to communicate their clinical reasoning can help clarify different points of view. Being able to communicate our clinical reasoning clearly to others is important for justifying our decisions or persuading others of their credibility; it is also essential to patient safety (Levett-Jones, 2018).

Individuals' contexts are another source of differences. As well as our socialised professional discipline roles, each person involved in communication and collaboration brings personal experiences, situations, aspirations, fears, preferences and capabilities. At times the influence of personal situations can impact negatively on communication. For example, time pressure, family issues, tiredness, illness and financial needs can be impediments to engaging with different views and ways of doing things. Explaining our situation to others may be helpful when these influences are impacting on our ability to communicate and collaborate. Similarly, when colleagues respond in an unexpected manner, it may be helpful to explore and understand their situation.

When we are collaborating with colleagues from different disciplines, it can be important to remember that the way they interact with us may say more about who they are as a person or what is happening around them than it does about their profession as a whole. We need to take care that our interpretation of situations does not inadvertently reinforce any negative stereotypes we might have developed (or be in danger of developing) about that profession.

Collaborative structures and styles introduce another form of diversity to interprofessional collaboration. Collaboration occurs in a range of team structures, from formal teams (such as community health teams where healthcare professionals are specifically appointed to the team) to loose networks (such as wards where people work together according to their rosters and their patients' needs), and across a range of decision-making styles. Although inclusive consensus styles of decision making are commonly preferred, authoritarian styles may be appropriate for particular collaborative situations (particularly when there is a sense of urgency). As healthcare professionals, we need to be able to adjust the way we interact with others according to the requirements and opportunities of the situation. (See 'Further reading' at the end of the chapter.)

In the literature, the notion of collaboration is often categorised in terms of role clarity and boundary blurring. For example, the term *multiprofessional* (or *multidisciplinary*) commonly refers to disciplines working in parallel with distinct roles, *interprofessional* (or *interdisciplinary*) tends to refer to blurred discipline roles and *transprofessional* (or *transdisciplinary*) refers to healthcare professionals transcending discipline boundaries through role expansion or role release (Choi & Pak, 2006). In this chapter (while recognising the importance for some discussions of having different terms to reflect different collaborative styles), we are choosing to use the term 'interprofessional collaboration' to mean the intentional practice of people working together to achieve a common purpose, without implying the collaborative style in which they are doing this. What is important in practice is to establish the nature of boundary clarity and role blurring of the collaborative situations in which we work.

Person-centredness as impetus

Although *being together within difference* is not necessarily straightforward, person-centredness provides a powerful unifying purpose for communication and collaboration in healthcare. As an adjective, 'person-centred' embraces the notion of people in healthcare. An important quality of person-centredness for interprofessional collaboration is the *patient focus* that provides a shared purpose for people to pull together in the same direction. It takes into account that patients are more than just the sum of their diseases and health problems. Similarly, person-centredness also recognises that the healthcare professionals in their varied patient-care roles are also individuals. Our colleagues are more than just the professions they represent or the roles they undertake. If we are to work collaboratively, humanistic views of our patients as people need to be expanded to include our colleagues. As captured by an experienced clinician (see Box 6.1), person-centredness is enhanced by treating each other as *people as well as professionals*.

> Person-centredness embraces the patient as a person, recognising their values, situations, needs, interests and capabilities. They are viewed as people with will, agency and preferences rather than disease entities or objects for the delivery of services. Because healthcare professionals and other staff are affected by and affect patients' healthcare, they are key players in person-centred healthcare (based on Croker et al., 2016).

Obtaining consent before sharing information between healthcare professionals is another important issue to consider for person-centred collaborative practice: What will we be discussing with others? Does the patient know we will be doing this? Do we have the patient's permission to do so? There are different types of consent, including explicit (such as a signed permission) and implied (such as agreeing to attend an appointment). The type of consent required may depend on the situation, the nature of information shared and the extent to which the wider 'team' is an explicit part of treatment expectations.

Respect as core ingredient

> *Our openness to each other,*
> *Our multiplicity, our shared focus*
> *Presumed and comfortable within our synergy,*
> *Encompassed by a word—'respect'.*

(Croker, 2011, p. 231)

BOX 6:1   Caring, coffee and camaraderie

An experienced clinician captures how the person-centred focus of his team relies on meaningful interactions between team members:

> We might have different roles, but we are all human beings.
> We're all here to do the best thing for our patients.
> When we are working together to care for our patients, almost nothing bothers us.
> Camaraderie helps us to do it.
>
> Coffee is important, the time when you sit down together.
> The tea room becomes somewhere you talk and get to know each other.
> You see that we're all people. We have lives beyond here.
> During such sharing and relaxing, you get to see the human side of things.
>
> We all have different skills but we're part of the same team.
> We had a patient come back to visit us recently.
> A few months ago we didn't think he was going to make it.
> It needed everybody to get him right and get him home.
> It was good to see him.

Source: This text is derived from research currently being undertaken by Croker, Smith, Fisher and May at the University of Newcastle, Department of Rural Health.

Respect has long been recognised as a key ingredient of interpersonal communication and interprofessional collaboration. Respect is complex, encompassing intentions, attitudes and behaviours towards people. It can be a taken-for-granted notion, used in a broad sense without necessarily being clear about *what* is being respected and *why* this respect is granted. We need to bring the notion of respect 'into the spotlight' and 'unbundle its parts' if we are to understand its role in interpersonal communication for interprofessional collaboration.

Respect is related to people's differences as well as their inherent value as humans. When we discuss the notion of respect, we need to take into consideration the diversity of those involved in healthcare, including self, other healthcare professionals, support staff, patients and carers. Such diversity can relate to discipline knowledge and socialisation, as well as personal capabilities, experience, needs, fears and aspirations.

Respect needs to be accorded to the different professions and their contributions to healthcare, yet it also needs to be earned by individuals in their particular roles. People's confidence and self-esteem, in terms of their discipline roles and collaborative contributions, can be enhanced by receiving respect from others. However, respect for individuals can be lost if certain verbal and non-verbal behaviours and attitudes are displayed during interpersonal interactions and communication.

Although there are many different elements of this complex notion, the experience of respect tends to be unanimously valued. Respect is closely intertwined with its partners of *trust, mutuality* and *willingness to work with others*. Respect can be developed through communicating and working with people from different professions. Knowing the other healthcare professionals as *people*, as they perform their healthcare roles, forms a basis for gaining respect and trust. Time and proximity can also nurture respect.

Respect has a directional element, being received *from* others (being respected) and being provided *to* others (showing respect). Without the coherence provided by respect, people may be indifferent to

FIGURE 6.1
Respect: Different perspectives and experiences

Source: Croker, A., Trede, F. & Higgs, J. (2012). Collaboration: What is it like? Phenomenological interpretation of the experience of collaborating within rehabilitation teams. *Journal of Interprofessional Care, 26*(1), pp. 13–20.

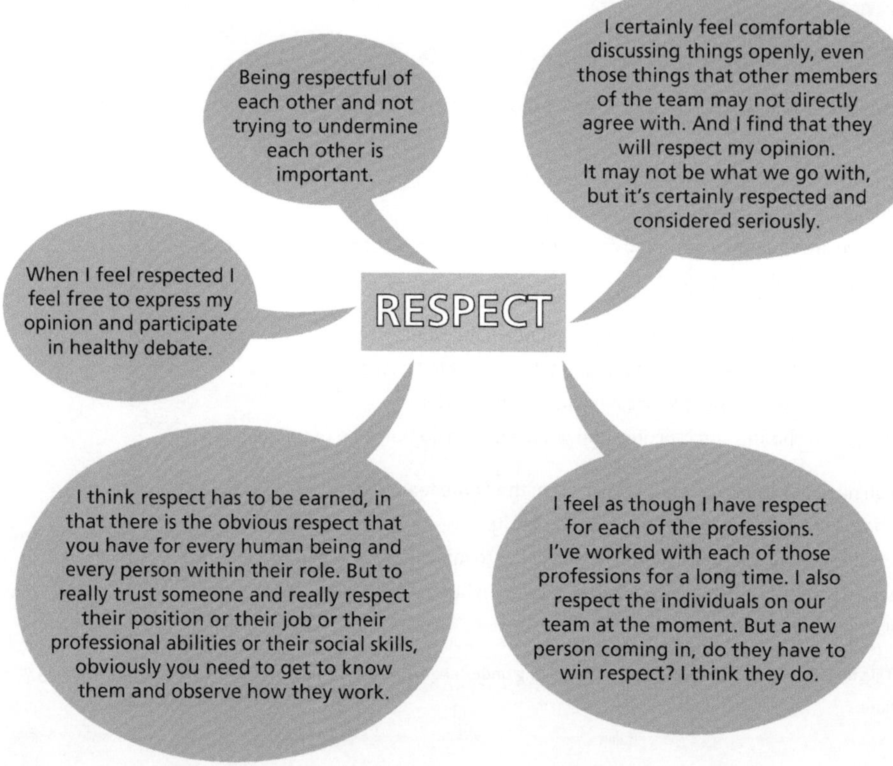

the value of each other's differences and the need to engage with others. Through such indifference, people forgo a key facilitator of collaborating and an important source of momentum.

Figure 6.1 provides a compilation of quotes to highlight different perspectives of, and experiences with, the notion of respect. Take time to consider the messages within the quotes and, as you do, reflect on the following questions:

- What is it about my role that I would like other healthcare professionals to understand and respect?
- What do I do to help my role be understood and respected?
- What do I understand and respect about others' roles and contributions?
- How do other healthcare professionals earn my respect?
- How do I show respect to other healthcare professionals?

Communicating with others

Capability for communicating with other healthcare professionals in clinical situations includes the core skills of:

> … *attentive listening (to encourage speakers and hear their messages), questioning (to elicit information and understand the perspectives of others), providing information (to explain and inform through clear verbal explanations or written reports), responding (to provide feedback about messages received), clarifying (to check understanding and highlight areas of tension) and empathising (to create an appropriate communication climate).*

(Croker & Coyle, 2012, p. 286)

Key points of interpersonal communication that are particularly relevant to patient safety are honesty, accuracy, legibility, clarity, timeliness (including attention to urgency), sufficient detail, suitability of avenues for communication and a focus on issues not emotions. (See Chapter 3 for more detail about patient-safe communication behaviours.)

There are a variety of forms of interpersonal communication commonly used between different healthcare professionals in clinical settings. Some styles follow particular formats (e.g. case notes) or are framed by expectations and a collaborative culture (e.g. team meetings), while other styles are more ad hoc and opportunistic in nature. Opportunistic interactions can involve fleeting encounters between healthcare professionals as they write in patient records or access electronic medical records, as well as more in-depth corridor chats or discussions in shared office spaces. The speed and flexibility of such communication enables healthcare professionals to keep up to date with issues and respond to them as they arise. They are also able to pick up subtleties that may not be available from written records (as shown in the following quotes):

'I just grab them and have a chat with them or I'll ring them upstairs, depending on how urgent it is.'

(Croker, 2011, p. 247)

'I think that being in the same location is pretty much what makes it work actually; the fact that we do all work within close proximity of one another. There's a lot of informal contact between people. Everyone has morning tea in the same room and lunch in the same room. And it's not far to walk to one another's offices.'

(Croker, 2011, p. 248)

'I'll hang around the nurses' station and listen to what's happening, talk to them informally about what's going on. If there is a problem, an issue, I'll grab them and talk to them formally about it.'

(Croker, 2011, p. 248)

'If it's something that we don't talk about at the meeting we can talk about it the following day or we talk about it as it arises.'

(Croker & Coyle, 2012, p. 17)

It is important to remember that outcomes of ad hoc forms of communication may need to be formally documented. Efficiency, flexibility and situational relevance of interpersonal communication for interprofessional collaboration are all enhanced when healthcare professionals are capable of using a range of communication styles in interrelated and appropriate ways.

Awareness of self, others and situations

Compare these quotes:

'There's flexibility to support each other when someone is snowed under.'

'We really do go the extra distance for our patients and for each other.'

'I have made conscious decisions about how I should work with [my colleagues].'

with these:

'We need to tread carefully with her, plan what we are going to say, and how to say it and have all the reasons worked out beforehand.'

'Her participation seems to be at a superficial level. She doesn't take our opinions on board. I know she is busy, but she can get a bit impatient!'

(Croker, 2011)

Experienced clinicians are usually well aware that different healthcare professionals have differing capabilities with regard to communication and collaboration. In this section we propose a framework for making sense of people's differing capabilities for collaborating with others based on the notions of *reflexivity*, *reciprocity* and *responsiveness* (Croker et al., 2016). These notions represent a higher level of abstraction than the requirements for communication discussed in the previous section (such as listening, questioning and responding).

Introducing the 3 Rs of collaborating

Being able to monitor our own contributions and actions, and make appropriate adjustments is important for successful collaborating. As healthcare professionals, we need to be able to consider:

- 'How am I going with my collaborative interactions?' We need to critically reflect on self and change according to these reflections (reflexivity).

- 'What can I do for you and you do for me as we both work towards providing the best care for our patients?' We need to be aware of the mutual 'give and take' of working with others towards a shared purpose and realign ourselves in order to do so (reciprocity).

- 'In light of the particular context we are working in, what do we need to take note of and what adjustments are required?' We need to be aware of our surroundings and make situationally appropriate adjustments (responsiveness).

The three interrelated capabilities of *reflexivity*, *reciprocity* and *responsiveness* are the 3 Rs of collaborating (see Figure 6.2, based on Croker et al., 2016).

The 3 Rs can be compared to a virus protection program running in the background of a computer; just as the virus protection aims to keep the computer running efficiently and safe from threats, so too do the 3 Rs facilitate the smooth running of collaboration and ensure that people work together for safe person-centred healthcare. They are integral to dealing with the collaborative ambiguities, uncertainties and subtleties often faced by healthcare professionals.

FIGURE 6.2
The 3 Rs of collaborating

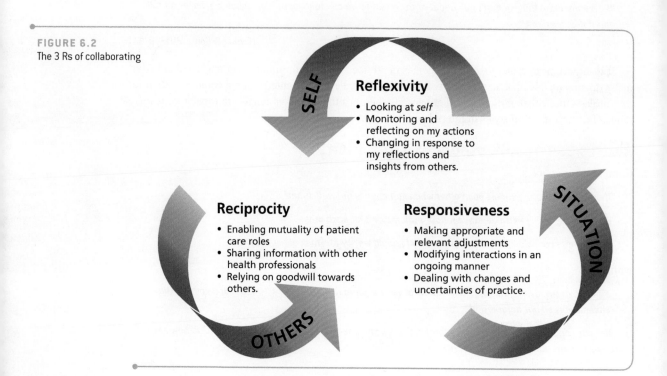

Reflexivity
- Looking at *self*
- Monitoring and reflecting on my actions
- Changing in response to my reflections and insights from others.

Reciprocity
- Enabling mutuality of patient care roles
- Sharing information with other health professionals
- Relying on goodwill towards others.

Responsiveness
- Making appropriate and relevant adjustments
- Modifying interactions in an ongoing manner
- Dealing with changes and uncertainties of practice.

SELF

SITUATION

OTHERS

Different levels of capabilities for reviewing

Unfortunately, capabilities for reviewing collaboration are not consistent across all healthcare professionals. Although the 3 Rs are interdependent, *reflexivity* plays a key role in this interdependence. High levels of reflexivity can enable healthcare professionals to contribute reciprocally to shared goals, and to be responsive to changing situations and the needs of people and contexts. If healthcare professionals are not able to critically reflect on self, their low levels of reflexivity are likely to affect levels of both reciprocity and responsiveness.

Interestingly, the Rs are often more obvious when they are missing than when they are fully present. Healthcare professionals who are constantly 'prickly' or 'tricky' during collaborative interactions may have low levels of capability for reviewing self, others and situations; or perhaps they lack opportunities to reflect on their collaborative practice. It can be challenging to work with people who are unaware of the influence of their actions, their contributions and the need for adjustments. To ensure that we are not 'that tricky person in the team', it is important for each of us to develop our capability for reviewing our collaboration. In this way, our colleagues' energy can be directed to patient care rather than dealing with 'us' as challenging members of the healthcare team.

Conclusion

We bring more than our particular professional roles to healthcare. We also bring different ways of seeing the world, different ways of interacting with others, and different personal and professional experiences. Respecting each other as we seek the best care for our patients brings us together, and helps us embrace and overcome differences. An awareness of self, others and situations is important for how we communicate with each other to provide collaborative person-centred care. Being open to working with professional, personal and situational difference can enhance the safety, scope and nature of care provided for our patients. Let us aspire to work *together* within difference.

Critical thinking activities

The following scenario is a cautionary one, reminding us of the importance of a *patient focus* in collaborative person-centred care. Read the scenario and reflect on what can happen when team members collaborate more closely with themselves than they do with the patient.

One voice against many: 'You are not listening to me …'

This scenario is based on a couple's actual experience at an early pregnancy clinic in a tertiary hospital. Lisa and Ben are meeting the consultant for the first time. They had been in contact with various team members during the previous week. The team had been discussing the case when they enter the room.

> Consultant: *'The team has told me all about you. You are obviously very anxious, Lisa. We will do the scan, show you the heartbeat, then you can get back to work.'*

> Lisa: *'I am not sure you understand. I am really worried about …'* Her words were cut off.

> The consultant interjected: *'We have discussed it. Your previous scan was normal and after a normal scan the blood tests don't matter.'*

> Lisa: *'But you're not listening to me …'*

If the team members in the room that day had listened, they would have heard Lisa say:

We've been getting mixed messages from the team. I don't think you've got the whole story. I think the previous scan was abnormal because the sonographer told me there was something wrong. I had a miscarriage three months ago and now my pregnancy symptoms have disappeared like last time. I am spotting and cramping. Over the last week my blood levels have been rising but not quickly enough, which I found very worrying. Some of the nurses who rang with the results seemed concerned, and others didn't and said I was being too anxious and should stop worrying. The last nurse told me, 'It is not looking good', and asked me to come in today for a scan. I was relieved that someone was taking me seriously. But since arriving here you have implied that I am

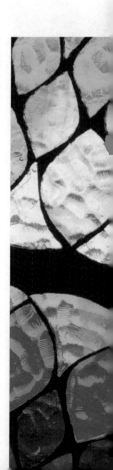

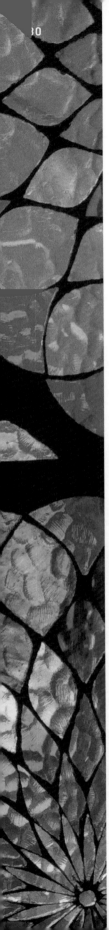

wasting your time being here and that I should be at work, that I am being unreasonably anxious. What I need you to hear is that I am scared and confused. The team's messages are mixed and I am feeling very judged, not understood.

But Lisa was not able to explain. She was allowed no voice.

With her story untold, the scan was performed. No foetal heartbeat was found. A stunned silence ensued. All present were surprised, except Lisa and Ben. They knew the whole story. But no one had listened. As their sadness and frustration turned to anger, their fear for future pregnancies was escalated by their sense of disempowerment. They felt the team was against them; theirs was one voice against many.

Issues of patient safety are not confined to physical harm. The patient's emotional safety is also important. Team members need to take time to ensure they have the full picture. Care needs to be taken not to act on unintegrated snippets of information and on other team members' unsubstantiated assumptions.

1   How did Lisa come to be framed as an overly anxious patient?
2   What mixed messages did Lisa and Ben receive from the team?
3   How might these mixed messages have come about?
4   What were the implications of the team's mixed messages for Lisa and Ben?
5   If the team had heard Lisa's story, how could the couple have been better supported?
6   What should the team do now?
7   How can we ensure that our patients are 'one voice with many' rather than 'one voice against many'?

Teaching and assessment activities

'Me and my perceptions'

We do not enter our healthcare professional roles, or education towards these roles, as 'blank slates'. We enter with a range of experiences, expectations and assumptions about our chosen profession, as well as other healthcare professions. These experiences, expectations and assumptions can influence our readiness to work with other healthcare professionals. The following personal reflective activity is adapted from the published insights of healthcare students as they grappled with learning to work with other professions (Tinlin, Croker & Wakely, 2016). Educators can provide students with opportunities to discuss these reflections and facilitate story telling about working positively with other professions.

1   **Early collaboration is learning about roles**. 'A five-minute exercise in a hospital and seeing people from different professions working towards a common goal was more powerful for learning about communication, negotiation and engaging with others (about their roles) than an hour lecture' (p. 239).

    Discussion questions

    a.   What opportunities do I have to see people from different professions working collaboratively?
    b.   How can these opportunities be facilitated?
    c.   What can I learn about others' roles in these opportunities?

2   **Our learning about other health professions is socialised**. 'Part of how we approach collaboration depends on the perceptions we build of participating professions. Our experiences growing up, our prior socialisation and current interactions all ultimately form our impressions of health professions' (p. 240).

    Discussion questions

    a.   What previous experiences might be influencing my current perceptions of particular professions?
    b.   What are the implications of these perceptions for working with these professions?

3   **Learning about other healthcare professions is difficult and complex**. '[On clinical placement] without confidence in our newly-forming skills we have good reason to steer clear of people we are nervous about communicating with (because we don't sufficiently understand their roles)' (p. 241).

    Discussion questions

    a.   How can I balance developing skills in my own role with learning about the skills and roles of others?
    b.   To what extend is collaborating with others integral to the value of the clinical placement?

4   **Sorting through similarities and differences**. 'At university it was easier to talk about the similarities, in the same bioscience or anatomy courses that we were taking. The differences, how we varied in our treatments or theoretical underpinnings, were less talked about' (p. 243).

Discussion questions

a. What opportunities do I have to understand the differences between my profession and other professions?
b. In what ways are we different?
c. What do I need to understand in order to truly value these differences?

Further reading

Croker, A., Higgs, J. & Trede, F. (2016). *Collaborating in Healthcare: Reinterpreting Therapeutic Relationships.* Rotterdam, The Netherlands: Sense Publishers.

Croker, A., Trede, F. & Higgs, J. (2012). Collaboration: What is it like? Phenomenological interpretation of the experience of collaborating within rehabilitation teams. *Journal of Interprofessional Care, 26*(1), 13–20.

Higgs, J., Croker, A., Tasker, D., Hummell J. & Patton, N. (2014). *Health Practice Relationships.* Rotterdam, The Netherlands: Sense Publishers.

Web resources

Canadian Interprofessional Health Collaborative (CIHC) framework.
<https://www.mcgill.ca/ipeoffice/ipe-curriculum/cihc-framework>

Western Health Sciences. Interprofessional Education and Research.
<http://www.ipe.uwo.ca/>

References

Ajjawi, R., Higgs, J. & McAllister, L. (2012). Communicating clinical reasoning. In J. Higgs, R. Ajjawi, L. McAllister, F. Trede & S. Loftus (Eds), *Communicating in the Health Sciences* (3rd edn, pp. 206–15). South Melbourne: Oxford University Press.

Choi, B. & Pak, A. (2006). Multidisciplinary, interdisciplinary and transdisciplinary in health research, services, education and policy: 1. Definitions, objectives, and evidence of effectiveness. *Clinical Investigative Medicine, 29*(6), 351–64.

Croker, A. (2011). Collaboration in Rehabilitation Teams. Unpublished PhD thesis. Charles Sturt University.

Croker, A. & Coyle, J. (2012). Communicating in teams. In J. Higgs, R. Ajjawi, L. McAllister, F. Trede & S. Loftus (Eds), *Communicating in the Health Sciences* (3rd edn, pp. 280–9). South Melbourne: Oxford University Press.

Croker, A., Higgs, J. & Trede, F. (2016). *Collaborating in Healthcare: Reinterpreting Therapeutic Relationships.* Rotterdam, The Netherlands: Sense Publishers.

Levett-Jones, T. (2018). Clinical reasoning: What it is and why it matters. In T. Levett-Jones (Ed.), *Clinical Reasoning: Learning How to Think Like a Nurse* (2nd edn, pp. 2–13). Melbourne, Australia: Pearson.

Tinlin, L., Croker, C. & Wakely, L. (2016). Students' experiences of learning to work with other professions: If we read enough patients' notes will we learn to collaborate? In A, Croker, J. Higgs & F. Trede, *Collaborating in Healthcare: Reinterpreting Therapeutic Relationships* (pp. 237–44). Rotterdam, The Netherlands: Sense Publishers.

World Health Organization. (2010). *Framework for Action on Interprofessional Education and Collaborative Practice.* Health Professions Networks Nursing and Midwifery Office, Human Resources for Health, Geneva.

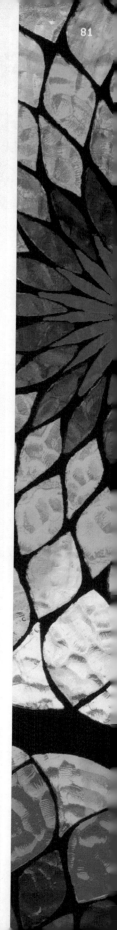

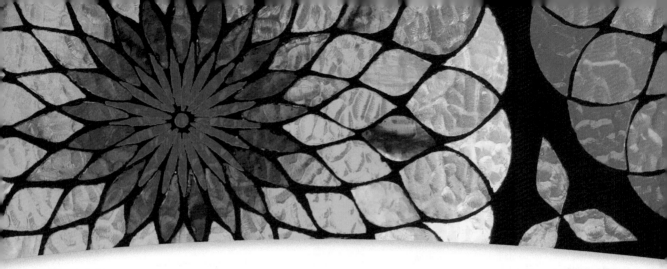

CHAPTER 7

CLINICAL HANDOVER

Tracey Moroney

LEARNING OUTCOMES

Chapter 7 will enable you to:

- [ ] describe the attributes of an effective clinical handover

- [ ] discuss the advantages and disadvantages of the bedside handover process

- [ ] outline potential risks associated with clinical handover practices

- [ ] define some of the mnemonics used to structure a clinical handover.

KEY CONCEPTS

clinical handover | patient rounds | handover protocols | ISBAR

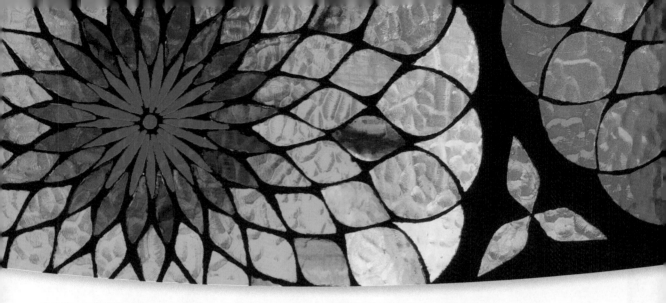

'The quality of a clinical handover directly influences patient safety, especially in the shift that follows.'

(Garling, 2008)

INTRODUCTION

Clinical handover is the 'transfer of professional responsibility and accountability for some or all aspects of care for a patient … to another person or professional group on a temporary or permanent basis' (Australian Medical Association, 2006, p. 8). An accurate clinical handover is important to continuity and safety of care so that healthcare professionals are well informed about the patients in their care at all times. When clinically relevant information is not transferred in an accurate or timely manner, adverse events can occur. There may be delays in patient diagnosis and treatment, inappropriate treatment, omissions in care, or poor care outcomes. This may result in lower satisfaction for healthcare professionals and the people they treat, increased costs, longer lengths of stay for patients and unplanned readmissions (Patterson & Wears, 2010).

Clinical handovers have been found to be time-consuming, inconsistent, and varied in style and format. In addition, many healthcare professionals receive little or no formal training in the handover process. As a consequence of this, clinical handover can be a 'vulnerable process' (Smeulers, Lucas & Vermeulen, 2014) and a high-risk area for patient safety.

Clear communication is the key to ensuring effective clinical handover between a person receiving care, their families and healthcare professionals. It is especially important during high-risk times, such as shift handover, transitions of care or when a person's condition or clinical care changes.

The National Safety and Quality Health Service (NSQHS) Standards (Australian Commission on Safety and Quality Health Care [ACSQHC], 2017) recognise the need for effective communication throughout a person's care journey. Standard 5 *Communicating for Safety* focuses on effective and coordinated communication systems to support continuous and safe care, and emphasises that structured communication processes should be used whenever care is transferred between healthcare professionals or clinical areas.

AN EXAMPLE OF A CLINICAL HANDOVER

Consider the communication interaction below. This exchange was recorded during a handover project conducted between 2007 and 2008 (Iedema et al., 2009). A number of clinical handovers were filmed and the video footage used as a feedback resource so that staff could reflect on the effectiveness of their handover communication practices with a view to improvement. The extract below is a transcript from one of the handovers in an emergency department (ED). DR1 is the night (junior) doctor who presents a handover to the senior day doctor (DR2) about a patient who had been involved in a motor vehicle accident and who he had cared for during the night. DR3 is a registrar.

> DR1: Well he … he … when he came in he was writhing around on the floor. He was just in referred pain. So he had indomethacin and about twenty morphine in five milligrams lots. About twenty morphine in five milligram lots too.
>
> DR2: How long ago did he have the morphine?
>
> DR1: Uh, I'm not sure when his last one was is – it – he took twenty basically straightaway to get him down.
>
> DR2: Uh, what time vaguely?
>
> DR1: Ah, probably about one o'clock would've been.
>
> DR2: So he's been pain free for si …
>
> DR1: Oh, he had fi … he went to sleep then he had five sometime between now and then, um …
>
> DR2: So he's had repeated doses?
>
> DR1: Just one.
>
> DR2: Oh, okay.
>
> DR1: There's not much else to do in terms of that.
>
> DR2: Mm …
>
> DR1: Wait for the CT.
>
> DR2: Is the pain completely gone?
>
> DR1: Yeah. Last we checked, yeah. He is being seen by the urologist, um [who was seeing him] about a month ago [and he knew that there was something bilaterally]. So we'll see what's going on at the moment.
>
> DR3: Is he having indomethacin for this?
>
> DR1: Yes, he has.
>
> DR3: Yeah, yeah right, and that didn't work much and that's why he had a whole lot of morphine.

The transcript shows that the junior doctor (DR1) sounds quite tentative in his responses ('Uh, I'm not sure …'). He is also not specific about the drugs he administered ('he had indomethacin and about twenty morphine in five milligrams lots'). The senior doctor asks, 'So he's had repeated doses', but we are not clear as to which drug this comment applies. The junior doctor's reply to this question is 'Just one'. In the absence of clarification of which drug is at issue, it is unclear whether this means the indomethacin was administered separately and only once, or whether it contradicts the junior doctor's earlier comment about the 'five milligram lots'. Overall, the junior doctor seems vague and confused. In addition, the video showed that those attending the handover did not seem very interested and engaged, and some had even started their own conversations while this part of the handover was unfolding.

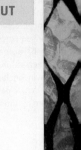

Reflecting on this scenario, there are several issues to be considered, including:

- why the junior doctor did not refer to some handwritten notes while delivering the handover
- why the junior doctor could not remember something as important as the exact details pertaining to the morphine
- the structure underpinning this handover communication.

On being shown this footage, the healthcare professionals in question were very critical of the process in general and of its execution more specifically. One person commented, 'All this is so inefficient!' Another asked the question, 'What are we all doing standing there? By the time we have handed a patient over they will already have moved out of the department!' This question referred to the apparent disjunction between the rapid pace of care in the ED and the comparatively slow pace of the clinical handover. All those who were present reflected that it should be possible to conduct clinical handovers in a better way.

Source: Handover Enabling Learning in Communication for Safety (HELiCS): A report on achievements at two hospital sites. Iedema, R., Merrick, E., Kerridge, R., Herkes, R., Lee, B., Anscombe, M., White, L. (2009). © 2009 Medical Journal of Australia. Reproduced with the permission of Wiley Publishing, Inc.

Effective handover practices

Handover practices are highly variable and differ markedly between institutions, health professional groups and healthcare professionals themselves. However, increasingly, handover is being under-taken in a person-centred way during patient rounds, with patients and their families contributing to decision-making and care-planning processes. In other situations, handover may be held away from patients, in staffrooms or conference rooms for example. While these situations present an opportunity for staff to come together as a team, the shift handover process generally includes only one professional group, such as nurses or doctors. Because of this, a holistic approach is often missing and information handed over is frequently incomplete or inaccurate.

The NSQHS Standard 5 (ACSQHC, 2017) indicates that healthcare professionals should use a structured clinical handover process that includes:

a. preparing and scheduling clinical handover
b. having the relevant information at clinical handover
c. organising relevant clinicians and others to participate in clinical handover
d. being aware of the patient's goal and preferences
e. supporting patients, carers and families to be involved in clinical handover, in accordance with the wishes of the patient
f. ensuring that clinical handover results in the transfer of responsibility and accountability for care.

The Australian Medical Association, in its 'Safe Handover: Safe Patients' document (2006), outlined a number of aspects of effective handover practices, stating that:

Good handover does not happen by chance. It requires work by all those involved, including organisations and individuals, and in some cases a change in culture. To achieve this:

- *shifts must cross-over*
- *adequate dedicated time must be allowed*
- *handover should have clear leadership*
- *adequate information technology support must be provided*
- *support for the handover process must come from all levels of the healthcare team.*

Sufficient and relevant information should be exchanged to ensure patient safety so that:

- *the clinically unstable patients are known to the senior and covering health professional/s*
- *junior members of the team are adequately briefed on concerns from previous shifts*
- *tasks not yet completed are clearly understood by the incoming team.*

For further information and examples that focus on effective and not so effective clinical handover practices (and the consequences of each), access Mark Green's story and Gavin Sinclair's story at <www.ipeforqum.com.au/modules/>.

Handover is of little value unless action is taken as a result and:

- *tasks are prioritised*
- *plans for further care are put into place*
- *unstable patients are reviewed in a timely manner.*

Source: *Australian Medical Association (2006). Safe Handover: Safe Patients, p. 7. Accessed January 2019 at <https://ama.com.au/sites/default/files/documents/Clinical_Handover_0.pdf>.*

Bedside handover

There are various methods and places to communicate information from one healthcare professional to another, but the bedside handover is increasingly recognised as one method to improve the accuracy and quality of communication transferred (Tobiano et al., 2017). More importantly, a bedside handover includes the person receiving care; it has been shown to improve patient care and reduce patient complaints (Whitty et al., 2017). See Figure 7.1 for an overview of the bedside handover process and Box 7.1 for an example of a bedside handover.

FIGURE 7.1
The bedside handover process

Source: Reproduced with permission from *Standard Operating Protocol for Implementing Bedside Handover in Nursing,* developed by the Australian Commission on Safety and Quality in Health Care. ACSQHC: Sydney, 2008.

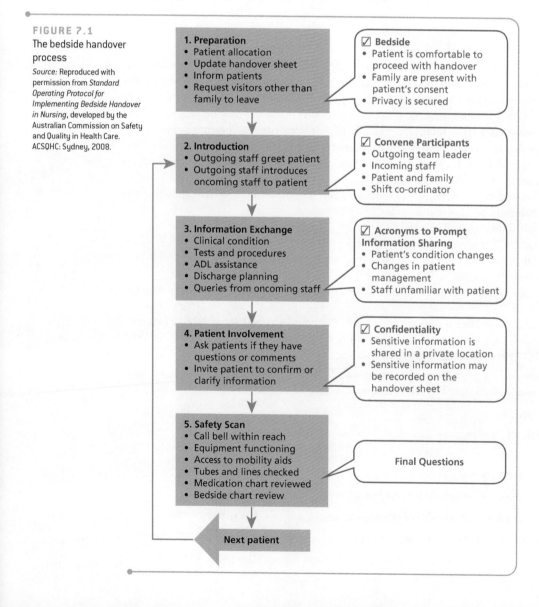

1. Preparation
- Patient allocation
- Update handover sheet
- Inform patients
- Request visitors other than family to leave

☑ **Bedside**
- Patient is comfortable to proceed with handover
- Family are present with patient's consent
- Privacy is secured

2. Introduction
- Outgoing staff greet patient
- Outgoing staff introduces oncoming staff to patient

☑ **Convene Participants**
- Outgoing team leader
- Incoming staff
- Patient and family
- Shift co-ordinator

3. Information Exchange
- Clinical condition
- Tests and procedures
- ADL assistance
- Discharge planning
- Queries from oncoming staff

☑ **Acronyms to Prompt Information Sharing**
- Patient's condition changes
- Changes in patient management
- Staff unfamiliar with patient

4. Patient Involvement
- Ask patients if they have questions or comments
- Invite patient to confirm or clarify information

☑ **Confidentiality**
- Sensitive information is shared in a private location
- Sensitive information may be recorded on the handover sheet

5. Safety Scan
- Call bell within reach
- Equipment functioning
- Access to mobility aids
- Tubes and lines checked
- Medication chart reviewed
- Bedside chart review

Final Questions

Next patient

BOX 7.1	An example of a bedside handover

Preparation	RN Annie is a team leader. She reads the patient's medical record before handover ensuring she is up to date with the medical decisions recorded in the doctors' notes. She checks the bedside chart to ensure everything in the handover is accurate.
	Towards handover time, RN Annie gets the team members together to update the handover sheet. Annie tells the patient that handover will occur shortly, ascertains whether the patient wishes family to be present during the handover and ask non-family members to wait outside for a short while.
	All oncoming staff members are given a handover sheet.
Introduction	'Mr Smith, good afternoon. This is Sylvia, an RN, Cindy an EN and Susan, a nursing assistant. They will be taking care of you in the evening shift.'
Information exchange	RN Annie keeps her voice low but ensures that Mr Smith and the oncoming staff can hear her.
S: Situation	S: Mr Smith came to the ED complaining of chest pain and shortness of breath. He was placed on O_2 via nasal cannula at 2l/min. He is on an antihypertensive, aspirin and a beta blocker (medication record shown to Nurse Sylvia).
B: Background	B: Mr Smith has a history of chest pain over the past two days, which radiated down his left arm. He has prn anginine at home. Over the past 6 months he has had several bouts of chest pain, and has been followed by his GP. Today, prior to being admitted, he developed chest pain but is currently pain free.
A: Assessment	A: This afternoon, his BP = 130/86, Temp = 38.0 and Heart Rate = 76. He is currently pain free.
R: Recommendations	R: Doctor Jones has arranged a cardiac echo for him. He has had an ECG today with no significant changes. Blood tests all attended and are waiting on results.
	RN Sylvia then asks about any treatment for his raised temperature and also questions about mobility. Nurse Annie responses: 'Dr Jones is aware and has asked to be notified if it goes above 38.5.' Mr Smith can mobilise with assistance but only toilet and shower privileges.
Patient involvement	Nurse Annie asks 'Mr Smith, have you been to cardiac echo?' Mr Smith says 'yes'. Nurse Annie then asks, 'Did the doctor say anything to you?' Mr Smith says, 'She said, I may need a cardiac catheter' Nurse Sylvia then asks 'Do you have any questions Mr Smith?' Mr Smith states 'Can you find out if I need the cardiac test?'
Safety scan	EN Cindy undertakes a safety check of the equipment, including checking that the call bell is within reach, the suction and oxygen equipment are functioning.
	RN Sylvia and RN Annie review the bedside chart, checking the following: care plan, observation chart, medication chart, fluid balance chart, and the pressure ulcer assessment. RN Sylvia asks 'Has Mr Smith needed any GTN recently?' RN Annie said 'Oh, I forgot, Mr Smith had chest pain around 9:30 am and took one GTN sublingually. This was relieved within 5 minutes. Yes. I will sign for the med now.'
Handover completed	Nurse Annie said 'Mr Smith, we have finished the handover, do you want to add anything before we leave?' Mr Smith said, 'No, I'll wait to hear about that other heart test.'
Confidentiality	After finishing the handover in the 4 bed room, all staff went out the room in the corridor, nurse Annie said 'I have to hand over some sensitive information related to Mr Smith; he has hepatitis C, so make sure you adhere to universal precautions when undertaking his care.'

Source: Reproduced with permission from *Standard Operating Protocol for Implementing Bedside Handover in Nursing*, developed by the Australian Commission on Safety and Quality in Health Care. ACSQHC: Sydney, 2008.

Engaging people in their care is integral to person-centred practice. Evidence suggests that patients strongly support bedside handover processes because they provide a genuine opportunity for active involvement (Whitty et al., 2017). This partnership is recognised as one method of promoting safe care and has been found to improve the standard of care and documentation by allowing for early visualisation of people and their records, as well as the transfer of accurate and detailed information (Kerr, Lu & McKinlay, 2014). Bedside handover also assists healthcare professionals to ensure clinical activities have been completed and to plan for the forthcoming shift. Importantly, the bedside handover is an opportunity to ask questions and clarify concerns.

However, despite the benefits of bedside handover, it should be acknowledged that there have been some reservations expressed. For example, one study suggested that too many healthcare professions clustered around the beside could be a barrier for engagement with patients and families, or that patients can feel overwhelmed or disempowered, especially when steps are not taken to invite active engagement (Whitty et al., 2017). Additionally, there is sometimes a perception that patients do not want others to hear about their condition or treatment, and issues of confidentially are cited as being a barrier to the bedside handover (Tobiano et al., 2017). Some nurses also believe that patients may feel too disempowered to speak up or that their condition might impact on being involved in the process. Healthcare professions have also expressed concerns that people may be anxious or distressed on hearing about their condition. Further, in some instances there are concerns that the flow of handover might be interrupted by noise, the patient or family members, and that this can increase the time taken for handover (Tobiano et al., 2017).

The success of bedside handover is contingent on people being invited to engage in two-way communication and healthcare professionals using methods that enable people to participate. The human connection (Tobiano et al., 2018), where there is a welcoming atmosphere, genuine interest and attention to building the therapeutic relationship, is critical to handover success.

Several practical steps can be undertaken to promote the participation of patients and to demonstrate an equal partnership. These include maintaining eye contact and sitting down at the bedside rather than standing over the person. Healthcare professionals should introduce themselves and ask the patient how they wish to be addressed. It is important that patients and families know what to expect from the beside handover so it would be helpful to provide information about the process and how they can be involved. Patients and their families should be invited to comment on their care and to clarify any issues related to their condition or treatment. While some may not wish to be involved in handover, they should at least be invited to participate (Manias & Watson, 2014).

Risks associated with clinical handovers

A systematic review by Wong, Yee and Turner (2008) identified some of the high-risk patient handover processes that can result in discontinuity of care, adverse patient outcomes and legal claims of malpractice. They include:

- **Interprofessional handover:** for example, between operating theatre and the post-anaesthesia care (recovery) staff, and between ambulance staff and emergency department staff.

- **Interdepartmental handover:** between emergency department and intensive care staff, and emergency department and ward staff (especially where interdepartmental boundaries/responsibilities are unclear).

- **Shift-to-shift handover:** risks related to the lack of a clear structure, policy or procedures for handover, interruptions, and information overload caused by overly long and detailed handovers.

- **Hospital to community and hospital to residential care handover:** risks related to poor hospital to community discharge processes and incomplete or inaccurate communication, resulting in clinical errors and re-hospitalisations.

- **Providing verbal handover only:** depending on memory causes a loss of information or inaccurate information transfer.
- **The use of non-standard abbreviations:** causing misunderstandings between health professionals.
- **Patient's characteristics:** complex patient problems receive poorer quality handover than more defined patient conditions.

Source: Adapted from Wong, Yee and Turner (2008).

Miscommunication during clinical handover is a major risk and is linked to adverse events, including longer stays, lack of continuity of care, duplication of services and dissatisfaction of both staff and patients (Spooner et al., 2013). The actual content of the clinical handover can be inconsistent and lacking in detail, which has the potential to result in poor clinical decision making. Moreover, the information presented during clinical handover is often subjective without the detail necessary for planning of care.

Despite international and national recommendations for clinical handover, the practice continues to be variable and often differs between clinical settings. The involvement of patients is also inconsistent; one study finding that, out of 532 handovers, only 45 per cent were found to include active involvement of patients (Chaboyer, McMurray & Wallis, 2010). This is despite recommendations that suggest actively involving patients in clinical handover improves participation, and allows for their needs, concerns and preferences to be better understood.

The lack of structure or procedures in clinical handover may result in the transfer of irrelevant or incorrect information; however, support for better structures that are flexible and responsive to person-centred practice are emerging. There are a number of tools and methods for adopting a structured approach to handover and their use has been shown to reduce errors of omission. They also improve the reliability of information being transferred by decreasing the reliance on memory and focusing on the important aspects of care. For example, processes such as ISBAR (Introduction, Situation, Background, Assessment and Recommendations) have provided clearly structured approaches to transfer information (see Figure 7.2).

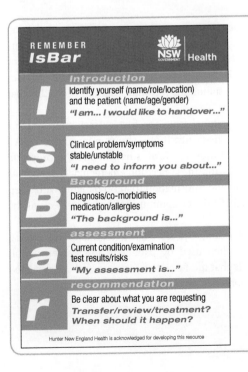

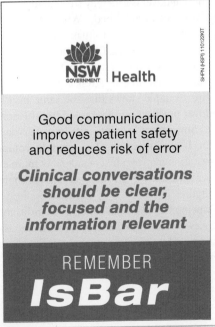

FIGURE 7.2
ISBAR

Source: © New South Wales Ministry of Health for and on behalf of the Crown in right of the State of New South Wales. Hunter New England Health is acknowledged for developing this resource. Reproduced by permission, NSW Health © 2019.

Improving handover practices

Not long after the clinical handover outlined earlier in this chapter occurred, the same junior doctor provided another handover, this time using ISBAR. In this extract, he (DR1) presents a handover to the medical night shift doctor (DR2) and two other doctors (DRs 3 and 4) using ISBAR:

> DR1: Um, she's [the patient being discussed] got disruptive sleep apnoea and asthma. She's on seretide for her asthma. Med reg has reviewed and is going to chat to the cardiologist that she's seen before.
>
> …
>
> Chest pain started at six o'clock this evening. The pain was more like a dull heaviness. Two out of ten. There's no radiation, no associated symptoms. She's had similar pain about six years ago. Had a stress ECG which was normal six years ago. At the moment she's stable, all the bloods are normal. Chest x-ray's normal. We're just waiting for an eight hour which is due at two o'clock in the morning.
>
> DR2: All done?
>
> DR1: Nods.
>
> DR3: Risk factors?
>
> DR4: She's low risk.
>
> DR1: Low risk.
>
> DR4: Just need to get a stress test organised by his GP.
>
> DR3: So if that's normal she can go home. Stress test.
>
> DR4: Huh?
>
> DR3: Stress test?
>
> DR4: Yeah absolutely.
>
> DR1: Nods.

This handover is generally structured according to the ISBAR protocol (patient identification having previously been established). When DR1 states that the patient has 'disruptive sleep apnoea' he sets out the present situation (Situation). The information about the registrar having reviewed the patient provides the background (Background). Then, when DR1 explains the chest pain problem he provides a current assessment (Assessment). Then, instead of DR1 stating his recommendation, DR4 adds that the patient 'needs to get a stress test' (Recommendation).

This example shows that the same healthcare professional from the first extract improved his handover practices and presented information more systematically. It also shows how simple ISBAR is and how easy it is to integrate into everyday practice. However, ISBAR is not the most appropriate approach in all situations. For example, complex patients and those needing emergency care such as resuscitation may require considerably more explanation and information than do patients with sleep apnoea and asthma. In these situations, more detailed handover communication processes will be required.

Mnemonics like IMIST-AMBO (Identification, Mechanism, Injuries, Signs, Treatment and Trends, Allergies, Medications, Background, Other issues) are often used by paramedic-to-emergency staff handover. They are *prescriptive* about the clinical details that are to be handed over and are designed to ensure clear communication across different institutions (Iedema et al., 2012) (see Figure 7.3).

IMIST-AMBO Handover Protocol

FIGURE 7.3
IMIST-AMBO
Source: © Ambulance Service of New South Wales.

IMIST-AMBO covers the standard way paramedics hand over information about patients to ED clinicians

I – **Identification**

M – **Mechanism / Medical complaint**

I – **Injuries / Information related to the complaint**

S – **Signs**

T – **Treatment and Trends**

A – **Allergies**

M – **Medication**

B – **Background history**

O – **Other information**

IMIST-AMBO aligns with the ISBAR mnemonic for handover.

Ambulance paramedics are asked to:

1. Review handover details pre-arrival
2. Maintain a 20-30 second period where the patient remains on the stretcher and deliver IMIST information uninterrupted
3. Encourage questions on completion of IMIST and again at the end of AMBO
4. Treating paramedic to remain with the patient during handover

ED clinicians are asked to:

1. Ensure the handover remains interruption free
2. Ask questions during the two provided opportunities, between IMIST and AMBO and upon completion of IMIST-AMBO
3. Observe 'Hands off, Eyes on', a 20-30 second period provided when the patient stays on the Ambulance trolley until the IMIST information is delivered
4. Identify team leaders

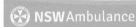 NSW Ambulance   www.archi.net.au/resources/safety/clinical/nsw-handover   NSW Health

Conclusion

Clinical handover is as important as other clinical work, and a critical, pervasive and dynamic part of everyday and ongoing clinical activity. The use of tools to standardise the practice of clinical handover has been shown to reduce miscommunication and adverse events (Spooner et al., 2013). Clinical handover tools such as ISBAR can help healthcare professionals determine what to communicate about their patients. Additionally, the bedside handover is a method of engaging people in their own care and is integral to the practice of person-centred care. This practice improves the accuracy and quality of communication, and provides a genuine opportunity for patient involvement.

Critical thinking activities

1   Reflect on the last clinical handover you witnessed; describe its general features: who spoke to whom, who wrote anything down, and so forth.
2   Can you remember the *structure* of that handover, or was it ad hoc? Would a structured handover format have made it easier for you to understand and remember what was communicated?
3   Did the person who communicated the information to you take account of your background knowledge, experience, and level of responsibility for the tasks that were handed over to you?
4   Reflect on your own handover practices. Do they promote patient safety? Do you use a structured approach? Is there 'room for improvement'?

Teaching and assessment activities

1   Provide an opportunity for students to review a selection of handover tools and, in small groups, critique their applicability to practice.
2   Facilitate a role play of a bedside handover, with students assigned to different roles. After the role play, discuss what was missing, what could be improved and how the handover may have (or not have) impacted safe patient care.

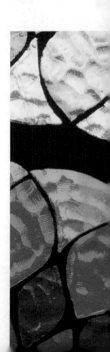

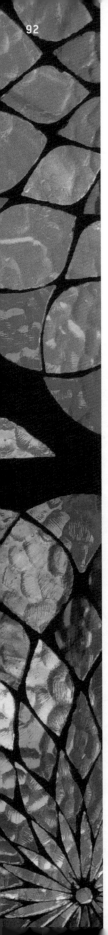

3 At the conclusion of the role play, students can also reflect on how it felt to be the 'person' who was the recipient of care as well as the healthcare professional giving the handover.

4 Integrate an oral communication assessment (e.g. ISBAR) as a component of a clinical skills examination or Objective Structured Clinical Exam (OSCE).

Further reading

Chaboyer, W., McMurray, A., Wallis, M. & Chang, H. Y. (2008). *Standard Operating Protocol for Implementing Bedside Handover in Nursing*, Griffith University, Australia. Accessed December 2018 at: <https://www.safetyandquality.gov.au/wp-content/uploads/2012/02/SOP-Bedside-Handover.pdf>.

Jorm, C., White, S. & Kaneen, T. (2009). Clinical handover: Critical communications. *Medical Journal of Australia, 190*(11), S108–9.

Web resources

Australian Commission on Safety and Quality in Health Care. The OSSIE Guide to Clinical Handover Improvement. <https://www.safetyandquality.gov.au/wp-content/uploads/2012/01/ossie.pdf>

The eHealth Services Research Group. A structured evidence-based literature review regarding effectiveness of improvement interventions in clinical handover. <https://www.safetyandquality.gov.au/wp-content/uploads/2008/01/Clinical-Handover-Literature-Review-for-release.pdf>

References

Australian Commission on Safety and Quality in Health Care. (2017). *National Safety and Quality Health Service Standards* (2nd edn). Sydney, Australia.

Australian Medical Association (2006). Safe Handover: Safe Patients: Guidance on clinical handover for clinicians and managers. Accessed December 2018 at: <https://ama.com.au/sites/default/files/documents/Clinical_Handover_0.pdf>

Chaboyer, W., McMurray, A. & Wallis, M. (2010). Bedside nursing handover: A case study. *International Journal of Nursing Practice, 16*, 27–34.

Garling, P. (2008). Final report to the Special Commission of Inquiry. Acute care services in NSW Public Hospitals. Overview Online. Accessed December 2012 at: <www.lawlink.nsw.gov.au/acsinquiry>.

Iedema, R., Ball, C., Daly, B., Young, J., Green, T., Middleton, P., … Comerford, D. (2012). Design and evaluation of a new ambulance-to-emergency department handover protocol: 'IMIST-AMBO'. *BMJ Quality and Safety, 21*(8), 627–33.

Iedema, R., Merrick, E., Kerridge, R., Herkes, R., Lee, B., Anscombe, M., … White, L. (2009). Handover—Enabling Learning in Communication for Safety (HELiCS): A report on achievements at two hospital sites. *Medical Journal of Australia, 190*(11), S133–6.

Kerr, D., Lu, S. & McKinlay, L. (2014). Towards patient-centred care: Perspectives of nurses and midwives regarding shift-to-shift bedside handover. *International Journal of Nursing Practice, 20*, 250–7.

Manias, E. & Watson, B. (2014). Moving from rhetoric to reality: Patient and family involvement in bedside handover. *International Journal of Nursing Practice, 51*, 1539–41.

Patterson, E. S. & Wears, R. L. (2010). Patient handoffs: Standardized and reliable measurement tools remain elusive. *Joint Commission Journal on Quality & Patient Safety, 36*(2), 52–61.

Smeulers, M., Lucas, C. & Vermeulen, H. (2014). Effectiveness of different nursing handover styles for ensuring continuity of information in hospitalised patients (Review). *Cochrane Database of Systematic Reviews 2014*(6). Article No.: CD009979. doi: 10.1002/14651858.CD009979.pub2.

Spooner, A. J., Chaboyer, W., Corley, A., Hammond, N. & Fraser, J. (2013). Understanding current intensive care unit nursing handover practices. *International Journal of Nursing Practice, 19*, 214–20.

Tobiano, G., Bucknall, T., Sladdin, I., Whitty, J. A. & Chaboyer, W. (2018). Patient participation in nursing bedside handover: A systematic mixed-methods review. *International Journal of Nursing Studies, 77*, 243–58. doi: 10.1016/j.ijnurstu.2017.10.014

Tobiano, G., Whitty, J. A., Bucknall, T. & Chaboyer, W. (2017). Nurses' perceived barriers to bedside handover and their implication for clinical practice. *Worldviews on Evidence-Based Nursing, 14*(5), 343–9. doi: 10.1111/wvn.12241

Whitty, J. A., Spinks, J., Bucknall, T. & Tobiano, G. (2017). Patient and nurse preferences for implementation of bedside handover: Do they agree? Findings for a discrete choice experiment. *Health Expectations: An International Journal of Public Participation in Health Care & Health Policy, 20*(4), 742–50. doi: 10.1111/hex.12513

Wong, M., Yee, K. & Turner, P. (2008). A structured evidence-based literature review regarding effectiveness of improvement interventions in clinical handover. *The eHealth Services Research Group*, University of Tasmania/ACSQHC, Australia. Accessed December 2012 at: <www.achs.health.nsw.gov.au/clHoverLitReview.pdf>.

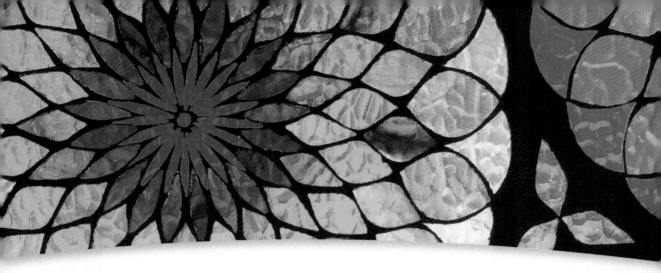

CHAPTER 8

OPEN DISCLOSURE

Rebekkah Middleton

LEARNING OUTCOMES

Chapter 8 will enable you to:

- discuss the background to and imperative for open disclosure

- describe the main elements of the Australian Open Disclosure Framework

- discuss the type of explanation that patients and families require when an error occurs and/or they are harmed while undergoing healthcare

- outline why a sincere apology is a critical component of open disclosure.

KEY CONCEPTS

patient safety incident | open disclosure | apology | Australian Open Disclosure Framework

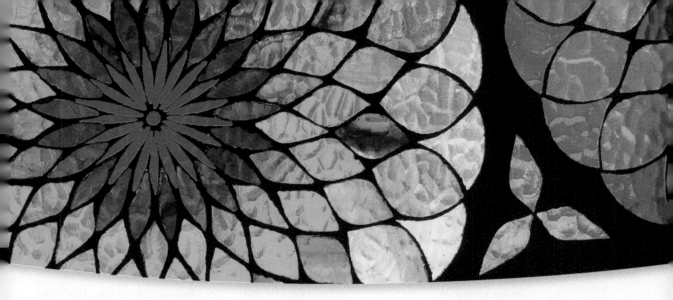

It was just the most powerful thing I've ever seen, this [clinician] saying 'I really don't know what happened. I really can't explain what happened, but it shouldn't have happened, and I have to take the responsibility for that. I was the one that had the responsibility for it.' You could see he was gutted and the family responded to that. This was a human, and their loved one was not well and really nobody knew how things were going to progress. But the patient did wake up, and the relationship that was formed between the patient and her partner and the clinician was really quite phenomenal and they both learnt such a lot from that whole episode.

(Iedema et al., 2008)

INTRODUCTION

This chapter introduces the background to, justification for and critical components of open disclosure in healthcare. 'Open disclosure is a process for ensuring that open, honest, empathic and timely discussions occur between patients and/or their support person(s) and health service professionals following a patient safety incident' (NSW Health, 2014, p. 1). Open disclosure involves healthcare professional(s) providing a person with a factual explanation of what happened and an apology. The person or people who experienced harm should also be provided with time to relate their experience, and a plan for immediate management and prevention of recurrence should be outlined (Australian Commission on Safety and Quality in Health Care [ACSQHC], 2013). This chapter will outline why open disclosure is important and how a clear explanation should be provided to patients and their families following an adverse incident.

Open disclosure—the background and the imperative

Development of the open disclosure policy in Australia began in 2001. This was a time when there were many pressures to improve the quality and safety of healthcare. In part, this pressure resulted from the publication of the Quality in Australian Health Care (QAHC) study in 1995 (Wilson et al., 1995). The QAHC study revealed that between 10 and 16 per cent of acute care episodes resulted in adverse patient outcomes, errors and failures that were directly attributable to the care process. Extrapolating its findings to healthcare services across Australia, the QAHC study estimated that more than 18 000 patients could die or be permanently disabled each year as a result of adverse incidents.

The results of this and other studies resulted in much greater attention being given to improving the quality and safety of healthcare generally. The introduction into Australia of open disclosure was a radical strategy in that it acknowledged the importance of a person's right to error-free healthcare, while at the same time advocating for healthcare professionals to be transparent about service shortcomings and serious about service improvement.

Extensive national consultation occurred in 2002, and in 2003 the Australian Open Disclosure Standard (Australian Council for Safety and Quality in Health Care, 2003) was published. The Council convened a group of clinicians, consumers, policy makers, insurers and lawyers to develop principles to guide healthcare professionals charged with communicating unexpected outcomes to patients. Following a review of the standards in 2012, the Australian Commission on Quality and Safety in Health Care issued an updated Open Disclosure Framework (ACSQHC, 2013).

The Australian Open Disclosure Framework

The Australian Open Disclosure Framework (ACSQHC, 2013) was designed to provide a nationally consistent approach for respectful communication following adverse events in all healthcare settings (see Figure 8.1). The Framework is part of the National Safety and Quality Health Service Standards, 2nd edition (ACSQHC, 2017a). This means that healthcare organisations are formally accredited for their adherence to and performance on incident disclosure, and that healthcare professionals need to be competent in open disclosure communication. The Framework is arguably the most important document regarding open disclosure at a national policy level, with each state and territory incorporating it into its own health and quality policies.

The Framework can be contextualised for rural settings, sub-acute areas, primary and community health, mental health, and smaller and solo practices. It is intended for use in different healthcare settings, including 'pharmacies, clinics, outpatient facilities, hospitals, patients' homes, community settings, practices and clinicians rooms' (ACSQHC, 2013, p. 11).

What type of explanation do patients and families require 'when things go wrong'

Open disclosure discussions occur in response to unplanned or unintended events or circumstances relating to a person's health while in a healthcare environment, whether that environment is acute, community or long-term care. The Australian Open Disclosure Framework (ACSQHC, 2013) outlines eight guiding principles that are directly applicable to acute healthcare settings. The eight principles that need to be considered as part of the open disclosure process are:

- open and timely communication
- acknowledgement
- apology/expression of regret
- support for the person harmed, along with family and carers
- support for healthcare professionals involved
- integration of clinical risk management and systems improvement
- good governance
- confidentiality.

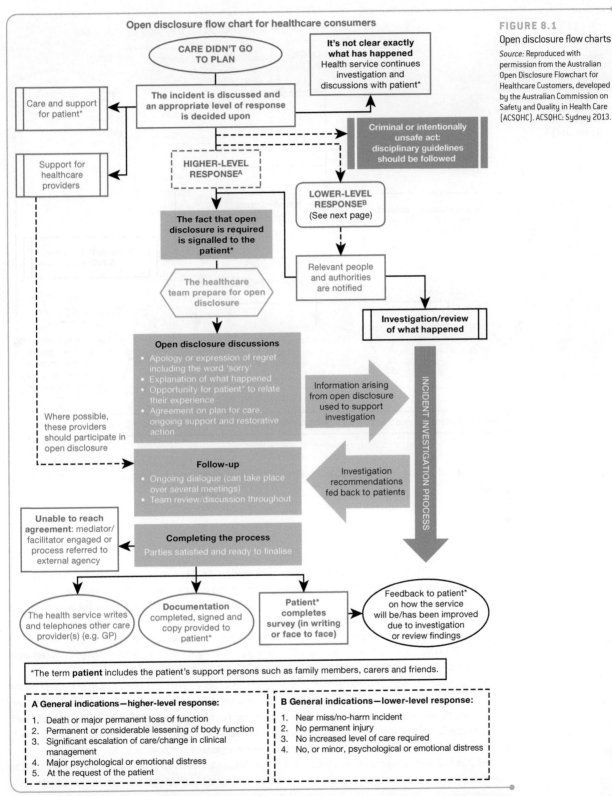

FIGURE 8.1

Open disclosure flow charts

Source: Reproduced with permission from the Australian Open Disclosure Flowchart for Healthcare Customers, developed by the Australian Commission on Safety and Quality in Health Care (ACSQHC). ACSQHC: Sydney 2013.

(Continued)

FIGURE 8.1
Open disclosure flow charts

Source: Reproduced with permission from the Australian Open Disclosure Flowchart for Healthcare Customers, developed by the Australian Commission on Safety and Quality in Health Care (ACSQHC). ACSQHC: Sydney 2013. (Continued)

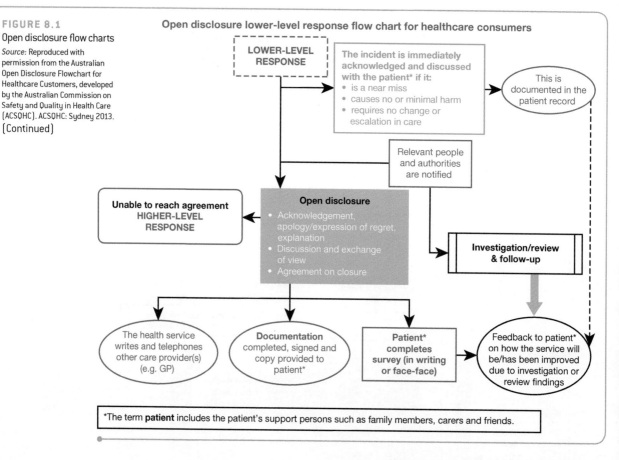

Open disclosure lower-level response flow chart for healthcare consumers

*The term **patient** includes the patient's support persons such as family members, carers and friends.

Consider the story below, as recounted by Ben (pseudonym) and his wife, in light of these guiding principles.

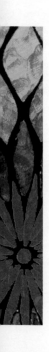

BEN'S STORY

Ben was admitted to hospital for scheduled surgery for bladder cancer. His surgery lasted much longer than expected and he experienced pain in his sides post-operatively. He was diagnosed with compartment syndrome and the following day his legs began to swell. He was taken back to surgery to have 'his legs cut open to reduce the swelling'. After the surgery, Ben lost feeling in his legs and the swelling spread to his whole body. He then developed kidney failure and required dialysis. Ben was put into an induced coma. His right leg, which was the worst affected, was put into a brace. This caused blistering of Ben's right heel. He was transferred to the rehabilitation unit and given 40 cycles or 'dives' of pressurisation inside a hyperbaric chamber.

Ben can no longer walk. The reason for the swelling of Ben's legs was not explained to him or his wife by the healthcare organisation or the healthcare professionals responsible for his care. Ben believes that it may have been caused by his 'length of time on the table', but he still has not been given a clear explanation. That said, both Ben and his wife feel that they were well supported by the hospital. For example, Ben's wife was permitted to help him shower and the required modifications to his house were organised and paid for by the hospital.

Ben has had several meetings with the healthcare professionals involved in his care to try and understand the adverse effects of his surgery. Overall, Ben feels that they have been honest with him. He and his wife both said that they were advised before the surgery of the risks involved. They have also found out that the surgeon has since changed his procedures.

Iedema et al. (2011) conducted research in Australia with 100 people who had been involved in incidents resulting in harm. The results found a number of concerns conveyed by people, including a lack of acknowledgement to the person involved and not providing adequate details of the incident. These issues can be seen in Ben's story above. When people go into hospital their care may be compromised by unexpected outcomes, which can result in other unexpected and undesirable outcomes. In Ben's story, it was clear that he and his wife were concerned that there may have been a problem with the surgery, leading to the swelling of his legs. Equally, the swelling necessitated other treatments, and these treatments either led to further complications or were unsafe or problematic in themselves because Ben is now unable to walk.

Confounding this further, the healthcare professionals delivered a number of inconsistent messages, leaving Ben and his wife confused. For instance, the surgeon later changed a procedure relevant to Ben's care, but no one has explained what this change was, why it was initiated and what this means about the quality and safety of Ben's care before the procedure change. Likewise, the hospital offered to support Ben through rehabilitation, but has thus far not been willing to explain how Ben ended up needing rehabilitation in the first place.

Overall, Ben and his wife were left with several questions about what had happened. They do not know whether the care following on from the surgery served to address complications arising from Ben's inability to recover, or whether it sought to compensate for a less than successful surgery. Ben is left without an accurate understanding of his own body's role in this whole episode, depriving him of knowledge that is critical to enabling him to make decisions about any kind of care he may need in the future.

Explaining potential risks associated with healthcare

When people go into hospital, they expect the treatments they receive to improve their situation. If there are risks related to the procedure or the medications administered, the treatment received can potentially exacerbate a person's condition. Known risks are to be communicated to people before they agree to treatment through a process referred to as 'informed consent'. Informed consent requires clinicians to discuss the various ways in which treatments may or may not produce improvements for the patient. However, informed consent generally targets only a narrowly defined scientific subset of the relevant risks and issues, generally ones deemed relevant by the healthcare professional delivering the information (Hanson & Pitt, 2017). This can mean that the practical or 'mundane' risks inherent in the care that is undertaken in a specific institution are overlooked (Agledahl, Førde & Wifstad, 2011).

These 'mundane risks' are frequently left unaddressed by healthcare professionals because they refer to practices that tend to be 'taken as given', unchangeable and a part of the culture. Typical examples include teamwork undertaken by healthcare professionals who do not know one another, supervisors granting junior clinicians unsafe levels of independence and documentation that is not maintained according to existing procedures.

When things go wrong as a result of such substandard practices, healthcare professionals are now obliged by the National Standards to offer explanations and apologies. That is because open disclosure is an integral part of clinical governance, which falls within the remit of the National Standards (ACSQHC, 2017a).

The open disclosure policy means that people receiving care and their families will expect and deserve a more reasoned, and a more reasonable, explanation—not one that just says, 'This is what we always do' (Agledahl et al., 2011). For example, they will want to know, and need to be told, why the team members did not introduce themselves and work collaboratively (and by so doing, create a risk for the patient), why the supervisor allowed junior clinicians to make dangerous and inappropriate decisions on their own, and why documentation was not maintained properly.

The main issue for patients and families

Below is an excerpt from an interview conducted with the wife of a person who died in hospital. In this part of the interview, she describes how the open disclosure meeting enabled her to explain that the intensive care unit drug overdose was not 'the main issue'. She wanted to convey to the healthcare

For further information and an example of open disclosure related to a medication error, access Young-Min Lee's story (video recording) at <www.ipeforqum.com.au/modules/>.

professionals that it was the failure of the emergency department's registrar and nurse to listen to her, and their dismissal of her concerns about her husband, that started off a cascade of failures and inappropriate actions:

> *The doctor that was in charge of the registrar who made the error said in the meeting that he was very busy. They were all very busy that day which, to me, that's your job, I'm afraid. You are busy. But … he said that he was very busy looking after the registrar who made the error and she was very upset. Well, yes, she should be more than upset. But my problem was that that registrar was going to be alive at the end of the day or at the end of the shift, but my husband wasn't [crying] and they still didn't even tell us that he was dying. And I can't understand why the doctor said that to me, I can't understand that. The drug error isn't the important issue. I thought, well, it's horrible that you have given 20 times the dose, but that's not the important issue. The issue is how is my husband? And that he's either died, or is dying. How come they don't just see that they need to tell you that? Instead, to have somebody come over and say, 'You tell me when you want your husband "turned off".' I still can't comprehend how that happened. We had the meeting here with the patient safety manager and I said to him that there was a conversation missing. He said he was going to come back and tell us. He said, 'Yes, there was a conversation missing, we should have come back and explained the sepsis and explained your husband's condition and that the outcome was not going to be good. Instead, we went from "We've made a drug error" to "You tell me when".' … I still can't fathom how somebody doesn't understand … yes, they deal with death every day, but we don't. We don't. That's my husband who is dying. I just don't get that. And this last meeting, to me, was an opportunity to convey that to the doctor who couldn't see that 20 times the drug error wasn't the main issue and I still don't see how he doesn't understand that.*

This woman further explained that the clinicians kept focusing on fixing an intravenous catheter that was inserted into the patient's arm instead of taking note of the wife's concerns about her husband's breathing and sweating. She was advised to go home that night by the healthcare professionals, even though her husband's condition was deteriorating. He was sent to the intensive care unit but the seriousness of the situation was not communicated to his wife, and when it was recognised that he was dying this was also not communicated to his wife. Instead, a nurse reportedly said, 'Tell me when you want me to turn him off.'

If we consider what open disclosure might mean in a context such as this, we realise that it may not be a situation in which healthcare professionals simply provide technical–clinical information to the people involved. Instead, open disclosure is an opportunity for the person receiving care and/or their relatives to raise questions about the care that was provided, and to challenge healthcare professionals about their version of events and their understandings of what went wrong. Further, open disclosure is an opportunity for healthcare professionals to expand their understanding of what is a healthcare incident and demonstrate that they are capable of improving their methods of working in ways that satisfy those who have been harmed.

How we think about open disclosure depends on whose perspective we take. Do we take the perspective of healthcare professionals and accept their profession-specific and scientifically delineated notions of what constitutes an incident? Or do we take the perspective of the person involved or their family, and acknowledge that culturally encrusted ways of working can generate a sense of 'unsafeness', and that clinicians' cavalier attitudes towards communication can put people they are caring for in danger?

Framed thus, open disclosure becomes much more than a post-incident, fact-provision exercise. Indeed, open disclosure may enable healthcare consumers to directly intervene in the cultures and practices of healthcare. In demanding that open disclosure be conducted as a two-way dialogue, those affected may be able to inject renewed impetus into clinical practice improvement, quality and safety training, and professional codes of conduct to promote transparency and openness.

Conclusion

Open disclosure promotes honesty and transparency. It allows errors to be reduced and the people who have been harmed to be properly cared for (Finlay, Stewart & Parker, 2013). Open disclosure is critical for reassuring patients and families that clinicians fully understand and have comprehensively thought through the care that they provide. It is critical for enhancing patients' and family members' trust in the clinical expertise and professionalism of clinicians.

Research shows that despite legal and ethical mandates, open disclosure does not always happen when it should (Iedema et al., 2008, 2011). Not being offered an apology and being excluded from the process of open disclosure following an adverse event is very difficult for patients and their families, as it ties them up in the process of seeking explanations (see Chapter 4). It also denies them the opportunity to grieve about what has happened and to come to terms with the harm incurred or their loss. Non-disclosure can limit a person's confidence about subsequent healthcare treatment and decisions. It is also reported anecdotally that people are motivated to litigate by a sense that information is being withheld, or that communication has been insufficient or inappropriate after adverse events. Healthcare professionals often perceive potential medico-legal consequences associated with open disclosure. However, open disclosure is not a legal process and there is nominal evidence suggesting either an increase or decrease of medico-legal risk when open disclosure occurs (ACSQHC, 2013).

Finally, it is evident that people are generally more informed about inappropriate care and incidents than healthcare professionals are willing to acknowledge (Iedema et al., 2011). Perhaps then, as healthcare professionals, we should be considering how patients could be more actively involved in incident investigation and practice-improvement processes. This is particularly relevant since *Partnering with Consumers* forms the second of the NSQHS Standards (ACSQHC, 2017b), and it would enhance our capacity as healthcare professionals to share decision making and partner more effectively with healthcare consumers.

Open disclosure is about 'doing the right thing' for everyone involved—not only the person to whom harm occurred and their family, but also healthcare professionals and administrators. When open disclosure occurs, it helps to facilitate the process of restoring trust by all people involved in the health system. Open disclosure has policies and processes to guide communication. When implemented and practised effectively, open disclosure works towards enabling a culture of openness and transparency.

Critical thinking activities

1   Ask your friends and family whether they have ever experienced an adverse incident while undergoing healthcare. If they have, ask them whether the incident was explained to them. If it was, ask how the explanation was given, whether they received an apology, and whether the discussion met their expectations and satisfactorily addressed their concerns. If it was not, ask the person how they felt about being denied an appropriate explanation. Consider what this means to you as a healthcare professional and how you think the situation could have been managed better. Write down key principles you will bring to your practice based on your reflection.

2   Imagine you are a patient in a case where your care does not result in the outcome that was intended and you are denied discussion about why you are not getting better. Describe how you would feel about the situation and about the healthcare professionals caring for you.

3   'Open Disclosure is about "doing the right thing" when a patient has been harmed while receiving healthcare. It enables staff to communicate with empathy—to walk in another's shoes—and to say sorry for what has happened.' (Clinical Excellence Commission, 2014, p. 12)

    What feelings does this statement evoke in you as a healthcare professional? Does it tell you anything about your attitudes to providing open disclosure? What do you need to do in order to practise open disclosure with empathy?

4   Imagine that you made a medication error and you have to tell the person affected. What kind of apology might you use? Answer this question after reading the excerpt in Box 8.1 from the new National Open Disclosure Framework about 'saying sorry'.

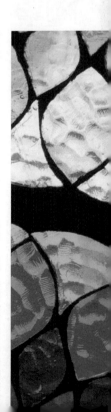

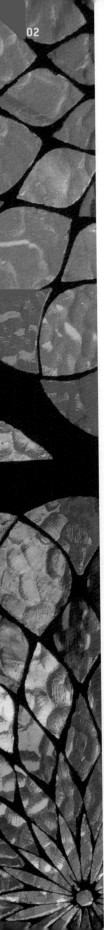

BOX 8.1   Saying sorry

Apology and/or expressions of regret are not only key components of open disclosure but also the most sensitive. 'Saying sorry' must occur with great care. The exact wording and phrasing of an apology (or expression of regret) will vary in each case, but the following points should be taken into consideration:

- The words 'I am sorry' or 'we are sorry' should be included.

- It is preferred that, wherever possible, people directly involved in the adverse event also provide the apology or expression of regret.

- Sincerity is the key element for success. The effectiveness of an apology or expression of regret hinges on the way it is delivered, including the tone of voice, as well as non-verbal communication such as body language, gestures and facial expressions. These skills are often not innate and may need to be practised (refer to Chapter 2). Training in open disclosure is therefore essential to both undergraduate students and practising clinicians.

- The apology or expression of regret should make clear what is regretted or being apologised for, and what is being done to address the situation.

- An apology or expression of regret is essential in helping patients, their families and carers cope with the effects of a traumatic event. It also assists healthcare professionals in their recovery from adverse events in which they are involved.

It is important to note that an apology or expression of regret alone is insufficient and must be backed up by further information and action to ensure effective open disclosure.

Source: Reproduced with permission from the Australian Open Disclosure Framework—Consultation Draft, developed by the Australian Commission on Safety and Quality in Health Care (ACSQHC). ACSQHC: Sydney 2012.

5   The NSQHS Standard 2 *Partnering with Consumers* (ACSQHC, 2017b, p. 14) specifies that healthcare organisations should enable people to be involved in their own healthcare journey to the extent they choose. How do you consider this partnership would influence adverse incidents?

6   In small groups, discuss the type of situation in which you would or would not consider disclosing an incident when no harm has occurred, or there has been a near miss.

Teaching and assessment activities

1   Access and work through the three open disclosure case studies from Victorian Government Health Information, available at: <http://vhimsedu.health.vic.gov.au/opendisclosure/topics/topic3/page1.php> (accessed December 2018).

        As a group, discuss the cases and what you have learned about the importance of open disclosure.

2   Read the Iedema et al. (2011) article, available at: <https://www.bmj.com/content/343/bmj.d4423> (accessed December 2018).

        The authors of this paper concluded that healthcare organisations and providers should strengthen their efforts to meet patients' and family members' needs and expectations. Consider strategies you can use to ensure this occurs in your practice along with the potential challenges to this occurring.

Further reading

Berlinger, N. (2005). *After Harm: Medical Error and the Ethics of Forgiveness*. Baltimore: Johns Hopkins Press.

Truog, R., Browning, D., Johnson, J. & Gallagher, T. (2011). *Talking with Patients and Families about Medical Error: A Guide for Education and Practice*. Baltimore: Johns Hopkins Press.

Web resource

Iedema et al. (2008). The National Open Disclosure Pilot: Evaluation of a policy implementation initiative. <https://www.mja.com.au/journal/2008/188/7/national-open-disclosure-pilot-evaluation-policy-implementation-initiative>

References

Agledahl, K., Førde, R. & Wifstad, A. (2011). Choice is not the issue. The misrepresentation of healthcare in bioethical discourse. *Journal of Medical Ethics, 37*, 212–15.

Australian Commission on Safety and Quality in Health Care. (2017a). *National Safety and Quality Health Service Standards* (2nd edn). Sydney, Australia: ACSQHC.

Australian Commission on Safety and Quality in Health Care. (2017b). Partnering with consumers factsheet. Accessed April 2018 at: <https://www.safetyandquality.gov.au/wp-content/uploads/2017/11/Partnering-with-Consumers.pdf>.

Australian Commission on Safety and Quality in Health Care. (2013). *The Australian Open Disclosure Framework*. Sydney, Australia: ACSQHC.

Australian Council for Safety and Quality in Health Care. (2003). *Open Disclosure Standard: A National Standard for Open Communication in Public and Private Hospitals Following an Adverse Event in Health Care*. Commonwealth of Australia, Canberra.

Clinical Excellence Commission. (2014). *Open Disclosure Handbook*. Sydney: Clinical Excellence Commission. Accessed April 2018 at: <http://www.cec.health.nsw.gov.au/_data/assets/pdf_file/0007/258982/cec_open_disclosure_handbook.pdf>.

Finlay, A. J. F., Stewart, C. L. & Parker, M. (2013). Open disclosure: Ethical, professional and legal obligations, and the way forward for regulation. *Medical Journal of Australia, 198*(8), 445–8. doi: 10.5694/mja12.10734

Hanson, M. & Pitt, D. (2017). Informed consent for surgery: Risk discussion and documentation. *Canadian Journal of Surgery, 60*(1), 69–70. doi: 10.1503/cjs.004816

Iedema, R., Allen, S., Britton, K., Grbich, C., Piper, D., Baker, A. … Gallagher, T. H. (2011). Patients' and family members' views on how clinicians enact and how they should enact incident disclosure: The '100 Patient Stories' qualitative study. *British Medical Journal, 343*, d4423.

Iedema, R., Mallock, N., Sorensen, R., Manias, E., Tuckett, A., Williams, A., … Jorm, C. M. (2008). The National Open Disclosure Pilot: Evaluation of a policy implementation initiative. *Medical Journal of Australia, 188*(2008), 397–400.

NSW Health. (2014). Open disclosure policy, PD2014_028. Sydney, Australia: Ministry of Health. Accessed April 2018 at: <http://www1.health.nsw.gov.au/pds/ActivePDSDocuments/PD2014_028.pdf>.

Wilson, R., Runciman, W., Gibberd, R., Harrison, B., Newby, L. & Hamilton, J. (1995). The Quality in Australian Health Care study. *Medical Journal of Australia, 163*(9), 458–71.

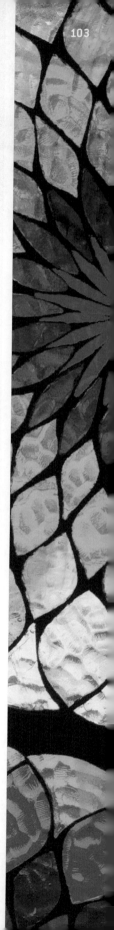

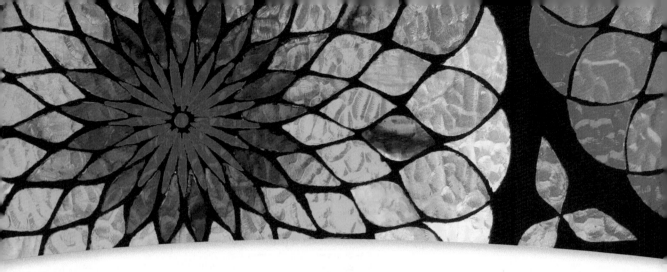

CHAPTER 9

DISCHARGE PLANNING AND CONTINUITY OF CARE

Ashley Kable   Dimity Pond

LEARNING OUTCOMES

Chapter 9 will enable you to:

- discuss the importance of comprehensive and accurate multidisciplinary discharge planning

- outline the risks and benefits associated with discharge planning

- identify strategies that healthcare professionals can use to improve communication associated with continuity of care in the post-discharge period.

KEY CONCEPTS

discharge planning | continuity of care | written communication | electronic communication

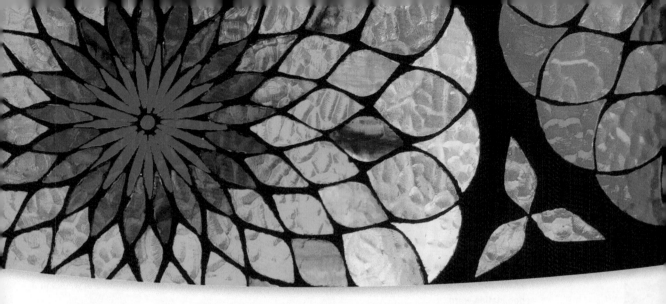

> 'Being discharged from the hospital can be dangerous.'
>
> (AHRQ PSNet, 2017)

INTRODUCTION

When patients are discharged from hospital or transferred from an acute health service to community-based care, they often need additional health services to sustain continuity of care and support their recovery. These services may include rehabilitation and ongoing therapy, medications, specialised clinics, home visits/community nurse support, general practitioner (GP) follow-up, specialist referral or post-discharge consultations. Discharge planning should commence at an early stage of the hospital admission as it may require extensive planning and modification because of the patient's needs and any actual or potential complications that may develop. Unfortunately, when patients are discharged, the plan for their management does not always eventuate as intended.

There are two critical forms of communication that occur at the time of discharge: the information provided to the patient, and the information provided to healthcare professionals who will deliver ongoing care. When the former fails, patients are often confused about what they are required to do, have inadequate mechanisms to access additional information or to clarify details and, sometimes, find that their needs have not been adequately considered (e.g. transport, co-morbid conditions, disability, carer arrangements). Consequently, they can experience significant delays in the provision of further healthcare. When the latter fails, healthcare professionals who are intended to provide continuing care may not receive the information they need or may receive inadequate information. Additionally, they may not be aware of the importance of scheduling/prioritising appointments to suit the person's needs, make adequate provision for the individual needs of the patient and recognise that the patient is inadequately informed. These types of communication breakdown impact on patient safety and result in a failure in continuity of care, sometimes described as 'falling between the cracks'.

If discharge planning and the provision of post-discharge care fail, recovery may be delayed, complications may ensue and readmission to hospital is likely. This affects both the patient and the patient's caregivers, who frequently assume de facto responsibility for coordinating

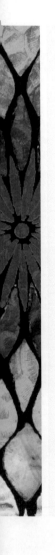

post-discharge management, following treatment plans and instructions, and monitoring for potential indications of developing complications. The impact can include stress, depression and anxiety, which further complicate the post-discharge experience and can impede healing (Broadbent et al., 2003; Gouin & Kiecolt-Glaser, 2011). 'Safe patient transitions depend on effective communication and a functioning care coordination process' (Johnson et al., 2012, p. i98).

JOANNE'S STORY

Joanne, a woman in her mid-50s, suffered a fractured femur as a result of falling at a bowling alley. The fracture was stabilised with a femoral nail and five screws, and she was hospitalised for several weeks in a rehabilitation ward.

Prior to Joanne's discharge, she had a home assessment by the occupational therapist to determine how she would manage at home. She had been working with the physiotherapist on her mobility but had not made as much progress as they had hoped due to continuing pain, and she required additional rehabilitation following discharge. Post-discharge appointments were arranged for Joanne to attend physiotherapy and for follow-up with her surgeon. Prior to discharge, she experienced urinary frequency and urgency; mid-stream urinalysis results were documented as 'pending' on the discharge summary. Joanne was discharged home on crutches in the care of her elderly parents who moved in with her temporarily. Joanne lived in a second-storey unit with an internal staircase.

At the time of her discharge, Joanne's mobility was poor and she was quite unstable on crutches. She was provided with analgesic medications sufficient for two days but she was still suffering significant pain in her leg and it was very swollen. Joanne's urinary tract infection presented significant challenges as a result of her compromised mobility and she was having a number of 'accidents' on the way to the toilet. She needed a prescription for antibiotics and further analgesic medications; however, she had not been advised that it would be necessary to follow up with the general practitioner (GP) about these issues immediately after discharge. The day after her discharge, Joanne phoned for an appointment with her GP and the receptionist added her to a very full appointment schedule. She negotiated the stairs at home on her bottom and her parents drove her to the appointment. She had to wait for approximately two hours, during which time Joanne described her pain as 'excruciating'.

When the GP saw Joanne, she was in significant pain and distress. He observed that her leg was very swollen and painful, and her mobility was quite poor. He arranged for a Doppler scan to be conducted and this detected a very large deep vein thrombosis (DVT) in her leg. Joanne was sent to the emergency department for further assessment. Although she was not readmitted at this time, she did require treatment for the DVT, her urinary tract infection and the unremitting pain. Joanne's recovery was slow and difficult, and she was unable to return to work for six months. She also remained on opioids for pain relief for a number of months.

In Joanne's story there were several failures of communication. Although the discharge team conducted a home visit, Joanne's mobility in hospital as well as her pain levels should have been thoroughly assessed and planned for prior to discharge. Joanne's symptoms of urinary frequency and urgency compounded by her mobility problems posed a significant risk of falls. The management plan should have been developed in consultation with Joanne and then clearly communicated to the healthcare professionals involved in her ongoing care. Joanne should also have had a clear explanation that she would be discharged with a two-day supply of pain medications, and that she would need to see the GP for prescriptions within 24 hours. This is vital, as GPs appointments are often difficult to organise at short notice. Indeed, the appointment would have been better made by the nursing staff prior to her discharge.

Furthermore, a contact number for someone from the hospital or community services to provide advice or assistance if necessary might have saved Joanne a good deal of discomfort and distress. A comprehensive discharge summary would have provided valuable information for the healthcare professionals who provided post-discharge services, particularly if it had been sent electronically at the time of her discharge so there was no delay in the provision of this information.

A full discharge assessment of Joanne would have uncovered the following issues that should have been documented on the discharge summary:

- poor mobility and instability on crutches
- limited ability to perform activities of daily living
- significant pain on mobilisation despite opioid medication
- significant swelling of the leg
- symptoms of urinary frequency and urgency that, because of her poor mobility, placed her at significant risk of falls
- living in a small home unit with stairs
- the ability of Joanne's elderly parents to care for her.

Professionals who were or could have been involved in Joanne's discharge planning include:

- a physiotherapist to provide advice about how to improve stability during mobilisation or how to maximise safety during activities requiring mobility, such as walking on crutches or stair climbing
- an occupational therapist to make recommendations about the need to install rails in the bathroom and modified strategies for negotiating internal stairs when Joanne had to attend appointments
- nursing staff to explore Joanne's symptoms of urinary frequency and urgency, and make appropriate recommendations regarding follow-up treatment
- a medical officer to review Joanne's pain, leg swelling and DVT; additionally, the MSU results and drug sensitivities should have been reviewed and correct antibiotics prescribed
- a social worker to assess Joanne's need for home care
- a community pharmacist to review Joanne's need for further medication
- a discharge planner to coordinate the above healthcare professionals, to ensure the development of an appropriate plan of care and to make appropriate referrals for post-discharge services so that Joanne did not experience unnecessary delays
- possibly a variety of community services, including home and community care services to assist with personal care, home care and transport, and so on.

Discharge documentation

In Joanne's situation, a comprehensive discharge summary would have provided documentation and information about her surgery, and an up-to-date list of medications, including strength, dose and when last administered. The summary should have specified the issues that the GP might need to follow up on, such as pain assessment and MSU results. A copy of the most recent pathology tests taken prior to discharge would have also been helpful.

Discharge summaries can be provided in several ways. It may be that the patient is given a paper copy of the summary with instruction to give it to their GP. This requires the patient to remember to take it to their next appointment. Alternatively, the summary can be faxed or emailed to the GP using a secure email system. Community pharmacists may also need to receive the discharge medication list.

The risks and benefits associated with discharge planning

When discharge planning fails, there may be serious consequences for the patient. Post-discharge complications may be as high as 63 per cent (Kable, Gibberd, & Spigelman, 2004) and adverse events have been reported to be nearly 20 per cent (Forster et al., 2003). In a study of over 11 million patients, inadequate discharge planning was identified as a primary reason for 20 per cent of readmissions (Jencks, Williams & Coleman, 2011). Increased risks associated with early discharge include pending test results at the time of discharge (reported to be 40% in a study of 2644 discharged patients) (Roy et al., 2005); and unresolved medical issues including diagnostic workups, referrals and laboratory tests (reported to be 28% in a study of 693 discharged patients) (Moore, McGinn & Halm, 2007).

Further, patients' understanding of the information provided to them at the time of discharge is often inadequate. A recent study that interviewed 305 older veterans discharged from the ED reported that 50 per cent did not understand their expected course of illness, 43 per cent did not understand their contingency plan and 25 per cent did not understand how soon they should follow up with their primary care provider (Hastings et al., 2012). Additionally, some patients think that medical records are shared across systems and thus may not volunteer information to the healthcare providers they see following discharge (Flink et al., 2012).

A review of 73 studies about communication and information transfer between hospital-based and community-based doctors identified some major deficits in these processes. Direct communication between these doctors was infrequent (3–20%) and the availability of a discharge summary at the first post-discharge visit was only 12–34 per cent. These factors affected the quality of care in approximately 25 per cent of follow-up visits (Kripalani, Jackson et al., 2007). In addition, the quality of documentation on discharge summaries is often poor, including missing test results (33–63%), inadequate treatment or hospital course (7–22%), missing discharge medications (2–40%), test results still pending at discharge (65%), inadequate patient or family education (90–92%) and inadequate follow-up plans (2–43%) (Kripalani, LeFevre et al., 2007). This is consistent with the results of another study of 1501 discharge documents, where 30 per cent were incomplete, 47 per cent mentioned pending test results and only 11 per cent included post-discharge management and follow-up plans (Gandara et al., 2009). Inadequate discharge communication can result in misinformation, duplication of tests or interventions, poor continuity of care and patient harm (Groene et al., 2012). Conversely, a systematic review of 18 studies reported that discharge planning and increased continuity of care are associated with improved patient outcomes and satisfaction (van Walraven et al., 2010).

Traditionally, there has been an expectation that GPs should take the lead in ensuring continuity of care (Flink et al., 2012; Gobel et al., 2012; Groene et al., 2012; Hesselink et al., 2012; Philibert & Barach, 2012); however, this may be an unreasonable expectation because the patient may not see the same GP, particularly in large practices. In some practice settings, this role is adopted by advanced practice nurses (Moore, 2012).

A recent consultation report from the Australian Commission on Safety and Quality in Health Care (ACSQHC) has identified multiple safety issues occurring during transitions in care (ACSQHC, 2017b). These include:

- poorly defined models of person-centred care
- poorly defined responsibility and accountability for communication at transitions of care
- inadequate engagement of patients in care planning and communication
- limited access to complete and current health and social information
- limited opportunities for medication reconciliation
- inadequate discharge planning (pp. 9–10).

The report emphasised the need for team-based communication and a particular focus on high-risk patient groups. It specifically identified that discharge communication is 'often left to the most junior member of the team' (p. 7) and that there are inadequate processes for acknowledging handover of responsibility regarding investigations where results are not available prior to discharge (ACSQHC, 2017b). The report also recognised that the quality of information in discharge summaries is often variable and information may be missing, inconsistent, poorly presented or irrelevant; and that the health and social needs of patients may not be described at discharge. Furthermore, discharge summaries frequently omit critical information about medication changes during hospitalisation, as well as current medications at discharge. It is important to remember that the discharge summary is the key communication mechanism for the primary health team to use after a patient is discharged from hospital.

Strategies that support discharge planning and enhance continuity of care

The following strategies can be used to make sure the discharge of a patient from one health-care context to another goes smoothly and is comprehensive. These strategies can contribute to improved continuity of care, timely provision of post-discharge services, improved communication with patients and healthcare professionals, and reductions in readmissions and the development of complications.

- Discharge planning meetings should be conducted to make sure that the patient's needs are adequately addressed following discharge. These planning meetings should be attended by key healthcare professionals involved in the patient's care (Gobel et al., 2012). Patients and family members should also be involved in discharge planning and their individual needs should be taken into consideration (Flink et al., 2012; Hesselink et al., 2012; Philibert & Barach, 2012). Shared decision making is considered to be the most useful approach to discharge planning, as it facilitates a person-centred approach (Hesselink et al., 2012; Moore, 2012). It is also recommended that the roles of clinicians who are responsible for communication at the time of discharge should be defined (ACSQHC, 2017b).

- Discharge documents provided to the patient should include clear and specific written instructions about continuation of treatment after discharge. They should include contact information for the relevant services and healthcare professionals, and the frequency and location of ongoing treatments and therapies. Medications should be listed accurately, with specific details about dosage and times they should be taken. Instructions about medications should be consistent with those of the written prescription. All information should be clear and consistent, and in a form that patients can understand, taking into account their level of health literacy (see Chapter 2), understanding of the English language, reading level and any sensory loss (e.g. impaired eyesight).

- Post-discharge referrals are frequently required and follow-up appointments may be made with the surgeon, other specialists or the GP. If the patient needs appointments within a few days of discharge, it is important that they are organised prior to discharge.

- Early discharge programs are common in acute healthcare services, and if complications (such as pain) occur, they are more likely to develop after discharge. Undiagnosed problems, such as infection or DVT, increase the potential for readmission. Education prior to discharge helps patients to recognise symptoms that may indicate potential complications, what they should do and who they should contact.

Seven strategies have been identified by Coleman (2011) to ensure continuity of care and patient safety following discharge. These include:

1 Fostering increased engagement of patients
2 Elevating the status of family caregivers as essential members of the care team
3 Implementing performance measurement
4 Defining accountability during transitions

5   Building professional competency in care coordination

6   Exploring technological solutions to improve cross-setting communication

7   Aligning financial incentives to promote cross-setting collaboration.

Coleman et al. (2005) has also developed the 15-item Care Transitions Measure® (The CTM-15®) for patients to rate their continuity of care experiences (see the tool at <https://caretransitions.org/wp-content/uploads/2015/08/CTM-15.pdf>); it is being used in a study by the World Health Organization.

Some issues require particular attention by healthcare professionals when discharging patients. For example, when patients are discharged immediately prior to the weekend, adequate planning is needed to ensure that their needs will be met over the weekend and until they can attend appointments and access further support.

Some elderly people have hearing or sight impairment, limited mobility, reduced capacity to manage activities of daily living and social isolation. They may also have complicated medical treatments, particularly polypharmacy, and require strategies to cope effectively with these challenges. Well-maintained hearing aids, current prescription glasses, documents in large type, provision of home care services and Webster packs are all examples of strategies that can support these needs effectively. Unrecognised cognitive impairment may also be an issue at the time of discharge for some older people and this requires a comprehensive assessment. Older people with pre-existing cognitive impairment may develop delirium in hospital and are at significant risk if discharged home without support. (Refer to Chapter 12 for further information about communicating with older people.)

Some patients may be particularly vulnerable due to language difficulties or limited social resources (Groene et al., 2012). When vulnerable patients are expected to assume an active role in transferring information between healthcare providers, or following and coordinating treatment plans independently, they may be at particularly high risk for having an unsatisfactory or inadequate transition between acute and primary care services.

Some patients may have cultural issues and/or literacy difficulties that should also be recognised and responded to appropriately. This requires awareness and sensitivity from healthcare professionals to make sure that the patient and their family are provided with appropriate advice and support.

Medications can be a particular challenge. When patients are discharged with their new medications as well as the medications they were prescribed prior to hospitalisation, they need clear discharge instructions. The recent consultation report about Safety Issues at Transitions of Care (ACSQHC, 2017b), recognised inadequate medication reconciliation as a major patient safety risk because patients, families and carers can be confused about which medications have been stopped, changed or continued while they were in hospital. This presents a risk for patients missing or duplicating medicines, or taking medicines inappropriately. The National Safety and Quality Health Service (NSQHS) Standards (2nd edn), include a Medication Safety Standard that requires health service organisations to establish processes to provide patients with a current medicines list and the reasons for any changes on discharge (ACSQHC, 2017a). In addition, some patients may routinely take complementary and alternative medicines and other over-the-counter preparations that may be contraindicated or may reduce the therapeutic action of their prescribed medications. A medication reconciliation may be recommended prior to or following discharge to determine whether patients understand their medication requirements and routines (Groene et al., 2012). This can be undertaken by a medical officer or a pharmacist.

Finally, it is important to listen to patients' concerns, problems, needs and preferences; and to determine whether a patient feels prepared for discharge (Hesselink et al., 2012; Moore, 2012). Frequently, patients can trigger clinical questions that can assist healthcare professionals to identify potential problems, and prevent post-discharge complications, deterioration and readmission to hospital.

Conclusion

At the time of discharge, healthcare professionals have a responsibility to ensure that adequate communication and collaboration has occurred with both the patient and the post-discharge service providers. If this is done from a person-centred perspective and with thoughtful consideration of the issues the patient may encounter following discharge, continuity of care is likely to ensue. This approach also minimises risks associated with early discharge programs and promotes patient safety. Healthcare professionals who address these issues will improve the experience of transition from one health service to another and significantly reduce the anxiety and uncertainty that patients commonly experience when they are discharged.

Critical thinking activities

Oliver (a thin, 60-year-old man who lived alone) had a small bowel resection and spent five days in hospital, during which he had an uncomplicated recovery. He was involved in the discharge planning process and provided with appointments for a dietician and post-operative assessment with his surgeon at six weeks. He was given some medications to manage minor pain and advised that there was no need to have the sutures in his wound removed. He went home in good spirits with printed discharge instructions. Four days later he noticed that his wound was becoming painful, swollen and red around the suture line. He started to feel quite nauseated and thought he had 'a bit of a temperature'. The pain medications did not seem to be very effective so he went to bed to try and 'sleep it off'. When he woke hours later, he said he 'felt pretty crook'.

1   What types of potential complications is a patient such as Oliver at risk of, following discharge?
2   On discharge, what advice should Oliver have been given about potential post-operative wound complications?
3   If you were one of the healthcare professionals involved in Oliver's discharge, who would you have advised him to contact should he have concerns about his recovery?

Teaching and assessment activities

The following patient story can be used for classroom discussion or as a stimulus for an assignment.

Mrs Andrews, aged 72, has been discharged from hospital following an operation to repair a fractured neck of femur and requires six weeks in rehabilitation. She is the only carer for her husband, aged 84, who has Parkinson's disease with dementia, and he was admitted at the same time as her because he could not care for himself. Mrs Andrews sustained the fracture while attempting to prevent her husband from falling. Mr Andrews is a fiercely independent man who has rejected home care of any sort in the past. Mrs Andrews is not allowed to drive for a further 6 weeks after discharge.

1   Describe the potential factors that put Mrs Andrews at risk (e.g. social issues, self-care issues, health literacy, communication deficits/difficulties [including being from a culturally and linguistically diverse or non-English-speaking background], medications that require monitoring, cognitive/developmental/residual disability/impairment, carer needs, mental health problems, rural/remote locations, and chronic and complex needs).
2   Identify the members of the primary healthcare team and other relevant people/healthcare professionals who may require information about Mrs Andrews at the time of discharge, as well as the type of information they will need to support her adequately after discharge.
3   Develop a list of strategies that should be adopted by the healthcare team to minimise the risk of discontinuity of care and poor outcomes after discharge.
4   Consider the organisational and system deficits that may present barriers to achieving the list of strategies you have developed.
    For more information about these issues, read the article by Kable, A., Chenoweth, L., Pond, D. & Hullick, C. (2015). Health professional perspectives on systems failures in transitional care for patients with dementia and their carers: A qualitative descriptive study. *BMC Health Services Research*. 15:567.

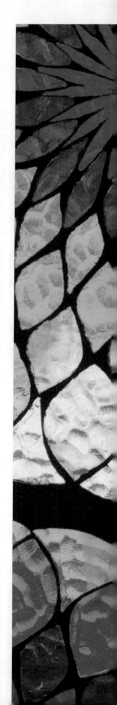

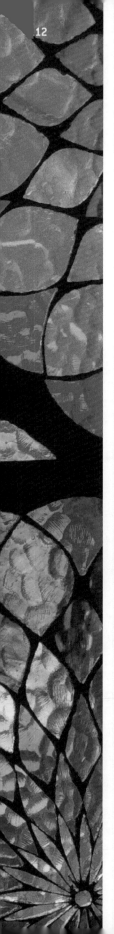

Further reading

Chenoweth, L., Kable, A., Pond, D. (2015). Research in hospital discharge procedures addresses gaps in care continuity in the community, but leaves gaping holes for people with dementia: A review of the literature. *Australasian Journal on Ageing*, *34*(1), 9–14.

Coleman, E. (2011). What will it take to ensure high quality transitional care? Accessed May 2018 at: <https://search.proquest.com/docview/905649636?pq-origsite=gscholar>.

Kable, A., Pond, D., Baker, A., Turner, A. & Levi, C. (2018). An evaluation of discharge documentation after hospitalization for stroke patients discharged home in Australia: A cross sectional pilot study. *Nursing and Health Sciences*, *20*(1), 24–30.

Kable, A., Pond, D., Hullick, C., Chenoweth, L., Duggan, A., Attia, J. & Oldmeadow, C. (2017). An evaluation of discharge documentation for people with dementia discharged home from hospital—A cross sectional pilot study. *Dementia: The International Journal of Social Research and Practice*, 1–13.

van Walraven, C., Oake, N., Jennings, A. & Forster, A. (2010). The association between continuity of care and outcomes: A systematic and critical review. *Journal of Evaluation in Clinical Practice*, *16*, 947–56.

Web resources

UpToDate is an evidence-based, clinical decision support resource that healthcare professionals can use to inform their point-of-care decisions.
<https://www.uptodate.com/contents/hospital-discharge-and-readmission>

Safety Issues at Transitions of Care: This document presents a summary of the outcomes of consultations undertaken by the ACSQHC (2017b) on safety issues and 'pain points' relating to clinical information systems at transitions of care. It is accompanied by a summary of the literature.
<https://www.safetyandquality.gov.au/wp-content/uploads/2018/03/Safety-issues-at-transitions-of-care-consultation-report.pdf>

References

AHRQ PSNet. (2017). Readmissions and adverse events after hospital discharge. *Patient Safety Primers.* Accessed December 2018 at: <https://psnet.ahrq.gov/primers/primer/11/readmissions-and-adverse-events-after-discharge>.

Australian Commission on Safety and Quality in Health Care. (2017a). *National Safety and Quality Health Service Standards* (2nd edn). Sydney, Australia: ACSQHC.

Australian Commission on Safety and Quality in Health Care. (2017b). *Safety Issues at Transitions of Care*. Sydney, Australia: ACSQHC.

Broadbent, E., Petrie, K., Alley, P. & Booth, R. (2003). Psychological stress impairs early wound repair following surgery. *Psychosomatic Medicine*, *65*, 865–9.

Coleman, E. (2011). What will it take to ensure high quality transitional care? *Patient Education and Counseling.*

Coleman, E. A., Mahoney, E. & Parry, C. (2005). Assessing the quality of preparation for posthospital care from the patient's perspective: The care transitions measure. [Comparative Study Research Support, Non-U.S. Gov't, Research Support, U.S. Gov't, P.H.S.]. *Medical Care*, *43*(3), 246–55.

Flink, M., Ohlen, G., Hansagi, H., Barach, P. & Olsson, M. (2012). Beliefs and experiences can influence patient participation in handover between primary and secondary care: A qualitative study of patient perspectives. *BMJ Quality and Safety*, *21*, i76–i83.

Forster, A., Murff, H., Peterson, J., Gandhi, T. & Bates, D. (2003). The incidence and severity of adverse events affecting patients after discharge from the hospital. *Annals of Internal Medicine*, *138*, 161–7.

Gandara, E., Moniz, T., Ungar, J., Lee, J., Chan-Mcrae, M., O'Malley, T. & Schnipper, J. (2009). Communication and information deficits in patients discharged to rehabilitation facilities: An evaluation of five acute care hospitals. *Journal of Hospital Medicine*, *4*(8), E28–E33.

Gobel, B., Zwart, D., Hesselink, G., Pijnenborg, L., Barach, P., Kalkman, C. & Johnson, J. (2012). Stakeholder perspectives on handovers between hospital staff and general practitioners: An evaluation through the microsystems lens. *BMJ Quality and Safety*, *21*, i106–i113.

Gouin, J., & Kiecolt-Glaser, J. (2011). The impact of psychological stress on wound healing: Methods and mechanisms. *Immunol Allergy Clin N Am*, *31*, 81–93.

Groene, R., Orrego, C., Sunol, R., Barach, P. & Groene, O. (2012). 'Its like two worlds apart': An analysis of vulnerable patient handover practices at discharge from hospital. *BMJ Quality and Safety*, *21*, i67–i75.

Hastings, S., Stechuchak, K., Oddone, E., Weinberger, M., Tucker, D., Knaack, W. & Schmader, K. (2012). Older veterans and emergency department discharge information. *BMJ Quality and Safety*, *21*, 835–42.

Hesselink, G., Flink, M., Olsson, M., Barach, P., Dudzik-Urbaniak, E., Orrego, C., ... Wollersheim, H. (2012). Are patients discharged with care? A qualitative study of perceptions and experiences of patients, family members and care providers. *BMJ Quality and Safety*, *21*, i39–i49.

Jencks, S., Williams, M. & Coleman, E. (2011). Rehospitalizations among patients in the Medicare fee-for-service program. *New England Journal of Medicine*, *360*(14), 1418–28.

Johnson, J., Farnan, J., Barach, P., Hesselink, G., Wollersheim, H., Pijnenborg, L., ... Arora, V. (2012). Searching for the missing pieces between the hospital and primary care: Mapping the patient process during care transitions. *BMJ Quality and Safety*, *21*, i97–i105.

Kable, A., Gibberd, R. & Spigelman, A. (2004). Complications after discharge for surgical patients. *ANZ Journal of Surgery*, *74*, 92–7.

Kripalani, S., Jackson, A., Schnipper, J. & Coleman, E. (2007). Promoting effective transitions of care at hospital discharge: A review of key issues for hospitalists. *Journal of Hospital Medicine*, *2*(5), 314–23.

Kripalani, S., LeFevre, F., Phillips, C., Williams, M., Basaviah, P. & Baker, D. (2007). Deficits in communication and information transfer between hospital-based and primary care physicians. *Journal of American Medical Association*, *297*(8), 831–41.

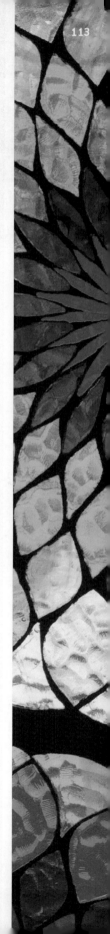

Moore, C., McGinn, T. & Halm, E. (2007). Tying up loose ends: Discharging patients with unresolved medical issues. *Archives of Internal Medicine, 167*(12), 1305–11.

Moore, S. M. (2012). The European HANDOVER project: The role of nursing. *BMJ Quality and Safety, 21*, i6–i8.

Philibert, I. & Barach, P. (2012). The European HANDOVER project: A multi-nation program to improve transitions at the primary care-inpatient interface. *BMJ Quality and Safety, 21*, i1–i6.

Roy, C., Poon, E., Karson, A., Ladak-Merchant, Z., Johnson, R., Maviglia, S. & Gandhi, T. (2005). Patient safety concerns arising from test resullts that return after hospital discharge. *Annals of Internal Medicine, 143*(2), 121–8.

van Walraven, C., Oake, N., Jennings, A. & Forster, A. (2010). The association between continuity of care and outcomes: A systematic and critical review. *Journal of Evaluation in Clinical Practice, 16*, 947–56.

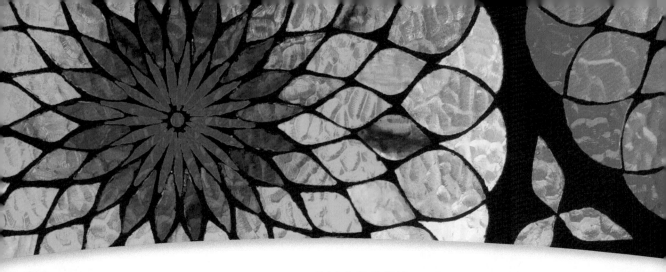

COMMUNICATING TO PROMOTE MEDICATION SAFETY

Elizabeth Manias

LEARNING OUTCOMES

Chapter 10 will enable you to:

- identify the relationship between medication safety and communication
- consider how communication is affected by the stages of the medication management process
- discuss attributes of actual communication encounters that occur in medication management
- identify model cases of medication communication encounters between healthcare professionals, patients and family members.

KEY CONCEPTS

stages of medication management | medication incidents | adverse drug reactions | medication safety

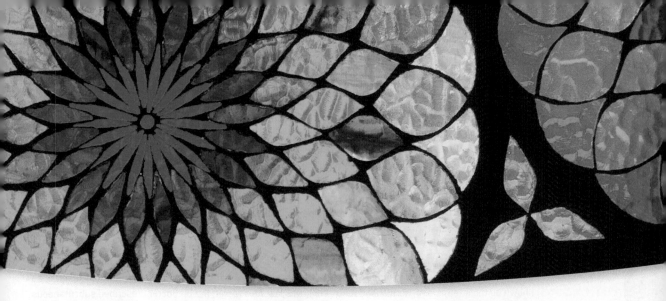

Words are, of course, the most powerful drug used by mankind.

(Rudyard Kipling)

INTRODUCTION

Medication incidents are very common in healthcare. Overall, between 2 per cent and 3 per cent of all hospital admissions result from medication incidents, which translate into over 230 000 hospital admissions in Australia each year (Roughead, Semple & Rosenfeld, 2013). While medication incidents within hospitals vary enormously due to the reporting methods used, in Australia between 1.6 and 5.8 medication prescribing errors occur per patient and between 1.0 and 2.5 medication administration errors occur per patient (Roughead, Semple & Rosenfeld, 2016). Furthermore, consistently high medication incident rates occur during transfer of care between hospital and community settings. Medication incidents can occur during the prescribing or ordering of medications, when medications are supplied to the practice setting from the pharmacy department; during patients' admission to and discharge from hospital; and when information is conveyed between healthcare professionals, patients and family members about how the medications are managed. Unsafe care is costly. Globally, the cost of medication incidents is estimated to be approximately US$42 billion annually (World Health Organization, 2017).

Medication incidents are particularly related to ineffective communication among healthcare professionals (such as doctors, nurses and pharmacists), and between healthcare professionals, patients and family members. However, efforts to improve interprofessional collaboration between healthcare professionals can reduce medication incidents (Manias, 2018; Manias et al., 2016). By creating a forum for good communication about the management of medications, it is possible to achieve enormous economic as well as health-related benefits (Walsh et al., 2017). It is, therefore, important for healthcare professionals to have a good understanding of the link between communication and medication safety, and of ways to improve communication with the aim of facilitating safe and high-quality management of medications.

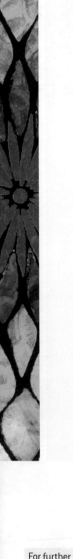

ALDO'S STORY

Aldo, an 80-year-old man on warfarin therapy for the treatment of a deep venous thrombosis (DVT), presented to the emergency department (ED) of a public hospital with dizziness and light-headedness. In the ED, Aldo was found to have a blood pressure (BP) of 80/40 mmHg, which appeared to explain his symptoms. On further examination, Aldo stated that his local doctor had recently increased the dose of perindopril arginine—an angiotensin converting enzyme inhibitor prescribed to treat hypertension.

The ED doctor was concerned that Aldo's BP might drop even further. She obtained an ampoule of 10 mg/1 mL of metaraminol and diluted it by adding 9 mL of sodium chloride. The metaraminol syringe was placed next to the patient's bedside so that it could be injected urgently if needed. The ED doctor did not tell the ED nurses about the metaraminol syringe.

Aldo's blood pressure improved without requiring any treatment and the plan was to discharge him on a lower dose of perindopril arginine. While he was in the ED, it was found that his level of anticoagulation, as shown by the international normalised ratio (INR), was low. As a result, the ED doctor prescribed subcutaneous low-molecular-weight heparin (LMWH), enoxaparin, on the discharge summary so that the patient could inject himself at home for three days to ensure adequate anticoagulation was obtained.

The ED pharmacist provided Aldo with an education session about how to give himself subcutaneous enoxaparin injections. These injections were to be administered two times daily. Aldo struggled to understand the instructions provided and how to go about giving himself the injections; however, the pharmacist was satisfied that he was able to go home. The pharmacist gave him six syringes that were pre-filled with the appropriate dose of enoxaparin. No information was given to Aldo about the need to take a lower dose of the antihypertensive, perindopril arginine.

As Aldo was packing up his belongings, he not only took the box containing the enoxaparin syringes, but also the syringe containing the metaraminol. The next morning, as he was about to inject himself with the metaraminol, Aldo was surprised at how different it looked from the other syringes. In a state of confusion, he contacted the ED and asked to speak to the pharmacist. After he spelled out to the pharmacist the label that was on the syringe, the pharmacist realised what had happened. She asked Aldo to discard the contents of the metaraminol syringe.

While this situation may be classified as a 'near-miss incident', since the patient was not harmed, there were several communication deficits that occurred at multiple levels. The ED doctor failed to inform the nurses that she had drawn up a syringe with metaraminol and so it was left by Aldo's bedside when it was no longer needed. No communication was made to Aldo about the need to reduce the dose of perindopril arginine and the reason for this reduction. There was an inadequate explanation provided to Aldo about how to use the enoxaparin syringes and, given his age and possible risk for further adverse events, it would have been appropriate to communicate with his GP and the hospital-in-the-home team about following up with him at home.

Stages of the medication management process and their links with communication

For further information about the relationship between medication safety and communication, view Eileen Poole's story at <http://www.ipeforqum.com.au/modules/>.

There are four major stages of the medication management process: supplying the medication; prescribing the medication; preparation and administration; and monitoring the medication (Bates, 2007; Bullock & Manias, 2016). All of these stages are associated with a number of interconnected steps that can cause medication incidents if communication problems occur. It is important that healthcare professionals are fully aware of these potential problems and take steps to prevent their occurrence.

Prescribing the medication

Prescribing the medication is the process of considering patient factors, such as age, coexisting medical illnesses and allergies, in deciding upon an appropriate medication for a clinical situation. This process also involves determining the route of administration, dose, frequency of administration and duration. The prescription needs to be documented in some permanent form using indelible ink and the prescriber's own handwriting (O'Connor, Gallagher & Omahony, 2012). With the move to electronic medical records, medication orders are more likely to be electronically generated, thereby reducing the chances of medication incidents caused by lack of legible writing. However, with the introduction of electronically generated prescriptions, problems can occur with incorrect entry of patient weight, inaccurate entry of the timing of drug levels and inaccurate information about patient doses (Ai et al., 2018; Tsyben, Gooding & Kelsall, 2016).

Problems with communication in prescribing can occur in many ways. Lack of interaction with the patient at the time of hospital admission or when first meeting the patient in a general practice consultation can mean insufficient details are collected about medication allergies or about various medications being taken concurrently, including complementary medicines and over-the-counter medicines. Asking the patient about various health conditions that could impact on their medication-taking behaviour is also important, such as pregnancy and past history of adverse drug reactions. An adverse drug reaction is a response to a medication that is harmful and unintended, and occurs at normal doses (Davies & O'Mahony, 2015; Hanlon et al., 2018).

Miscommunication can also result during telephone orders if unclear or insufficient directions are given. Telephone orders should always be followed up by documentation of the prescription within a defined period, which is usually around 24 hours. Past research involving a pre–post intervention approach has shown that the use of a clear protocol for taking medication orders by telephone led to a reduction in the number of telephone medication errors (Grant-Coke et al., 2015). Thus, when taking a telephone order from a prescriber, it is important that the healthcare professional repeats the patient's name, medication name (which includes spelling the name to avoid an error due to 'sound alike' medications), dosage (which includes pronouncing the amount in single digits—e.g. 15 mg should be read as one five), route and frequency (which includes stating the interval in full rather than using abbreviations—e.g. three times daily, not TDS).

Inadequate communication can occur in interactions with people who have special needs. These include individuals from cultural and linguistically diverse (CALD) backgrounds, individuals with cognitive impairment and those with sensory deficits such as sight or hearing loss. The risk of people with special needs having problems in following prescriptions is inherently increased in the presence of multiple chronic conditions, multiple prescribers and frequent changes to medication regimens (Eassey et al., 2017; Patricia & Foote, 2016; Weng et al., 2013). Strategies that can be used for people with special needs include the use of medication instructions using large lettering and in different languages, bilingual support people, and communication boards. After instruction has been given with the support of strategies, it is important to check that the individual has understood the information given about their medications.

Written forms of communication, as shown by documentation of prescriptions, can be illegible or ambiguous. Mistakes can also be made by pharmacists and nurses when reading these orders, leading to medication incidents. Prescribers should use generic medication names rather than brand names when writing out prescriptions, and an additional means of avoiding confusion is to include the indication for the medication. Brand names promote the corporate image of the pharmaceutical company as indicated by promoting similar-sounding names, and the use of brand names can lead to the prescription of duplicate orders if the prescriber is not familiar with them. Patients should also be encouraged to identify their medications by their generic names. Moreover, medication names can be displayed inconsistently in electronic systems, thereby increasing the likelihood of medication incidents (Quist et al., 2017).

Similarly, the use of certain types of abbreviations on a prescription can lead to miscommunication; for example, AZT has been interpreted as zidovudine or azathioprine and EPO can be interpreted as evening primrose oil or epoetin-alpha. For these reasons, it is important that medications are written out in full on the prescription and not abbreviated, and that only accepted abbreviations are used in providing directions for use. The Australian Commission on Safety and Quality in Health Care (ACSQHC; 2017b) has published recommendations for abbreviations used in medication documentation—see <https://www.safetyandquality.gov.au/publications/recommendations-for-terminology-abbreviations-and-symbols-used-in-medicines-documentation/>.

Prescriptions in hospital settings are often written during ward rounds and doctors' handovers where changes may be made to patients' medications. During these situations, nurses and pharmacists may not be present at the bedside, leading to delays in processing these changes. Medication incidents can arise from late administration of medications, delayed arrival of medications to the wards or inappropriate doses being administered. It is important that prescribers inform relevant members of the healthcare team about what medications have been ordered, and any changes to prescribed medications. Direct and active involvement of healthcare professionals from different disciplines has been shown to improve collaboration in prescribing practices. Improved involvement also facilitates better interactions with patients and family members (Liu, Gerdtz & Manias, 2016; Rathbone et al., 2016).

A further concern involving prescribing is the presence of multiple specialists involved in the patient's care, who may not individually know what each is prescribing. When patients have to seek out information from many different specialists, there is an increased chance that they will be prescribed several medications. In past research involving a retrospective review, collaboration between nurses and pharmacists identified medication-related problems and possible solutions to improve the quality of life for home-dwelling older people with functional limitations (Pherson et al., 2018). In another study examining polypharmacy and inappropriate medication use, investigators found a relationship between older patients being assigned to specialists and multiple prescriptions of unnecessary medications (Garfinkel & Mangin, 2010). Clearly, effective collaboration and communication are required between specialists, as with all members of the medication team.

Supplying the medication

Supplying the medication involves the process of the pharmacist delivering the medication from a central pharmacy department to a patient. In the process of supplying the medication, the pharmacist may have to prepare the medication in some way; for instance, an intravenous infusion may need to be made up. In addition, packaging, labelling, record keeping and the physical transfer of medication from one environment to another need to be undertaken. Supplying also involves incorporating medications into manually packaged dose-administration aids that are made available to older people situated in residential aged care settings and the community (Jackson & Welsh, 2017).

Sources of communication problems arising from supplying medications can relate to pharmacists being distracted by colleagues when preparing medications (Croft et al., 2017). As a result, an incorrect dose could be calculated in making a formulation, or a pharmacist could misread a prescribed dose due to illegible handwriting. This is a form of documentation miscommunication. In addition, if a doctor or nurse in a hospital ward does not convey to a pharmacist that a medication has been prescribed, the patient could be delayed in receiving the medication. The supply of incorrectly filled dose-administration aids has also been found to relate to the lack of adequate communication between aged care facilities and pharmacies. Past research has shown that patients' medication charts held by pharmacies filling the aids can often be outdated, in some cases leading to supply of ceased medications (Hussainy et al., 2012). These communication problems can be addressed by ensuring pharmacists are not distracted when completing their supply activities, by making sure pharmacists receive all medication changes promptly and by making certain that current and legible medication orders are provided. Development of a collaborative, person-centred model involving pharmacists, residents, carers, nurses and general practitioners can help to address these concerns (Elliott et al., 2017).

Preparation and administration

The actions of preparation and administration involve obtaining the medication and providing it to the patient in a form that is ready for consumption. Preparing may involve counting, calculating, mixing, labelling or formulating in some way. Administering comprises giving or taking the right medication for the right patient, in the right dose, by the right route, at the right time (Bullock & Manias, 2016).

Problems with communication commonly feature as the key reason for the occurrence of medication administration incidents. In a prospective study involving nine residential aged-care sectors and four nursing homes, a total of 188 249 medication administration attempts were analysed (Szczepura, Wild, & Nelson 2011). For the 345 residents observed, 90 per cent were identified as experiencing at least one preparation or administration incident. Nurses provided likely reasons for the existence of these incidents, which included interruptions during medication preparation and administration rounds (n = 43, 96%), and nurses feeling stressed during rounds due to miscommunication of orders (n = 23, 51%). Ensuring nurses are not interrupted during preparation and administration of medications can assist in reducing incidents (Johnson et al., 2018; Reed, Minnick & Dietrich, 2018).

Monitoring

Monitoring involves observing the patient to determine if the medication is working appropriately. The process includes checking that the medication is being used correctly and that therapeutic benefit is being achieved. It is also important to monitor that the medication is not actually harming the patient.

Communication failures can occur in monitoring if different healthcare professionals are involved in a patient's care. This situation may arise if patients move between hospital and community settings. Movements within hospital settings, as patients transfer from one hospital setting to another, can also set up a defective chain of events where communication failures occur. As patients move across various environments, aspects of the patients' monitoring need to be conveyed between healthcare professionals at handover (see Chapters 7 and 9). If inadequate information is conveyed, it is more likely that monitoring incidents will result. Patients also need to be informed about current and relevant aspects of their medication monitoring needs in the form of discharge education. If inadequate handover between healthcare professionals occurs or ineffective discharge education is provided to patients, a number of monitoring incidents can manifest. Such monitoring incidents include medications not being ceased once a treatment course is completed, or if a treatment course is clearly not helping the patient. In addition, monitoring incidents can relate to the full course of prescribed medication not being completed, medication levels not being measured, or medication levels being measured but not checked or acted upon by health professionals. Very little research has been conducted on the importance of communicating during monitoring of medications. A summary of how communication impacts on the medication management process is provided in Box 10.1.

BOX 10.1   Summary of how communication impacts on the medication management process

Prescribing

- Insufficient or inaccurate details collected about patients to enable appropriate decisions to be made about patients' medications.

- Unclear or insufficient directions given during telephone orders.

- Inadequate communication in interactions with people of special needs, including those from cultural and linguistically diverse (CALD) backgrounds, those with cognitive impairment and those with sensory deficits.

- Illegible or ambiguous documentation of prescriptions.

- Confusion due to the use of brand names and inappropriate abbreviations in medication orders.

- Delays in relaying information about medication prescription changes documented during ward rounds and handovers.

- Multiple specialists prescribing for the patient.

(Continued)

BOX 10.1   Summary of how communication impacts on the medication management process (Continued)

Supplying

- Distractions by colleagues when preparing medications in the central pharmacy department.
- Misreading of prescription doses due to illegible handwriting.
- Failure to notify the pharmacist of a medication order for a patient.

Preparation and administration

- Interruptions from colleagues during medication preparation and administration activities.
- Nurses feeling stressed due to miscommunication of orders, misinterpretation of orders or difficulties in reading orders.
- Time pressures associated with medication preparation and administration and competing activities.

Monitoring

- Different healthcare professionals involved in the care of patients as the patients move within hospital settings, and between hospital and community settings.
- Ineffective handover between healthcare professionals that fails to convey important information about patients' medication monitoring needs.
- Inadequate discharge education to patients that fails to convey important information about patients' medication monitoring needs.

REFLECTIVE THINKING QUESTION

As a healthcare professional, what strategies could you implement to address the communication problems arising from the medication management process? Consider these strategies from your own professional standpoint as well as from the perspective of other healthcare professionals.

Conceptualising the complexity of the actual communication encounter in the management of medications

Aside from examining how communication impacts on various stages of medication management, it is important to also consider the actual communication encounter. The communication encounter involves a number of interconnected and interdependent steps (Aronson, 2009), including the way in which healthcare professionals converse with each other, and with patients and family members about medications; how patients' and family members' beliefs, concerns and preferences are incorporated into information conveyed during communication encounters; and developing an awareness of how certain decisions dominate over others. In addition, the communication encounter involves determining who speaks, who is silent, what is said, what aspects of medication management are prioritised, the use of body language by all individuals involved, and the actual words and gestures used (Manias, 2010).

Various attributes need to be present in the actual communication encounter to demonstrate open and effective communication. Open and effective communication occurs if there is cooperation among healthcare professionals of different disciplines and varying levels of seniority involved with managing medications; and if there are opportunities for patients and family members to be involved in making shared decisions, and openly expressing their concerns (Coomber et al., 2018; Tudor Car et al., 2016). All healthcare professionals need to work together to carefully plan for the patient's transfer or discharge, and this process needs to commence from the patient's admission. In addition, all healthcare professionals should feel confident and reassured in offering their perspective about the patient's progress. Healthcare professionals from different disciplines must value the contribution of other team members and recognise their own responsibility in willingly contributing their expertise (Wilson et al., 2016).

What makes an open and effective communication encounter?

SOMETHING TO THINK ABOUT

- Encouraging active involvement of all health discipline groups during various communication forums, including bedside conversations, handover, ward rounds and team meetings.
- Encouraging the involvement of colleagues of varying levels of seniority in communications.
- Creating opportunities for patients and family members to be involved in communication, even if they choose to defer decision making to healthcare professionals.
- Encouraging healthcare professionals to focus on person-centred goals in planning, implementing and evaluating medication management activities, and in their communication with each other and with patients.

Conclusion

Healthcare professionals need to have a clear understanding of the link between communication and medication safety, and of ways to improve communication with the aim of facilitating excellent management of medications. Communication is a complex process that involves interactions between healthcare professionals, patients and family members during the stages of supplying, prescribing, preparing, administering and monitoring medications. Careful determination of the communication problems occurring during the various stages can help to identify strategies to resolve these problems. Also important is a consideration of the attributes of open and effective communication related to medication activities. Key attributes include collaboration among healthcare professionals from different disciplines and varying levels of seniority, and creating opportunities for involvement of patients and family members about medication management decisions.

Critical thinking activities

Mrs Smith is a 75-year-old woman, admitted to hospital for cardiac valvular surgery. Her surgery has gone smoothly and her post-operative recovery is progressing well. The healthcare professionals approach Mrs Smith's bed during the ward round to evaluate her progress and plan for hospital discharge. The consultant, nurse unit manager, bedside nurse, physiotherapist, social worker and pharmacist are in attendance. Mr Smith is very supportive of his wife. He is keen to hear about her progress and to ask questions at the ward round.

Medical consultant: *Hello, Mrs Smith. How are you feeling today? It is good that your husband is here as well.*

Mrs Smith: *I am feeling so much better today, doctor. Every day I seem to be feeling stronger and more able to get around.*

Mr Smith: *Yes, everything has been going very well, especially the last couple of days.*

Nurse: *Mrs Smith has been doing extremely well. She is able to attend to most things herself, with only minimal assistance from me.*

Nurse unit manager: *She has not experienced any problems with her diabetes since her medications were changed.*

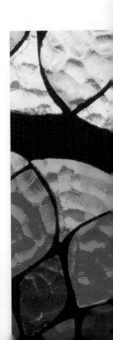

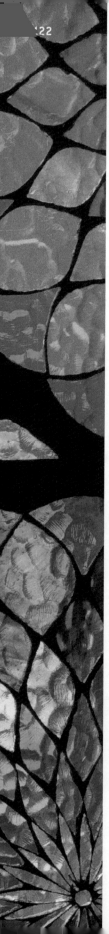

Pharmacist: Yesterday, we started going over the changes we have made to her diabetes medications. We also looked at the new medications she will be taking at home: the analgesic for pain and the warfarin for stopping blood clots forming around the valve. Mr Smith was there as well to get an idea of what was happening, weren't you?

Mr Smith: Yes, it was very helpful. It is good to know what she will need to take before she actually goes home.

Medical consultant: That's great. The surgery went very well and there have been no complications at all. Do either of you have concerns about anything?

Mrs Smith: Well, before yesterday, I wasn't sure about the changes made to my medications, but since the pharmacist has gone over these changes, I know what I have to do.

Physiotherapist: I saw Mrs Smith this morning, and she was able to do her coughing and deep breathing, and leg exercises extremely well, provided she has some analgesic beforehand.

Mrs Smith: Yes, the physiotherapist and I also went for a walk around the ward and I did some exercises around the bed just after I took my medications, and I didn't feel breathless or sore at all.

Medical consultant: We could possibly look at organising discharge home over the next day or so, if everyone is okay with that. What do you think, Mrs Smith?

Mrs Smith: I would love to go and I do feel well enough.

Nurse unit manager: That should give us ample time to organise her discharge.

Social worker: I can come and see you later today to see if you need additional support at home.

Pharmacist: We will go over your medications again later today, just to make sure you are clear about what they are for and how to take them. I will also draw up a medication list that I can go over with you.

1 In considering the communication that occurred between the various healthcare professionals, the patient and the family member, what examples of open and effective communication can you find?

2 How do you think planning occurred before the ward round to enable participation from the various healthcare professionals, the patient and the family member during the ward round?

3 What can the bedside nurse and pharmacist do in their communication with the patient and family member to ensure they have a good understanding about the medications before hospital discharge?

4 How does this situation compare with your own clinical practice in terms of creating opportunities for involving various individuals in a communication encounter?

Teaching and assessment activities

Mr Jonas, aged 68, has presented to hospital for exacerbation of chronic obstructive pulmonary disease (COPD). His past medical history includes depression, type 2 diabetes mellitus and hypertension. After stabilising his presenting complaint, the emergency department doctor prepares the letter to his general practitioner. The nurse and pharmacist provide counselling to Mr Jonas about his medications prior to discharge home. During these counselling sessions, Mr Jonas states that he has so many specialists managing his medications, and he is often confused about his medication regimen. As a result, he relies on his wife to help him with his medications. His medication regimen comprises the following:

- tiotropium inhaler: 18 micrograms, 1 puff once a day
- fluticasone propionate: 250 micrograms and salmeterol, 50 micrograms Accuhaler®, 1 puff two times a day
- salbutamol inhaler: 100 micrograms, 1–2 puffs when required for relief of respiratory symptoms
- metformin: 1 g, two times a day
- gliclazide: 60 mg, controlled-release tablet, once a day
- pravastatin: 20 mg, once a day
- aspirin: 100 mg, once a day
- ramipril: 10 mg, once a day
- amlodipine: 10 mg, once a day

- sertraline: 100 mg, once a day
- prednisolone: 30 mg, once a day for 7 days
- doxycycline: 100 mg, once a day for 7 days.

    Encourage students to undertake a role-play of this case scenario and to reflect on the following questions.

1 In what ways can Mr Jonas be included in the counselling sessions to improve his understanding of his medication regimen?
2 How can communication be facilitated with Mr Jonas' general practitioner following his discharge home?
3 What other healthcare professionals in the community can be identified to assist Mr Jonas with his medication regimen?
4 How can Mr Jonas' family be involved to support him to manage his medication regimen?
5 In examining the National Safety and Quality Health Service Standards (ACSQHC, 2017a) for medication safety, identify what medication information needs to be documented in an accurate and legally appropriate way in Mr Jonas' medical record?

Further reading

Britten, N. (2008). *Medicines and Society*. New York: Palgrave.

Tully, M. & Dean Franklin, B. (Eds). (2016). *Safety in Medication Use*. Boca Raton, USA: CRC Press-Taylor and Francis Group.

Web resources

Agency for Healthcare Research and Quality. Communication improvement.
<https://psnet.ahrq.gov/search?topic=Communication-Improvement&f_topicIDs=630>

Australian Commission on Safety and Quality in Health Care. Medication safety.
<http://www.transfusion.com.au/sites/default/files/NSQHS%20Standards%20%282%29.pdf>

Institute for Safe Medication Practices. Tools and resources.
<https://www.ismp.org/>

World Health Organization. Medication without harm. WHO's third global patient safety challenge.
<http://www.who.int/patientsafety/medication-safety/en/>

Patient Safety for Nursing Students: Medication Safety.
<https://patientsafetyfornursingstudents.org/resources/medication-safety/>

References

Ai, A., Wong, A., Amato, M. & Wright, A. (2018). Communication failure: Analysis of prescribers' use of an internal free-text field on electronic prescriptions. *Journal of the American Medical Informatics Association*. doi: 10.1093/jamia/ocy1003

Aronson, J. (2009). Medication errors: Definitions and classification. *British Journal of Clinical Pharmacology*, *67*(6), 599–604.

Australian Commission on Safety and Quality in Health Care. (2017a). *National Safety and Quality Health Service Standards* (2nd edn). Sydney, Australia: ACSQHC.

Australian Commission on Safety and Quality in Health Care. (2017b). *Recommendations for Terminology, Abbreviations and Symbols Used in Medicines Documentation*. Sydney, Australia: ACSQHC.

Bates, D. W. (2007). Preventing medication errors: a summary. *American Journal of Health-System Pharmacy*, *64*(14 Suppl 9), S3–S9.

Bullock, S. & Manias, E. (2016). *Fundamentals of Pharmacology* (8th edn). Melbourne, Australia: Pearson Australia.

Coomber, P., Clavarino, A., Ballard, E. & Luetsch, K. (2018). Doctor–pharmacist communication in hospitals: Strategies, perceptions, limitations and opportunities. *International Journal of Clinical Pharmacy*. doi: 10.1007/s11096-11018-10592-11091

Croft, H., Nesbitt, K., Rasiah, R., Levett-Jones, T. & Gilligan, C. (2017). Safe dispensing in community pharmacies: How to apply the SHELL model for catching errors. *Clinical Pharmacist*, *7*(9), 215–24.

Davies, E. A. & O'Mahony, M. S. (2015). Adverse drug reactions in special populations: The elderly. *British Journal of Clinical Pharmacology*, *80*(4), 796–807.

Eassey, D., McLachlan, A. J., Brien, J.-A., Krass, I. & Smith, L. (2017). 'I have nine specialists. They need to swap notes!' Australian patients' perspectives of medication-related problems following discharge from hospital. *Health Expectations*, *20*(5), 1114–20.

Elliott, R. A., Lee, C. Y., Beanland, C., Goeman, D. P., Petrie, N., Petrie, B., … Gray, J. (2017). Development of a clinical pharmacy model within an Australian home nursing service using co-creation and participatory action research: The visiting pharmacist (ViP) study. *BMJ Open*, *7*(11), e018722–e018722.

Garfinkel, D. & Mangin, D. (2010). Feasibility study of a systematic approach for discontinuation of multiple medications in older adults: Addressing polypharmacy. *Archives of Internal Medicine*, *170*(18), 1648–54.

Grant-Coke, M., Powell, D. L., Lyttle, J. & Hewitt, H. (2015). Establishing a telephone medication order policy and protocol for a small private hospital in Jamaica. *The West Indian Medical Journal*, *65*(2), 328–31.

Hanlon, P., Nicholl, B. I., Jani, B. D., McQueenie, R., Lee, D., Gallacher, K. I. & Mair, F. S. (2018). Examining patterns of multimorbidity, polypharmacy and risk of adverse drug reactions in chronic obstructive pulmonary disease: A cross-sectional UK Biobank study. *BMJ Open*, *8*(1), e018404–e018404.

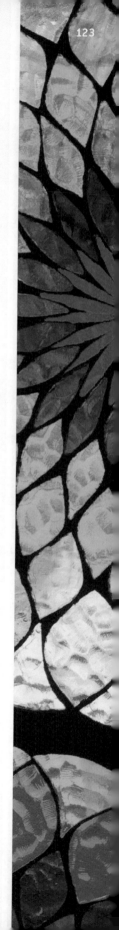

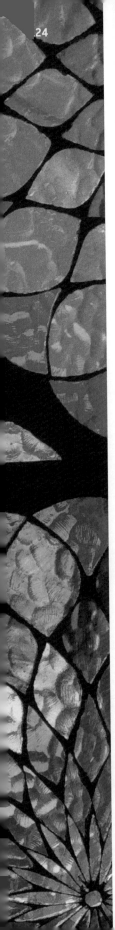

Hussainy, S., Marriott, J., van Koeverden, P. & Gilmartin, J. (2012). How accurate are manually prepared dose administration aids in residential aged care facilities? *Australian Pharmacist, 31*(4), 320–5.

Jackson, J. & Welsh, E. (2017). Medication charts in residential aged-care facilities. *Australian Prescriber, 40*(2), 20–2.

Johnson, M., Weidemann, G., Adams, R., Manias, E., Levett-Jones, T., Aguilar, V. & Everett, B. (2018). Predictability of interruptions during medication administration with related behavioral management strategies. *Journal of Nursing Care Quality, 33*(2), E1–E9.

Liu, W., Gerdtz, M. & Manias, E. (2016). Creating opportunities for interdisciplinary collaboration and patient-centred care: How nurses, doctors, pharmacists and patients use communication strategies when managing medications in an acute hospital setting. *Journal of Clinical Nursing, 25*(19–20), 2943–57.

Manias, E. (2018). Effects of interdisciplinary collaboration in hospitals on medication errors: an integrative review. *Expert Opinion on Drug Safety, 17*(3), 259–75.

Manias, E. (2010). Medication communication: A concept analysis. *Journal of Advanced Nursing, 66*(4), 933–43.

Manias, E., Gerdtz, M., Williams, A., McGuiness, J. & Dooley, M. (2016). Communicating about the management of medications as patients move across transition points of care: An observation and interview study. *Journal of Evaluation in Clinical Practice, 22*(5), 635–43.

O'Connor, M. N., Gallagher, P. & Omahony, D. (2012). Inappropriate prescribing: Criteria, detection and prevention. *Drugs and Aging, 29*(6), 437–52.

Patricia, N. J. & Foote, E. F. (2016). A pharmacy-based medication reconciliation and review program in hemodialysis patients: a prospective study. *Pharmacy Practice, 14*(3), 785.

Pherson, E., Roth, J., Nkimbeng, M., Boyd, C. & Szanton, S. (2018). Ensuring safe and optimal medication use in older community residents: Collaboration between a nurse and a pharmacist. *Geriatric Nursing and Home Care.* doi: 10.1016/j.gerinurse.2018.1003.1004

Quist, A. J. L., Hickman, T.-T. T., Amato, M. G., Volk, L. A., Salazar, A., Robertson, A., ... Schiff, G. D. (2017). Analysis of variations in the display of drug names in computerized prescriber-order-entry systems. *American Journal of Health-System Pharmacy: AJHP: Official Journal of the American Society of Health-System Pharmacists, 74*(7), 499–509.

Rathbone, A. P., Mansoor, S. M., Krass, I., Hamrosi, K. & Aslani, P. (2016). Qualitative study to conceptualise a model of interprofessional collaboration between pharmacists and general practitioners to support patients' adherence to medication. *BMJ Open, 6*(3), e010488–e010488.

Reed, C. C., Minnick, A. F. & Dietrich, M. S. (2018). Nurses' responses to interruptions during medication tasks: A time and motion study. *International Journal of Nursing Studies, 82*(June), 113–20.

Roughead, E., Semple, S., & Rosenfeld, E. (2016). The extent of medication errors and adverse drug reactions throughout the patient journey in acute care in Australia. *International Journal of Evidence-Based Healthcare, 14*, 113–22.

Roughead, E., Semple, S. & Rosenfeld, E. (2013). *Literature Review: Medication Safety in Australia.* Sydney: Australian Commission on Safety and Quality in Health Care.

Szczepura, A., Wild, D. & Nelson, S. (2011). Medication administration errors for older people in long-term residential care. *BMC Geriatrics, 11*(82). doi:10.1186/1471-2318-1111-1182

Tsyben, A., Gooding, N. & Kelsall, W. (2016). Assessing the impact of a newly introduced electronic prescribing system across a paediatric department—Lessons learned. *Archives of Disease in Childhood, 101*(9), e2–e2.

Tudor Car, L., Papachristou, N., Gallagher, J., Samra, R., Wazny, K., El-Khatib, M., ... Franklin, B. (2016). Identification of priorities for improvement of medication safety in primary care: A PRIORITIZE study. *BMC Family Practice, 17*(1), 160.

Walsh, E. K., Hansen, C. R., Sahm, L. J., Kearney, P. M., Doherty, E. & Bradley, C. P. (2017). Economic impact of medication error: A systematic review. *Pharmacoepidemiol Drug Saf, 26*(5), 481–97.

Weng, M. C., Tsai, C. F., Sheu, K. L., Lee, Y. T., Lee, H. C., Tzeng, S. L., ... Chen, S. C. (2013). The impact of number of drugs prescribed on the risk of potentially inappropriate medication among outpatient older adults with chronic diseases. *QJM: Monthly Journal of The Association of Physicians, 106*(11), 1009–15.

Wilson, A., Palmer, L., Levett-Jones, T., Gilligan, C. & Outram, S. (2016). Interprofessional collaborative practice for medication safety: Nursing, pharmacy and medical graduates' experiences and perspectives. *Journal of Interprofessional Care, 30*(5), 649–54.

World Health Organization. (2017). *Medication Without Harm—Global Patient Safety Challenge on Medication Safety.* Geneva: World Health Organization.

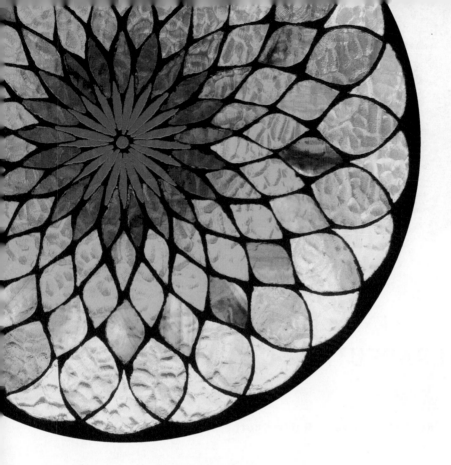

SECTION 3
Improving therapeutic communication to promote patient safety and wellbeing

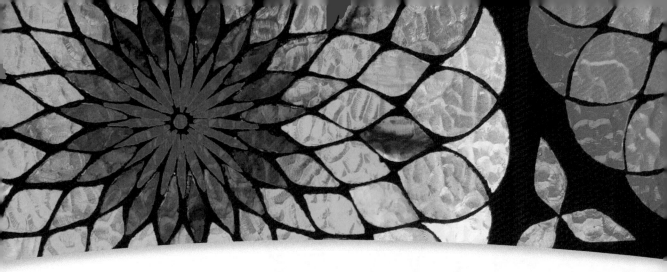

CHAPTER 11

KEY ATTRIBUTES OF
THERAPEUTIC COMMUNICATION

Rachel Rossiter   Robin Scott   Carla Walton

LEARNING OUTCOMES

Chapter 11 will enable you to:

- discuss the importance of therapeutic communication to patient safety and wellbeing
- explain the key attributes of therapeutic communication
- discuss barriers to therapeutic communication
- identify ways in which you can enhance your capacity to communicate in a therapeutic manner
- reflect upon your therapeutic communication skills.

KEY CONCEPTS

therapeutic presence | mindfulness | validation | empathy | self-awareness | non-judgmental stance | genuineness/authenticity

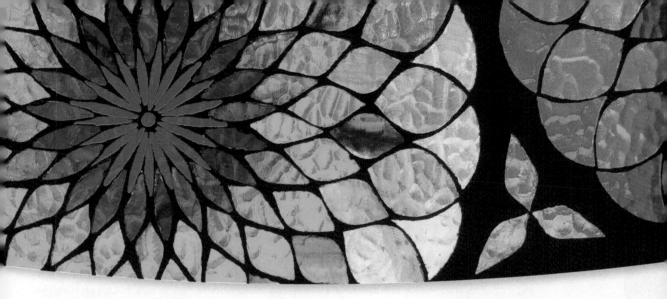

> What we are missing! What opportunities of understanding we let pass by because at a single decisive moment we were, with all our knowledge, lacking in the simple virtue of a full human presence.
>
> (Karl Jasper, cited in Sonneman, 1954, p. 375)

INTRODUCTION

As healthcare professionals, each of us devotes many hours to acquiring the specialist knowledge and clinical skills specific to our discipline. Our work may be situated in a broad range of clinical settings and across the entire spectrum of the life cycle. It encompasses not only the acute/urgent but also the provision of services such as primary healthcare, chronic care, forensic settings and end-of-life care where relationships with patients may continue for an extended period of time. Common to each of these contexts is the need for the essential skills of assessment, problem solving and clinical reasoning. However, to use these skills, we need to be able to obtain accurate and comprehensive information from the patient, and to understand the patient's perceptions of what is happening and what he or she is seeking from the health services. Thus, if we are to provide effective care and ensure patient safety, it is imperative that we strengthen our capacity for therapeutic communication. The challenge is to utilise our specialist knowledge and skills, and our capacity for assessment and decision making, while at the same time ensuring that we suspend our personal judgments and biases and authentically demonstrate respect and empathy for the person requiring our care. In other words, how do we as healthcare professionals 'be with' our patients in a way that is therapeutic and invokes trust and confidence? Remember, if your patients don't feel safe with you or don't trust you, they will not tell you everything; likewise, they may not follow through on your instructions for treatment.

Chapter 2 provided an introduction to communication skills and Chapter 3 highlighted the key attributes of patient-safe communication. This chapter explores the key attributes required for effective therapeutic communication and examines what the evidence says about barriers to being therapeutic. We then consider the ways in which we can strengthen our capacity to communicate in a therapeutic manner, as without these skills our practice will not be safe.

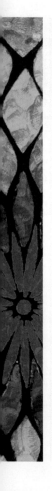

CLARA'S STORY

I had been a midwife for six years when I enrolled in postgraduate studies. I really believed I knew how to communicate with the women in my care. At least, I did until I enrolled in a course about therapeutic engagement and started learning strategies to improve my ability to communicate therapeutically and to understand more about the psychosocial interventions available for people who are struggling with emotional difficulties.

I was working on the antenatal ward when Clara, in the early weeks of her first pregnancy, presented repeatedly with painful uterine contractions. None of the tests or repeated assessments found a reason for her pain. When Clara was admitted yet again, I listened as colleagues talked about her as 'a druggy' while they continued giving analgesia, which had no impact on Clara's distress.

At this point, I decided to practise my 'new' therapeutic communication skills. Before speaking with Clara, I consciously focused on putting aside the 'druggy label'. When I sat down with her, I was mindful of putting aside any judgments and listening with openness and empathy. To my surprise, I discovered that the previous year Clara had experienced an episode of depression requiring medication and psychotherapy. She was no longer seeing the psychologist and had stopped her medication, as she had been feeling well and had wanted to have a baby.

I spoke with Clara about the potential impact of pregnancy and childbirth on emotional stability and about research that has found that recent discontinuation of mood-stabilising medications may increase the risk of postpartum psychosis (Khan & Lusskin, 2010). We discussed Clara's options and she decided that she would go back to see the psychologist and book an appointment with her primary care provider to review her mental health.

You know, I did not expect what happened next. For the remainder of that shift, Clara did not ask for any analgesia. In the weeks that followed, she did not re-present. Clara's outpatient notes showed that her pregnancy was progressing well and she had accessed psychological support with beneficial effect. For me, this experience strengthened my focus on using the therapeutic communication skills I was learning.

Source: The authors were given permission to use Clara's (pseudonym) story in teaching healthcare professionals about therapeutic communication.

Why is therapeutic communication important?

As healthcare professionals, we are accustomed to applying the term 'therapeutic' to a wide variety of interventions and treatments; but we may not have thought of the way in which we communicate with our patients as having the potential to be therapeutic or non-therapeutic. However, it is highly likely that we have observed communication behaviours that were non-therapeutic and disruptive for those on the receiving end. The impact of such non-therapeutic communication has widespread effects not only on patient care but also on relationships between healthcare professionals and treatment outcomes (Kinnersley & Edwards, 2008; Rosenstein, 2009). Most of us do not set out to be deliberately non-therapeutic, but unhelpful ways of communicating occur because we either lack the necessary skills or there are barriers that affect our capacity to communicate in an empathic and therapeutic manner.

Here, *therapeutic* means to have an outcome that is both beneficial and desirable.

While research indicates that therapeutic communication improves patient satisfaction, it also impacts patient safety and clinical outcomes. A common assumption is that patients will follow our instructions and that providing information is all that is required. Bennett et al. (2011, p. 54) suggest that this is a 'rarely met assumption … with at least four out of ten patients ignoring, forgetting, misunderstanding, or inaccurately following directives on appointments, prescriptions and lifestyle changes'. In contrast, patients who are satisfied with the quality of healthcare communication are more likely to adhere to treatment plans (Locke et al., 2011).

Person-centred and therapeutic communication has been demonstrated to increase patient satisfaction and adherence to treatment, and contribute to positive clinical outcomes for patients with chronic disease (Levinson, Lesser & Epstein, 2010). For example, it has been demonstrated that adherence to treatment in patients with diabetes is enhanced by the quality of the therapeutic communication from healthcare professionals (Rungby & Brock, 2010).

What is therapeutic communication?

Chapter 3 identified attributes that epitomise a person-centred clinician; that is, a clinician whose interactions are beneficial for the patient. Studies have also identified *understanding and empathy*, *being there and being available*, *being genuine* and *demonstrating self-awareness* as vital components in the development of a person-centred and therapeutic relationship (Dziopa & Ahern, 2009).

From the patient's perspective, a healthcare professional is seen as trustworthy if he or she demonstrates care, genuine concern, empathy and interest in the patient as a unique individual, by actively listening (hearing, understanding and believing the patient) (Levinson, 2011). The willingness and ability of healthcare providers to empathise in combination with effective communication skills have been shown to markedly improve patients' satisfaction with healthcare consultations (Schrooten & de Jong, 2017). Patients also highly value a healthcare professional who uses straightforward, understandable terms when providing explanations and information (Hancock et al., 2012; Salt, Rowles & Reed, 2012).

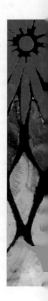

NANCY'S STORY

Nancy has lived with severe and life-threatening systemic lupus erythematosus (SLE) since she was 19 years old. She shares her experience of chronic illness and the therapeutic communication skills that she sought and valued in healthcare professionals:

> It was ... finding a doctor I could work with to help me to get well ... someone I would feel comfortable with asking questions and receiving answers back that I could understand. I wanted a doctor who would offer new and up-to-date alternative treatments and explain to me what was going on at different stages of my disease. I felt this doctor was caring, genuinely concerned and attuned to my feelings. I felt he was listening to what I had to say.

During the course of her illness, Nancy experienced many difficult times. She describes speaking to a nurse specialising in immunology about her struggles living with SLE:

> She listened and let me cry ... I felt safe and a sense of trust in being able to express my feelings without feeling labelled or judged and the confidence in knowing any discussion would be confidential.

Source: Kalevski, N. (2010). *Red Butterfly: Living with Lupus*. Newcastle, Australia: Self-published.

As we now examine therapeutic communication in closer detail, you may be tempted to skip this section, thinking that you already know what the terms mean or that this is not really relevant to your work. *If you are so inclined, we caution you to remember the relationship between therapeutic communication and patient safety!*

To communicate therapeutically, healthcare professionals need to pay attention to developing and strengthening the following attributes:

■ **Genuineness/authenticity:** Be human, be yourself. The patient quickly perceives whether you are genuine or just 'going through the motions'. Non-verbal indicators of inattention, your tone of voice and speed of communication, all give the person a sense of your genuineness.

■ **Empathy:** Empathy is defined as the capacity for participating in and understanding the feelings or perspectives of another person. It is important not to confuse empathy with sympathy, which can be seen as being about the healthcare professional, that is, 'sharing the suffering of another—I feel your pain' (Carkhuff & Berenson, 2009, pp. 3–6). It is impossible to understand another person's experience exactly; being empathic is to fully accept another person's experience and not make comparisons with our own experience. Every experience, like every person, is unique. We cannot assume that we truly know how another person feels in any situation. Remember,

SOMETHING TO THINK ABOUT

Empathy is a strange and powerful thing … There is no right way or wrong way to do it. It's simply listening, holding space, withholding judgment, emotionally connecting and communicating that incredibly healing message of 'you're not alone'.

(Brené Brown, 2015).

Mindfulness is now widely considered to be an inherent quality of human consciousness—a capacity of attention and awareness oriented to the present moment that varies in degrees within and between individuals (*known as dispositional mindfulness*) (Black, 2011, p. 1). Evidence is growing that intentional mindfulness (i.e. deliberately practising mindfulness) deactivates the 'default mode' that operates when a person is ruminating or worrying and instead 'activates areas of the brain that are associated with focused attention on present moment sensory experiences', thus contributing to improved psychological health (Wheeler, Arnkoff & Glass, 2017, p. 1484).

demonstrating empathy requires more than 'words'. A willingness to empathise and having the skills to empathise must be matched with an empathic attitude and communication that reflects your empathy for the person (Schrooten & de Jong, 2017).

- **Self-awareness:** Self-awareness denotes a deep awareness of our thoughts, feelings and behaviours, as well as the impact that they have on the manner in which we interact with others. Motivation (the desire to do the best you can) and moral agency (using the self to create a therapeutic relationship) are key aspects of self-awareness (Dempsey et al., 2009, pp. 245–6).

  Genuineness and authenticity, empathy and self-awareness are the platform from which we can utilise the following techniques to communicate therapeutically with the people in our care.

- **Mindfulness:** Mindfulness is focused attention and awareness. A well-known definition states that 'mindfulness is the awareness that emerges through paying attention on purpose, in the present moment, and non-judgmentally to the unfolding of experiences moment by moment' (Kabat-Zinn, 1994). In the information-rich and fast-paced environments that constitute health service delivery, mindfulness enables healthcare professionals to consider multiple perspectives while keeping the patient at the forefront of their attention (Anthony & Vidal, 2010).

  Mindfulness skills improve the capacity 'to be attentive, listen deeply to patients' concerns *and* respond to patients more effectively' (Beckman et al., 2012, p. 815). Research also suggests that mindfulness 'may enable healthcare professionals to work with compassion in stressful and demanding work environments' (Hunter, 2016, p. 918). For more information about mindfulness, see 'Further reading' and 'Web resources' at the end of this chapter.

- **Put aside biases and assumptions:** Although it may be hard to admit, it is often difficult to understand or relate to people who are different from us. We all have personal beliefs, biases and assumptions that influence the ways in which we respond to others. These may at times impede our ability to be empathic and therapeutic in our interactions with others. Add to this the tasks associated with working in an environment where resources are limited and demands are high, and it is apparent how a limited awareness of our own behaviours, feelings, emotions and thought processes may contribute to errors in patient care.

SOMETHING TO THINK ABOUT

'Begin challenging your own assumptions. Your assumptions are your windows on the world. Scrub them off every once in a while, or the light won't come in.'

(Alan Alda, n.d.)

REFLECTIVE THINKING QUESTION

Possessing bias is part and parcel of being human. And the more we think we are immune to it, **the greater the likelihood that our own biases will be invisible or unconscious to us!** (Ross, 2014)

Take a moment to identify a situation where you became aware of what had previously been an unconscious bias. How did your newly found awareness change your behaviour?

■ **Non-judgmental stance:** As human beings, we frequently use shorthand expressions when talking with each other as a faster way to communicate. For example, we might say, 'He's a great guy' or 'He's a bit of a creep'. In this brevity we can miss some of the important details. We don't really know what is meant by him being a 'great guy' or a 'creep'. As healthcare professionals we have conversations with our patients, with our colleagues and with ourselves about our patients (and our colleagues!). We will often reflect on our patients, what we are doing with them and what we can do differently. Our tendency to use shorthand judgments is so well practised that it is easy to use these judgments when we talk and think about our patients. When we do this, it often increases our emotions, closing off options in terms of thinking about how we can help.

What might we do differently? For example, if we are told that 'Sally is a really difficult patient', we may dread and even avoid interacting with Sally. Stop and reflect on what a statement like 'She's a really difficult patient' tells us about Sally. Does it tell us what she does (or doesn't do) that makes her difficult? A more useful way to communicate these shorthand judgments with our colleagues and our patients is to suspend our judgment and just state the facts and the consequences. If we just describe the facts, it opens up problem-solving options for how we might help. The facts about Sally are that her immune function is compromised and she walks around the general hospital instead of staying in her room. This places her at increased risk of infection and the nurses spend a lot of time trying to find her to bring her back to her room. Thinking in this way, our frustration is likely to lessen and we can move into a place of finding a solution.

■ **Validation:** To validate has been defined as 'to make valid, substantiate or confirm' (<www.websters-online-dictionary.org>). Telling a person, 'I understand how you feel', seldom assists the person to feel that you really do understand. You are much more likely to encounter a response such as, 'How could you possibly know what I'm feeling'. To validate requires us to 'communicate to the patient that their responses make sense and are understandable within their current … situation' (Linehan, 1993, pp. 222–3). Actively focusing on putting aside your biases and assumptions, and taking a non-judgmental stance, frees you up to be present with the person and to validate their experience. Actively employing these skills enables you to cultivate your ability to be present.

■ **Therapeutic presence** is described as the act of intentionally 'bringing one's whole self' into the interaction with a patient (Geller, Greenberg & Watson, 2010, p. 599). Once you are 'fully' present, you are then in a position to communicate in a way that is beneficial for the patient.

Take time now to review the pictorial representation of the relationship between these attributes and skills, and the desired outcome of effective therapeutic communication (Figure 11.1).

> 'If we could look into each other's eyes and understand the unique challenges each of us face, we would treat each other much more gently, with more empathy, patience, tolerance and care' (Marvin J. Ashton, n.d.).

> 'We cannot be fully present with others until we can be fully present and at home with ourselves … We cannot see or hear who others actually are or what they feel unless we are at home with ourselves and not living behind a veil of self-deception or ego' (Geller & Greenberg, 2012, p. 79).

ROBIN'S REFLECTION

I have been working in emergency mental health for many years. A vital part of my professional practice is regular participation in clinical supervision. This provides a safe environment where I can voice my concerns and frustrations and also describe the successful moments. The skills learnt in supervision are consciously used in my everyday work, especially to increase my mindfulness of my biases and assumptions and how these may negatively affect my capacity to genuinely engage and connect with people.

For example, a phone call from the emergency department (ED) says that a patient has re-presented and requires a mental health assessment. Sometimes this prompts immediate feelings of frustration: 'Oh no, not her again', 'Didn't she listen to or do the things we talked about the other day?' and 'What has she done this time?'. Now I acknowledge these feelings and make a conscious decision to put them aside. I spend the time walking to the ED thinking about how I can be of help to this person rather than becoming immersed in those unhelpful feelings. By the time I reach the ED, my mind is cleared to focus my attention fully towards the person.

Source: Robin Scott, personal reflection

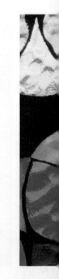

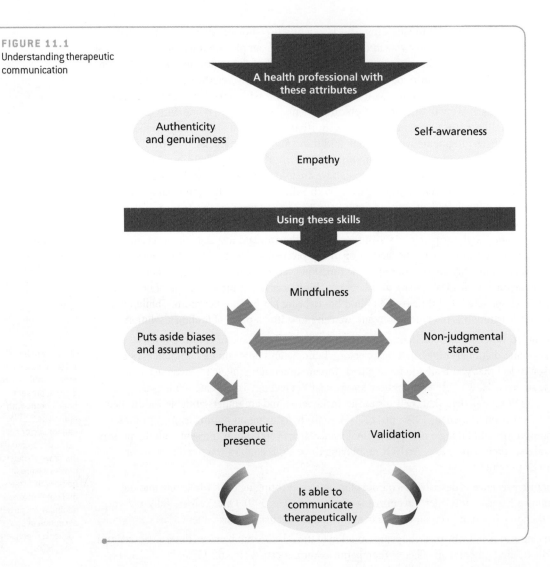

FIGURE 11.1
Understanding therapeutic
communication

What are the barriers to therapeutic communication?

As a starting point for considering the factors that impede our ability to be therapeutic, think of some of the obstacles that reduce the capacity to live our lives with ease outside of work, as it is likely that these obstacles will also impact on our functioning at work. Geller and Greenberg (2012, p. 76) suggest that factors such as 'stress, fatigue, burnout, lack of self-care, overwork, unresolved personal issues, lack of presence with others in daily life, and excessive busyness' are likely to reduce an individual's capacity to be therapeutic. Table 11.1 details barriers to therapeutic communication that have been identified in the healthcare setting. Keep in mind that without self-awareness, authenticity and empathy, it will be difficult to overcome these barriers to patient-safe and therapeutic communication.

So far, this chapter has examined some of the key aspects of therapeutic communication and identified some of the barriers that block therapeutic communication. Next we consider how you can improve your ability to engage in communication interactions that are therapeutic.

Barriers	Example	What helps?	Example	
Over-reliance on technology	'More mistakes are made from want of a proper examination than for any other reason' (Russell John Howard, 1875–1942).	Mindfulness; focused attention	Taking time to listen to the patient will provide invaluable information that would otherwise be missed.	**TABLE 11.1** Barriers to therapeutic communication
Limited time	'You know, my focus is on looking after the acute issues. I don't have time to waste being empathic.'	Empathy	'Of course, the legal, clinical and professional tasks have to get done, but doing them with a bit of ordinary humanity can make such a difference' (Kennard et al., 2007).	
The patient may get upset	'If I show the person that I care too much, they'll get all upset and then I've got to manage all of that emotion as well; it's easier to just keep moving right along.'	Self-awareness and empathy	'This is not all about me! I know it may be hard and perhaps painful to listen, but I can still choose to connect with this person and be empathic.'	
Fear that showing empathy will lead to burnout	'You know, I deal with people who are suffering all day long. If I let myself feel all that pain, I'll just end up exhausted and unable to do my job.'	Self-awareness, clinical supervision and reflection	'I can make sure that I talk to my clinical supervisor or mentor about these challenging moments.'	
Lack of knowledge and education	'I don't know what to ask and I'm scared that if I say the wrong thing I'll make things worse.'	Additional education	It is important to understand our limits, but that does not mean we cannot attempt to connect. If we do make mistakes, we should feel supported and not left to make decisions in isolation and without consultation.	
Relying on written patient information only	'I've given the patient the information. Why don't they do as they're told.'	Put aside assumptions	Check that the patient has understood the information provided and ask whether they have any questions or concerns.	

Source: Hardee & Platt (2010), p. 18; Haslam (2007); Levinson, Lesser & Epstein (2010).

What you can do to strengthen your therapeutic communication skills

There are many strategies that have been shown to enable healthcare professionals to build their capacity for therapeutic communication, for example:

1 Remind yourself to repeatedly ask, 'What would it be like to be in this person's place?' (Hojat, 2007, p. 192).
2 Ask yourself, 'What if this person was my mother, father, son, daughter, husband, wife …?'
3 Focus on 'listening with the third ear', seeking to 'understand the patient's experience *beyond the spoken words*' (Hojat, 2007, p. 192).
4 Practise 'viewing events with the third eye to understand the patient's experiences more completely' (Hojat, 2007, p. 192).
5 Take every opportunity to participate in professional development courses focusing on therapeutic communication.

6   Participate in regular clinical supervision[1] where the focus is on strengthening your therapeutic interactions (White & Winstanley, 2011).

7   For medical professionals and psychologists, seek out a Balint group[2] in your area and attend regularly (Lustig, 2008, pp. 263–4).

8   Make sure that you access a broad range of literature, art, music and film outside of your discipline to deepen your understanding and provide other perspectives of suffering and pain.

9   Take time to know the person's unique story. As we understand a little of a person's life, our ability to be empathic and compassionate is strengthened.

The growing body of research related to the impact of mindfulness and therapeutic presence on therapeutic communication includes suggestions that are helpful for all healthcare professionals. As a starting point, consider incorporating these recommendations to further strengthen your ability to communicate therapeutically:

1   Pay attention to looking after yourself. This will require an ongoing commitment to self-care. Remember that physical health is a tremendous aid to resilience, and the most consequential threats to safety are threats to the body. The common sense basics are as follows:
   • Have a balanced and nourishing diet.
   • Get a good night's sleep.
   • Take regular exercise.
   • Minimise or eliminate intoxicants.
   • Early intervention identifies and treats potential health problems (Hanson & Hanson, 2018, p. 91).

2   Ensure that you have 'a life' outside of your work.

3   Make regular time in your life to be with friends and family, with a focus on being non-judgmental, accepting of others and listening carefully.

4   Strengthen your commitment to personal growth and self-awareness. Your capacity to communicate therapeutically with patients is directly influenced by the extent to which you are comfortable with yourself and with close emotional contact with others.
   • Review your personal ethics and moral values on a regular basis.
   • Access professional workshops to enhance your communication and self-awareness capacity.

5   Make room in your life for 'quiet spaces', reflection and contemplation. Consider regular practices such as mindfulness, yoga and other similar practices (Geller & Greenberg, 2012). Regularly examine your motivation and commitment to providing person-centred, therapeutic healthcare.

Conclusion

This chapter has challenged you to ensure that the way in which you communicate is safe, therapeutic and beneficial to your patient's health and wellbeing. The key to success is finding within yourself the motivation and willingness to work on developing and strengthening your therapeutic communication skills. Just as all healthcare professionals need to make a commitment to ongoing professional development to ensure they are able to deliver evidence-based care, the same level of commitment is required to keep our therapeutic communication skills well honed.

In the chapters that follow (Chapters 12–20), the focus is on therapeutic communication with specific groups of patients. Remember that what you have learnt in this chapter will underpin your interactions with all of your patients.

---

1   Clinical supervision has been described as 'a support mechanism for healthcare professionals within which they can share clinical, organisational, developmental and emotional experiences with another professional in a secure, confidential environment in order to enhance knowledge and skills. This process is designed to enhance accountability and reflective practice' (Lyth, 2000, p. 728).

2   Balint group: 'experiential, small educational group in which practising clinicians meet regularly to discuss their own doctor–patient interactions' (Lustig, 2008, p. 263). 'Participants always report increased ability to cope with difficult clinician–patient interactions, psychologically challenging situations in general … and [with] mental health issues; reduction in work-related stress; and increased professional satisfaction' (drawn from <https://www.timothy.works/balint-groups/>).

Critical thinking activities

Levinson (2011) reminds us that to deliver safe care requires focused attention on strengthening our clinical and technical skills and knowledge *as well as* the same level of attentiveness to strengthening our therapeutic communication skills. As you consider Levinson's assertion, ponder this reflection:

Maria, an experienced renal dialysis clinician, reflected:

I am always very busy both physically and mentally when I am at work. I used to view this as a sign that I was a 'good nurse', highly organised and competent, until I realised that while I was getting the work done I was just providing 'lip-service' to 'being there' for my patients—in other words, to the concept of being present …

I began to pay closer attention to 'being present'. When I put my patients on the [dialysis] machine I now focus entirely upon them. If a staff member wants to speak to me (and it is not an emergency), where previously I would interrupt my patient and have a conversation with the staff member, I now ask them to wait until I have finished. I try to actively listen to my patients and don't attempt to think I can finish their conversation with words like 'Yes, I know' or 'But of course'. You know, if the truth be told, I really had no idea; and I was just wishing for them to finish so I could move on to the next patient.

I think in dialysis it is absolutely essential to have technical and clinical competence. But when I think about the time we spend with our patients, more consideration needs to be given to our interpersonal relationships and to fostering a culture that openly values the relationships developed with our patients.

One thing I totally did not anticipate—you could say it was an unexpected benefit of my study—I am enjoying work for the first time in a long time. Just by being present with my group of patients, I feel that I am working at a higher level and have developed effective therapeutic relationships with them.

Source: The authors were given permission to use Maria's reflection in teaching healthcare professionals about therapeutic communication.

1 Thinking about your own practice, how do you respond to interruptions when you are looking after a patient?
2 Do you think that there are aspects of Maria's story that are relevant to your clinical practice?
3 Imagine how your work context and capacity for therapeutic communication would change if your team tried Maria's experiment.
4 Review Clara's story (p. 126). Compare the midwife's actions against those illustrated in Figure 11.1. Identify the attributes and skills that the midwife specifically concentrated on in her interactions with Clara.
5 As a result of reading this chapter, what specific actions do you need to take to strengthen your capacity for therapeutic communication?

Teaching and assessment activities

Activity 1

Identifying and exploring the impact of assumptions upon patient care

This activity is based on Wolfe's (2016) feature article in the *Australian Medical Students Journal*.

Current assessment processes in healthcare use questions designed to identify factors that can increase the risk of poorer health outcomes for patients. As we undertake an assessment, we then group risk factors together and draw assumptions related to sociocultural risks. We tick boxes, for example: 'Do you have a history of previous intravenous drug use?', 'Do you identify as an Aboriginal or Torres Strait Islander?', 'Are you from a refugee or migrant background?', and 'Do you live in a rural or remote area?' (Wolfe, 2016, p. 60). We turn our attention to 'vulnerabilities' and 'high-risk groups' without much consideration of the impact of these questions and our subsequent assumptions on the person's individual health identity.

Ask students to respond to the following:

a. Consider some of the assumptions that may be linked to questions such as those above.
b. How might these assumptions influence further assessment and communication with the person?
c. Identify pros and cons associated with assumptions related to a person's socio-cultural risks.
d. Ponder how assumptions related to risk can impact upon the delivery of person-centred care and therapeutic communication.

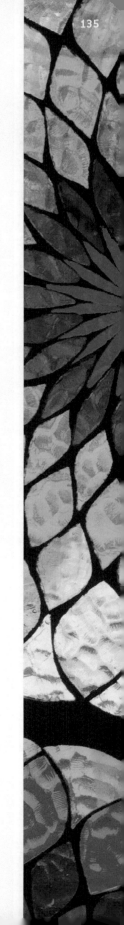

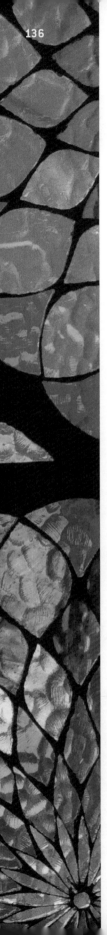

Activity 2

Exploring care, compassion and empathy (therapeutic communication) while practising nursing activities such as personal care

This activity is based on Richardson, Percy and Hughes' (2015) review (see references list).

Rather than focusing on therapeutic communication skills in isolation, consider extending the focus of learning activities to include questions that invite students to reflect beyond their technical competence. For example:

a. What must it feel like to be in this situation?

b. What would you do or think if you were the patient?

c. How would you like to be treated if you had this intervention undertaken on you? (Richardson et al., p. e4)

Further reading

Geller, S. & Greenberg, L. (2012). Preparing the ground for therapeutic presence. *Therapeutic Presence: A Mindful Approach to Effective Therapy* (pp. 75–91). Washington: American Psychological Association.

Hojat, M. (2016). *Empathy in Health Professions Education and Patient Care*. Switzerland: Springer International Publishing.

Hanson, R. & Hanson, F. (2018). *Resilient: How to Grow an Unshakable Core of Calm, Strength, and Happiness*. New York: Harmony Books.

Web resources

Balint Society of Australia and New Zealand
<http://www.balintaustralianewzealand.org/>

Black, D. (2011). A brief definition of mindfulness. Mindfulness Research Guide
<www.mindfulexperience.org>

'Does Mindfulness Really Work?' With Daniel Goleman and Richard Davidson
<https://www.youtube.com/watch?v=RBg2i7ZsXgk>

Openground mindfulness training
<http://www.openground.com.au/openground>

Harvard Neuro Blog: The neuroscience behind mindfulness
<https://harvardneuro.wordpress.com/2016/01/06/the-neuroscience-behind-mindfulness/>

REACHOUT.com: How to practice mindfulness
<https://au.reachout.com/articles/how-to-practice-mindfulness>

Andy Puddicombe: All it takes is 10 mindful minutes
<https://www.ted.com/talks/andy_puddicombe_all_it_takes_is_10_mindful_minutes?referrer=playlist-talks_to_help_practice_patienc>

References

Alda, A. (n.d.) Accessed December 2018 at <http://www.azquotes.com/quote/4257>.

Anthony, M. & Vidal, K. (2010). Mindful communication: A novel approach to improving delegation and increasing patient safety. *Online Journal of Issues in Nursing, 15*(2).

Beckman, H., Wendland, M., Mooney, C., Krasner, M., Quill, T., Suchman, A. & Epstein, R. (2012). The impact of a program in mindful communication on primary care physicians [Evaluation Studies Research Support, Non-U.S. Gov't]. *Academic Medicine, 87*(6), 815–19.

Bennett, J., Fuertes, J., Keitel, M. & Phillips, R. (2011). The role of patient attachment and working alliance on patient adherence, satisfaction, and health-related quality of life in lupus treatment. *Patient Education and Counseling, 85*(1), 53–9.

Black, D. (2011). A brief definition of mindfulness. *Mindfulness Research Guide*. Accessed January 2019 at <www.mindfulexperience.org>.

Brown, B. (2015). *Daring Greatly: How the Courage to Be Vulnerable Transforms the Way We Live, Love, Parent, and Lead*. New York: Penguin Random House.

Carkhuff, R. & Berenson, B. (2009). *The Heart of Empathy*. Massachusetts: HRD Press Inc.

Dempsey, J., Hillege, S., French, J. & Wilson, V. (2009). Thoughtful practice: Self awareness and reflection. In N. McKenzie & L. Jabbour (Eds), *Fundamentals of Nursing and Midwifery: A Person-Centred Approach to Care* (Australian and New Zealand edn, pp. 242–57). Philadelphia, PA: Wolters Kluwer/Lippincott Williams & Wilkins.

Dziopa, F. & Ahern, K. (2009). What makes a quality therapeutic relationship in psychiatric/mental health nursing? A review of the research literature. *Internet Journal of Advanced Nursing Practice, 10*(1), 1–19.

Geller, S. & Greenberg, L. (2012). Preparing the ground for therapeutic presence. In *Therapeutic Presence: A Mindful Approach to Effective Therapy* (pp. 75–91). Washington: American Psychological Association.

Geller, S., Greenberg, L. & Watson, J. (2010). Therapist and client perceptions of therapeutic presence: The development of a measure. *Psychotherapy Research, 20*(5), 599–610.

Hancock, R., Bonner, G., Hollingdale, R. & Madden, A. (2012). 'If you listen to me properly, I feel good': A qualitative examination of patient experiences of dietetic consultations [Research Support, Non-U.S. Gov't]. *Journal of Human Nutrition & Dietetics, 25*(3), 275–84.

Hanson, R. & Hanson, F. (2018). *Resilient: How to Grow an Unshakable Core of Calm, Strength, and Happiness*. New York: Harmony Books.

Hardee, J. & Platt, F. (2010). Exploring and overcoming barriers to clinical empathic communication. *Journal of Communication in Healthcare, 3*(1), 17–23.

Haslam, N. (2007). Humanising medical practice: The role of empathy. *Medical Journal of Australia, 187*(7), 381–2.

Hojat, M. (2007). Enhancement of empathy. In *Empathy in Patient Care: Antecedents, Development, Measurement and Outcomes* (pp. 173–200). New York: Springer.

Hunter, L. (2016). Making time and space: The impact of mindfulness training on nursing and midwifery practice. A critical interpretative synthesis. *Journal of Clinical Nursing, 25*(7–8), 918–29. doi:10.1111/jocn.13164

Kabat-Zinn, J. (1994). *Wherever You Go There You Are: Mindfulness Meditation in Everyday Life*. New York: Hyperion.

Kalevski, N. (2010). *Red Butterfly: Living with Lupus*. Newcastle: Self-published.

Kennard, D., Fagin, L., Hardcastle, M. & Grandison, S. (2007). Things you can do to make in-patient care a better experience. In M. Hardcastle, D. Kennard, S. Grandison & L. Fagin (Eds), *Experiences of Mental Health In-patient Care* (pp. 205–7). East Sussex: Routledge.

Khan, S. & Lusskin, S. (2010). Update on depression in pregnancy. *Female Patient, 35*(6), 27.

Kinnersley, P. & Edwards, A. (2008). Complaints against doctors. *British Medical Journal, 336*(7649), 841–2.

Levinson, W. (2011). Patient-centred communication: A sophisticated procedure. *BMJ Quality & Safety, 20*(10), 823–5.

Levinson, W., Lesser, C. & Epstein, R. (2010). Developing physician communication skills for patient-centered care. *Health Affairs, 29*(7), 1310–18.

Linehan, M. (1993). *Cognitive-Behavioral Treatment of Borderline Personality Disorder*. New York: Guilford Press.

Locke, R., Stefano, M., Koster, A., Taylor, B. & Greenspan, J. (2011). Optimizing patient/caregiver satisfaction through quality of communication in the pediatric emergency department. *Pediatric Emergency Care, 27*(11), 1016–21.

Lustig, M. (2008). Humanising medical practice: The role of empathy. *Medical Journal of Australia, 188*(4), 263–4.

Lyth, G. (2000). Clinical supervision: A concept analysis. *Journal of Advanced Nursing, 31*(3), 722–9.

Richardson, C., Percy, M. & Hughes, J. (2015). Nursing therapeutics: Teaching student nurses care, compassion and empathy. *Nurse Education Today, 35*(5), e1–e5. doi: 10.1016/j.nedt.2015.01.016

Rosenstein, A. (2009). Disruptive behaviour and its impact on communication efficiency and patient care. *Journal of Communication in Healthcare, 2*(4), 328–40.

Ross, H. J. (2014). *Everyday Bias: Identifying and Navigating Unconscious Judgments in Our Daily Lives*. United Kingdom: Rowman & Littlefield.

Rungby, J. & Brock, B. (2010). What can we do to improve adherence in patients with diabetes? In A. Barnett (Ed.), *Clinical Challenges in Diabetes* (pp. 155–61). Oxford: Atlas Medical Publishing Ltd.

Salt, E., Rowles, G. & Reed, D. (2012). Patients' perception of quality patient–provider communication. *Orthopaedic Nursing, 31*(3), 169–76.

Schrooten, I., & de Jong, M. D. T. (2017). If you could read my mind: The role of healthcare providers' empathic and communicative competencies in clients' satisfaction with consultations. *Health Communication, 32*(1), 111–18. doi:10.1080/10410236.2015.1110002

Sonneman, U. (1954). *Existence and Therapy: An Introduction to Phenomenological Psychology and Existential Analysis*. New York: Grune & Stratton.

Wheeler, M. S., Arnkoff, D. B. & Glass, C. R. (2017). The neuroscience of mindfulness: How mindfulness alters the brain and facilitates emotion regulation. *Mindfulness, 8*(6), 1471–87. doi:10.1007/s12671-017-0742-x

White, E. & Winstanley, J. (2011). Clinical supervision for mental health professionals: The evidence base. *Social Work & Social Sciences Review, 14*(3), 73–90.

Wolfe, N. L. (2016). Forget everything you thought you knew: How your assumptions are impacting the health outcomes of your patients. *Australian Medical Students Journal, 7*(2), 60–2. Accessed May 2018 at: <http://www.amsj.org/archives/5550>.

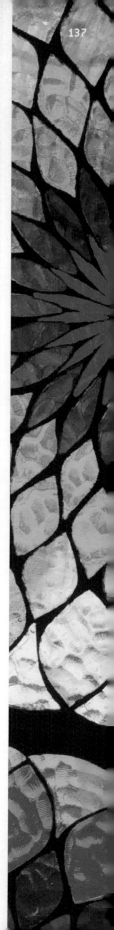

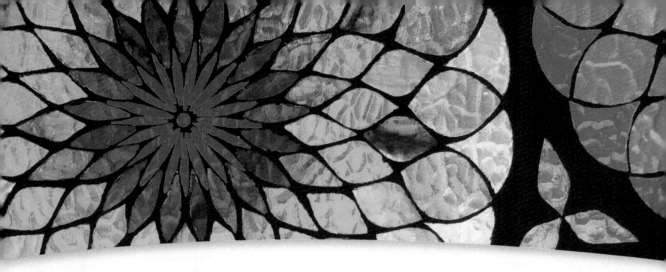

CHAPTER 12

COMMUNICATING WITH OLDER PEOPLE

Karen Watson   Joanne Lewis   Deborah Parker

LEARNING OUTCOMES

Chapter 12 will enable you to:

- discuss why older people are at increased risk of adverse events
- outline how delirium and dementia can lead to a loss of communicative ability
- engage in the critical conversations necessary to enhance high-quality, safe and person-centred care for older people
- discuss the importance of interprofessional communication and collaboration when caring for older people
- reflect on your capacity to communicate with older people in ways that promote safety and wellbeing.

KEY CONCEPTS

ageism | risk factors | vulnerability | preventable adverse events | person-centred care

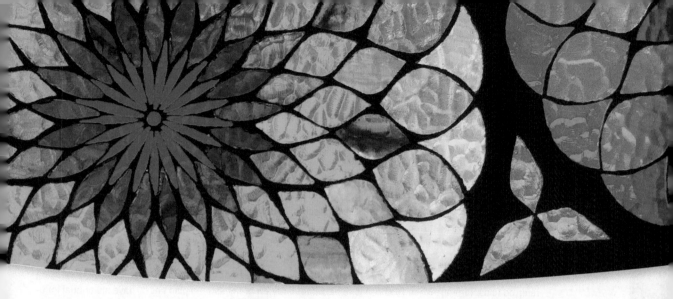

Morris says to his doctor, 'My right knee hurts.'

'How old are you now, Morris?' asks the doctor.

'I'm 101,' he replies.

'Well, what do you expect at your age?'

Morris pauses for a second, then rises in anger.

'The problem with that, Doc, is that my left knee

is also 101, and it doesn't hurt at all!'

(Robert N. Butler, MD, Founding Director, National Institute on Aging; President, International Longevity Centre)

INTRODUCTION

This chapter invites you to think about the 'critical conversations' needed to ensure safe and effective care of older people across contexts and settings. Although many older Australians are healthy and have a rich range of personal skills, knowledge, experiences and abilities that contribute to their wellbeing (Read & Maslin-Prothero, 2011), as people age their healthcare needs become more complex (Australian Institute of Health and Welfare, 2016). One of our key roles as healthcare professionals is to seek to understand the needs, perspectives and values of older people, as this can enhance communication and reduce the incidence of adverse events. Unfortunately, factors that impact on the health and wellbeing of older people are too often overlooked or dismissed (Liu et al., 2012).

Of particular concern is that ageist attitudes pose significant barriers to person-centred communication (Storlie, 2015) and are negative predictors of active ageing (Fernandez-Ballesteros et al., 2017). Additionally, the stress associated with negative stereotypes of ageism may increase the risk of morbidity and mortality (Allen, 2016). These factors, coupled with the older person's stoicism and perception that they are a burden to others (Australian Human Rights Commission, 2013), may conspire against the provision of safe and effective care for older people. For these reasons, effective conversations with older people and among healthcare professionals about their care needs are critical.

The beliefs and negative stereotypes held in relation to older people can interfere with communication. The perception that all older people have memory problems, are deaf or are unable to learn, process information or comprehend is incorrect and may lead to miscommunication and inappropriate decision making (Touhy, 2010).

THOMAS' STORY

Thomas is a 79-year-old man who lives alone in his own home. He has history of adult onset asthma and osteo-arthritis. Thomas walks every day and has recently begun swimming three times a week, as he finds this helps with his asthma and osteoarthritic pain.

Hearing loss has become an increasing issue for Thomas. He is having difficulty socialising as much as he once did due to his inability to follow conversations, particularly when a number of people are talking and there is background noise. He hasn't mentioned his concerns about his hearing to his daughter Susan or son Malcom, as he doesn't wish to concern them and is not sure that anything can be done to improve hearing loss associated with old age. Susan has become increasingly concerned about her father, as she has noticed that he responds inappropriately to her questions at times and has become more and more withdrawn over the last few months.

Thomas has been seeing the same GP for nearly 10 years but, although he likes and trusts him, he does not like the way that he calls him 'young Tommy boy', as he finds this condescending and has never liked being referred to as 'Tommy'. When Thomas visits his GP for a review of his asthma plan and to have his annual influenza vaccination, he mentions his hearing issues. His GP gives Thomas details for an audiometry clinic and states that it is common for people his age to lose their hearing. Thomas doesn't make an appointment to attend the clinic, as he believes from his conversation with his GP that nothing can be done to improve his hearing.

Susan and Malcom visit Thomas the following week and enquire how his visit to the GP went. Thomas states that he was told he was in good health for someone his age. Susan raises concerns with her father that she thinks there might be some problems with his comprehension, and maybe his memory, as she has noticed he appears confused in conversation at times and somewhat withdrawn. Thomas explains that this is probably because his hearing is becoming more difficult and that this is to be expected in old age.

The following day Thomas attends his regular bowls club where he has lunch with friends. Talking to his friends he discovers that others in the group had been for hearing checks and they encourage Thomas to book in. Thomas makes an appointment for an audiometry assessment the following day.

Why are older people at increased risk of adverse events?

As noted in previous chapters, much of the literature relating to communication and patient safety focuses on reportable events, including medication errors, absence of consent for procedures, and surgical errors (Watkin et al., 2012). Moreover, clinical complexity for disease burden and co-morbidity, reduced functional ability and poor care are considered causative factors contributing to adverse events (Long et al., 2013). Older people often feature in these events, since up to 70 per cent of hospitalised patients are older people with chronic, complex conditions (Schnitker et al., 2011). Indeed, up to 8.6 per cent of people over the age of 70 experience a reported adverse event while in hospital (Watkin et al., 2012). Older people also experience adverse events in the community, particularly in relation to errors with medication administration that often result in admission to hospital (Robinson, Howie-Esquivel & Vlahov, 2012).

Older people tend to seek healthcare advice only when they are concerned, and at this time they are often fearful and apprehensive. When, where and how they seek advice depends on critical conversations with a number of people, including family members, friends and healthcare professionals. Thomas' story reminds us that older people often remain socially and physically active in older age and wish to be treated respectfully. It demonstrates the importance of healthcare providers being knowledgeable about ageing and mindful of how ageist attitudes can influence their communication with older people. It is also important to note that older people often use the Internet to support healthcare decision making and to confirm information received from healthcare professionals.

Vulnerable older people are more likely to experience difficulty communicating. This group of people includes those who are frail (Gilleard & Higgs, 2011; Read & Maslin-Prothero, 2011), those who are cognitively impaired (Stanyon et al., 2018), those who have limited social support and live alone (Palmer, Newsom & Rook, 2016), and those being transferred between points of care such

See Eileen Poole's story to explore the relationship between communication and medication safety in community settings: <http://www.ipeforqum.com.au/modules/>.

as residential aged care facilities (RACFs) and hospital emergency departments (ED) (Rustad et al., 2016). Health literacy, which was outlined in Chapter 2, is at its lowest in the older population with poor health (MacLeod et al., 2017). Limited health literacy impedes the person's ability to understand and utilise healthcare information. This requires healthcare professionals to ensure that their communication is person-centred and individualised to the older person's level of health literacy (Medlock et al., 2015).

Box 12.1 presents some of the factors that can increase vulnerability in older people.

BOX 12.1   Factors that place older people at risk of an adverse event

Social changes, such as:

- isolation and lack of family contact
- loss of loved ones
- disruption to living arrangements.

Normal ageing physiology and age-related changes, including:

- sensory changes
- functional capacity.

Health and wellbeing, including:

- decreased activity levels
- absence/presence of disease.

Others:

- medication use/polypharmacy
- admission to hospital
- the need for long-term care
- low levels of health literacy
- being from a culturally and linguistically diverse background.

MR ALI'S STORY

Mr Ali is an 82-year-old who was transferred from a residential aged care facility to the emergency department (ED) via ambulance at 3 am. The ambulance officer informs the ED staff that Mr Ali has been transferred because of severe pain, possibly due to constipation; he also appears to be disoriented, which is believed to be caused by the pain and the time of day. The ED staff members are unhappy about the time of transfer and the reason. Following an initial assessment and examination, Mr Ali was given an enema, which had an immediate effect and he was discharged back to the residential aged care facility at 5:30 am the same day. At 5 pm that evening, Mr Ali re-presented to the ED confused, disoriented and extremely agitated. He was diagnosed with delirium.

Following examination and routine urinary analysis, Mr Ali was found to have a urinary tract infection and was started on oral antibiotics.

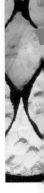

Delirium in older people

Delirium is an acute confusional state that 'develops over a short period of time (usually hours to days) and tends to fluctuate during the course of the day' (American Psychiatric Association, 2013). Delirium is:

- frequently preventable
- a common presentation during acute illness
- a medical emergency that is often undetected

- frequently not recognised or misdiagnosed
- falsely attributed to dementia or depression
- described by older people as terrifying (Australian Commission on Safety and Quality in Health, 2016; Inouye, Westendorp & Saczynski, 2014).

The prevalence of delirium in Australia ranges from 50 per cent for hospitalised older people up to 80 per cent for older people admitted to intensive care units (Traynor, Burns & Britten, 2016; Travers et al., 2013). Delirium is associated with:

- a range of undesirable consequences (see Box 12.2)
- sudden changes in 'reality', giving rise to fear, anxiety, anger and isolation
- loneliness, hopelessness and depression (Traynor et al., 2016; Partridge et al., 2012).

BOX 12.2 Consequences of delirium in older people

- Falls
- Pressure areas
- Institutionalisation
- Longer stays in hospital
- Increased mortality up to 12 months after hospital admission
- Death

Source: Traynor et al., 2016; Inouye et al., 2014.

Dementia in older people

Delirium is often confused with dementia; however, the two conditions differ both in causation and in manifestations. 'Dementia' is an umbrella term for a variety of progressive brain diseases that are categorised by loss of core abilities, including communication skills. More than 400 000 people in Australia live with dementia and it is the second leading cause of death nationally (Dementia Australia, 2018). One in four people with dementia are hospitalised each year (Alzheimer's Australia, 2014), with associated complications or co-morbidities. Of particular concern is the poorer health outcomes connected with the hospitalisation of people with cognitive impairment in comparison to other older people (Butcher, 2018).

The progressive loss of communicative ability in people with dementia is associated with memory loss, difficulty in expressing language and deficits in reasoning ability (Mendes & Palmer, 2018), and is a contributing factor in the inequity of care outcomes for hospitalised patients (Alzheimer's Australia, 2014). When healthcare professionals are not knowledgeable about dementia, miscommunication frequently occurs. This can frustrate the person with dementia and result in behavioural outbursts or noncompliance. Challenges to communication can also lead to misdiagnosis of symptoms, with hospital-acquired delirium often remaining undetected in this population (Butcher, 2018). Dementia Australia (2018) emphasises the importance of all healthcare professionals being knowledgeable about dementia so that they can communicate more effectively and provide safe patient care in all healthcare settings.

Key principles for effectively communicating with people with dementia include:

- providing an appropriate introduction (see Chapter 2)
- engaging empathically with patients/residents
- maintaining eye contact

- remaining composed
- involving family and carers
- limiting the number of choices presented
- use of appropriate body language
- use of short simple sentences to facilitate comprehension and encourage participation in healthcare decisions (Mendes & Palmer, 2018).

Critical questions for critical conversations

Critical conversations with older people, and particularly those living with dementia or experiencing delirium, are dependent on healthcare professionals asking the right questions, at the right time and with the right people. Box 12.3 presents a framework of questions that can be used both to reflect on our personal and professional values about older people, and to enhance communication with and about older people.

BOX 12.3   Framework of critical questions for critical conversations

For each clinician

- Are my beliefs, actions and behaviours consistent with valuing older people?
- How do the philosophies, theories, codes and standards of my profession guide my communication with older people and their families?
- Is my knowledge current, and sufficient to comprehensively assess, communicate with and minimise risk to the older person?
- Are there cognitive issues for the person such as delirium or dementia that I should consider?
- Are the goals of care directed by the patient and his/her family or by the health professionals?
- How can I improve the care I provide to older people?

With older people, their families and carers

- What is this older person's goal?
- What matters to this older person?
- What are the older person's wishes/preferences for care?
- What is the older person's understanding, perspective and experience of the situation?
- What are the family members' needs or concerns about the older person?

In interprofessional teams

- How is the individual and combined knowledge of healthcare professionals used to enhance the care of older people?
- How does the interprofessional team communicate effectively and efficiently among themselves and with other teams across contexts and settings?
- Within the team, is there awareness of each professional's scope of practice, skills, knowledge, responsibility and accountability?
- Does the team honour the rights of older people as both people and patients?
- What can the team do differently or better?
- Does the team's attitudes and behaviours convey respect to older people, their carers, team members and volunteers?

Applying the framework of questions to Mr Ali

While Thomas's situation was managed in the community, Mr Ali's situation was more challenging and required that he be transferred to the ED. The complexity of Mr Ali's situation required engagement of a range of healthcare professionals working across settings: residential care, primary care and the ED. Following Mr Ali's discharge and in order to improve the quality of care provided to other patients in the future, the ED staff used his experience as a stimulus to discuss the 'Framework of critical questions for critical conversations' outlined in Box 12.3. This enabled them to have critical conversations about care processes and the quality and safety of older people in the ED. The conversations revealed the following:

■ There was a perception among some staff that Mr Ali's transfer to the ED was not warranted, nor was the timing of the transfer appropriate. It is likely that assumptions were made about Mr Ali's constipation, pain and disorientation and that staff did not check these assumptions. For example, staff did not appear to look for other factors related to Mr Ali's presentation but instead assumed that he would have communication difficulties because of his age and assumed ethnic background.

■ Although an interprofessional team approach mandates communication across and within the team, the ED staff did not speak directly with the carers in the residential setting or with Mr Ali's family.

■ In the absence of critical questions and communication with carers and family members, important elements of Mr Ali's situation at the initial presentation were missed and were not linked to the possibility of delirium or the need to take active steps to prevent delirium. That he had an undiagnosed infection, was usually cognitively alert, may have had fluctuating levels of cognition associated with the constipation and/or the infection, and his disorientation were all cues to the potential for delirium.

■ In the absence of communication with the patient or family members, all treatment and care was directed by the healthcare professionals. However, a person-centred approach mandates that staff ask, 'What matters to Mr Ali?' Healthcare professionals also need to be aware of possible preconceptions or assumptions as they need to be tested or 'checked out' by attending to critical questions/conversations.

The healthcare professionals who participated in conversations about Mr Ali's situation identified a number of change initiatives, such as:

■ a review of information provided by the ED to ensure that the font size in documents was easily read, clear and succinct for older people and their carers

■ enhanced provision and documentation of supportive care aimed at preventing delirium, provided in partnership with older people and their carers

■ strategies to promote person-centred care

■ strategies to promote attitudinal change in the ED staff (e.g. promoting delirium- prevention activities as essential care, not simply 'giving old people a cup of tea')

■ regular meetings between ED staff and staff of residential care facilities.

Reflection on practices has since led the health professionals in the ED to:

■ have 'critical conversations' with each other about older people

■ have 'critical conversations' across healthcare settings about concerns

■ facilitate members of the healthcare team to think about older people positively and to appreciate that patient behaviours are a type of non-verbal communication

■ align the service to the older person's goals for health and care

■ develop interprofessional team communication processes to focus on detection and prevention of delirium in older people

■ improve care processes and systems to ensure that critical conversations occur across contexts and that these conversations are documented so that all staff are aware of the needs of the older person.

Most importantly, these health professionals have reinvigorated their commitment to person-centred care. They are re-learning to ask, 'What matters to you?', as well as 'What is the matter?' (Barry & Edgman-Levitan, 2012, p. 781).

Interprofessional communication and collaboration when caring for older people

When caring for older people and ensuring their safety, healthcare professionals need to apply evidence-based knowledge (Marcum, Vande-Griend & Linnebur, 2012), and use effective assessment and communication skills (Manias, 2012). Stereotyping older people can prevent the development of effective therapeutic relationships with older patients (Australian Human Rights Commission, 2013). Ageist attitudes also affect the ability to have meaningful conversations with older people, yet healthcare professionals' resistance to and lack of interest in working with older people continues to be reported in the literature (Eymard & Douglas, 2012).

As healthcare professionals, we all have a responsibility to ensure that our behaviours meet the standards and expectations of our profession. We are also required to ensure that our colleagues practise professionally. With this in mind, there may be times when we need to have a conversation with others about their approaches and practices when relating to and caring for older people.

The ways in which different professional groups interact to achieve person-centred care is a key factor in reducing adverse events (Prouty et al., 2016; Warh et al., 2013). Building collaborative approaches to service delivery that crosses the health and social care continuum is imperative, particularly for vulnerable populations such as older people (Hickman, Rolley & Davidson, 2010; Brown & Oliver-Baxter, 2016). The skills of the interprofessional healthcare team in the management of complex patient-care events are enhanced through collaboration, mutual respect and effective communication (Brown & Oliver-Baxter, 2016; Harris et al., 2016). However, in order to enhance patient/client/resident outcomes, staff need to work in ways that are person-centred rather than profession-centric (Hickman et al., 2010) (also see Chapter 6).

Most healthcare professionals have undertaken independent preparatory education, which reinforces preconceived professional roles and boundaries based on learned culture, beliefs and cognitive approaches (Henderson et al., 2013). Unfortunately, this often results in a poor understanding of each other's roles, leading to stress, anxiety, conflict and, at times, ineffective and unsafe healthcare delivery. By comparison, interprofessional teams that engage in collegial and respectful interactions and negotiations have a positive impact on patient outcomes and staff satisfaction.

Interprofessional groups work within and across care settings. Figure 12.1 identifies the transition points in people's healthcare experiences where conversations and communication between older people, their carers and healthcare providers in homes, primary care, residential aged care and hospitals are critical in order to anticipate and prevent adverse events. Partnership working, where interprofessional teams work with services external to the healthcare setting (such as voluntary and community sector organisations), helps to provide older people and their carers with choice regarding the provision of services (Brown & Oliver-Baxter, 2016; Hickman et al., 2010; Maslin-Prothero & Finney, 2011).

Critical conversations and reflections should occur:

• with each clinician
• with older people, their families and carers
• in the interprofessional team, within and across care settings.

FIGURE 12.1

Categories of health need and points of transition for older people

Source: Health Continuum, from Queensland Health, Queensland Health Guide to Health Service Planning, 2010, page 12.

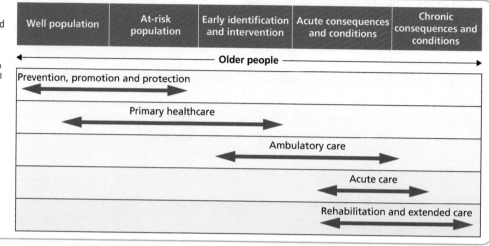

Well population	At-risk population	Early identification and intervention	Acute consequences and conditions	Chronic consequences and conditions

── Older people ──

Prevention, promotion and protection ←──→

Primary healthcare ←──────→

Ambulatory care ←──────→

Acute care ←──→

Rehabilitation and extended care ←──→

Conclusion

Communication with older people is often poor because of the attitudes, perceptions, beliefs, values and knowledge of healthcare professionals rather than because of deficits in older people themselves. Improved care and reduced risk requires a range of critical conversations at many levels. The role of healthcare professionals is to both communicate effectively with older people and their families/carers, and to work collaboratively with other healthcare providers to ensure that the needs, values and preferences of the older person are respected and upheld.

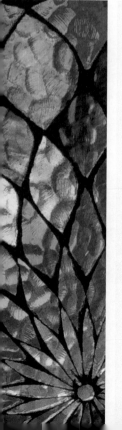

Critical thinking activity

Ida was an 86-year-old woman admitted to hospital with heart failure. Her doctors noted that she had iron deficiency anaemia and referred her to Dr James, the gastroenterologist on call. When Dr James arrived on the ward, some of the staff expressed their concern about Ida's anaemia and felt that it was contributing to her breathlessness and affecting her quality of life. They indicated that they felt Ida needed immediate investigation and treatment of her anaemia.

Dr James went to visit Ida. She explained to Ida the common causes of anaemia in older people, described the ways of investigating the anaemia and told her how anaemia could be affecting her wellbeing. Dr James also told Ida that she could arrange very quickly for an initial series of investigations to see what was happening.

Ida understood the information provided by Dr James and asked questions about her options. She then sat quietly for a few moments contemplating what she should do. When Dr James asked Ida what she would like and what mattered to her, Ida said that she had other issues to worry about at the moment. She would commence iron therapy but did not want the anaemia investigated right now. She agreed to see the gastroenterologist in the outpatient department in three months. Ida said what mattered most to her at this time was having her symptoms managed so that she was able to go on the two-month trip with her family that she had been planning for some time.

When Dr James told the staff about Ida's decision, one of them suggested that Ida's family should be consulted about her care. Dr James clarified with the staff member that Ida would share information with her family as she wished, and reminded the staff that Ida was a competent adult who could exercise informed choices about her healthcare.

1   Think about the issues that this situation raises for healthcare professionals who want to ensure safe and quality care for older people.

2   Reflect on how having critical conversations with older people recognises their rights and abilities, maintains the ideals of person-centred care and upholds professional and legal expectations.

3   Imagine that you are an older person. What difference is there between being asked 'What is the matter with you?' and 'What matters to you?'

Teaching and assessment activities

1   Watch *Barbara, the whole story* at the following link and reflect on the experience of living with dementia:

<https://youtu.be/DtA2sMAjU_Y>

Discuss the strategies and approaches that healthcare professionals could have used to provide person-centred care, and to communicate more effectively with Barbara and other people with dementia.

2   The following scenario can be role played with six students who take on the these roles:

- John, a man with moderate dementia
- Two nursing staff members
- Three boisterous residents in the dining room.

John wakes up to the noise of a nurse coming into his room. His bedroom light is switched on and the curtains pulled back. The nurse says, 'It's time to get up, John' and then leaves the room.

John feels confused. He doesn't know where he is and suddenly feels very frightened. He gets up and realises that he has soiled his pants. He tries to clean it up but makes a bigger mess.

The nurse returns to John's room and sighs. John tries to apologise but he has difficulty with his speech; he knows what he wants to say but can't find the right words out. The unit is short staffed this morning. The nurse quickly washes John and takes him down to breakfast providing little opportunity for him to participate in his care.

John is taken to the busy dining room and left in a chair. The breakfast room is loud with residents arguing over the breakfast menu and someone calling out for more juice.

a.   Reflect on how John might be feeling.

b.   Have there been opportunities for him to communicate his needs?

c.   Conduct the role play again, this time embedding some of the techniques from this chapter to facilitate effective communication.

Further reading

Barry, M. & Edgman-Levitan, S. (2012). Shared decision-making: The pinnacle of patient-centered care. *New England Journal of Medicine, 366*(9), 780–1.

Day, J., Higgins, I. & Keatinge, D. (2011). Orientation strategies during delirium: Are they helpful? *Journal of Clinical Nursing, 20*, 3285–94.

Higgins I. (2007). Issues in older person nursing. *Contemporary Nurse Journal, 26*(2), 161–3.

Harper, D. & McMillan, M. (2007). Towards innovation: The development of a person-centred model of care for older people in acute care. *Contemporary Nurse Journal, 26*(2), 164–76.

Phillipson, L., Goodenough, B., Reis, S. & Fleming, R. (2016). Applying knowledge translation concepts and strategies in dementia care education for health professionals: Recommendations from a narrative literature review. *Journal of Continuing Education in Health Practitioners, 36*(1), 74–81.

Web resources

Shared decision making
<https://www1.health.nsw.gov.au/pds/ActivePDSDocuments/GL2005_057.pdf>

Delirium guidelines and care pathways
<https://www.aci.health.nsw.gov.au/chops>
<http://www.health.gov.au/internet/publications/publishing.nsf/Content/delirium-care-pathways-toc>

Dementia communication
<https://www.dementia.org.au/national/support-and-services/carers/managing-changes-in-communication>

Rights of older people
Older Persons Advocacy Network (OPEN): <http://www.opan.com.au/>

Come into my world, come walk with me—person-centred care for a person with dementia
<nursing.flinders.edu.au/comeintomyworld/media/video.php?video=1>

References

Allen, J. (2016). Ageism as a risk factor for chronic disease. *The Gerontologist, 56*(4), 610–14.

Alzheimer's Australia. (2014). *Dementia Care in the Acute Hospital Setting: Issues and Strategies.* (Paper 40).

American Psychiatric Association. (2013). *Diagnostic and Statistical Manual of Psychiatric Disorders* (5th) (DSM-V). Washington: APA.

Australian Commission on Safety and Quality in Health Care. (2016). *Indicator Specification: Delirium Clinical Care Standard.* Sydney: ACSQHC

Australian Human Rights Commission. (2013). *Fact or Fiction Stereotypes of Older Australians.* (Research report). Sydney.

Australian Institute of Health and Welfare. (2016). *Australia's Health 2016.* Australia's health series no. 15. Cat. no. AUS 199. Canberra: AIHW.

Barry, M. & Edgman-Levitan, S. (2012). Shared decision making: The pinnacle of patient-centered care. *New England Journal of Medicine, 366*(9), 780–1.

Brown, L & Oliver-Baxter, J. (2016). Six elements of integrated primary healthcare. *Australian Family Physician, 45*(3), 139.

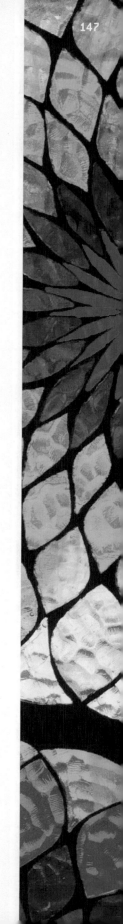

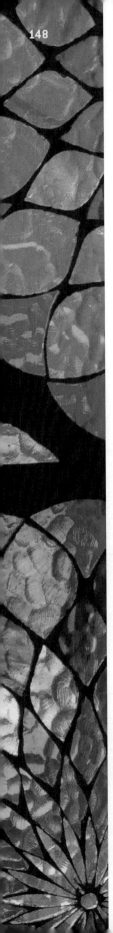

Butcher, L. (2018). Caring for patients with dementia in the acute care setting. *British Journal of Nursing*, *27*(7), 358–62.

Dementia Australia™. (2018). *Key Facts and Statistics*. Accessed January 2019 at <https://www.dementia.org.au/statistics>.

Eymard, A. & Douglas, D. (2012). Ageism among health care providers and interventions to improve their attitudes toward older adults: An integrative review. *Journal of Gerontological Nursing, 38*(5), 26–35.

Fernandez-Ballesteros, R., Olmos, R., Santacreu, M., Bustillos, A.,Molina, M. A. (2017). The role of perceived discrimination on active ageing. *Archives of Gerontology and Geriatrics, 71,* 14–20.

Gilleard, C. & Higgs, P. (2011). Frailty, disability and old age: A re-appraisal. *Health, 15*(5), 475–90.

Harris, M., Advocat, J., Crabtree, B., Levesque, J., Miller, W., Gunn, J., … Russell, G. M. (2016). Interprofessional teamwork innovations for primary health care practices and practitioners: Evidence from comparison of reform in three countries. *Journal of Multidisciplinary Healthcare, 9,* 35–46.

Henderson, J., Koehne, K., Verrall, C., Gebbie, K. & Fuller, J. (2013). How is primary health care conceptualized in nursing in Australia? A review of the literature. *Health and Social Care in the Community, 22*(4), 337–51.

Hickman, L., Rolley. J. & Davison, P. (2010). Can principles of the chronic care model be used to improve care of the older person in the acute care sector? *Collegian, 17*(2), 63–9.

Inouye, S., Westendorp, R. & Saczynski, J. (2014). Delirium in elderly people. *The Lancet, 383,* 911–22.

Liu, Y., While, A., Norman, I., & Ye, W. (2012). Health professionals attitudes towards older people and older patients: A systematic review. *Journal of Interprofessional Care, 26,* 397–409.

Long, S. J., Brown, K. F., Ames, D. & Vincent C. (2013). What is known about adverse events in older medical hospital patients? A systematic review of the literature. *International Journal for Quality in Health Care, 25*(5), 542–54.

MacLeod, S., Musich, S., Gulyas, S., Cheng, Y., Tkatch, R., Cemplin, D., … Yeh, C. (2017). The impact of inadequate health literacy on patient satisfaction, healthcare utilizations, and expenditures among older adults. *Geriatric Nursing, 38*(4), 334–41.

Manias, E. (2012). Complexities of pain assessment and management in hospitalised older people: A qualitative observation and interview study. *International Journal of Nursing Studies, 49*(10), 1243–54.

Marcum, Z., Vande-Griend, J. & Linnebur, S. (2012). FDA drug safety communications: A narrative review and clinical considerations for older adults. *American Journal of Geriatric Pharmacotherapy, 10*(4), 264–71.

Maslin-Prothero, S. & Finney, A. (2011). Long term conditions. In P. Linsley, R. Kane & S. Owen (eds), *Nursing and Public Health*. Oxford: Oxford University Press.

Medlock, S., Eslami, S., Askari, M., Arts, D. L., Sent, D., de Rooij, S. E. & Abu-Hanna, A. (2015). Health information–seeking behavior of seniors who use the Internet: A survey. *Journal of Medical Internet Research, 17*(1).

Mendes, A. & Palmer, S. (2018). Communicating effectively with a person living with dementia. *British Journal of Nursing, 27*(2), 101.

Palmer, A., Newsom, J. & Rook, K. (2016). How does difficulty communicating affect the social relationships of older adults? An exploration using data from a national survey. *Journal of Communication Disorders, 62,* 131–46.

Partidge, J., Martin, F., Harari, D. & Dhesi, J. (2013). The delirium experience: What is the effect on patients, relatives and staff and what can be done to modify this? *International Journal of Geriatric Psychiatry, 28,* 804–12.

Prouty, C., Mazor, K., Greene, S., Roblin, D., Firneno, C., Lemay, C., Robinsons, B. & Gallagher, T. (2014). Providers' perceptions of communication breakdowns in cancer care. *Journal of General Internal Medicine, 29*(8), 1122–30.

Read, S. & Maslin-Prothero, S. (2011). The involvement of users and carers in health and social research: The realities of inclusion and engagement. *Qualitative Health Research,* 21 May, 704–13.

Robinson, S., Howie-Esquivel, J. & Vlahov, D. (2012). Readmission risk factors after hospital discharge among the elderly. *Population Health Management, 15*(6), 338–51.

Rustad, E., Furnes, B., Cronfalk, B. & Dysvik, E. (2016). Older patients' experiences during care transition. *Dovepress, 10,* 769–79.

Schnitker, L., Martin-Khan, M., Beattie, E. & Gray, L. (2011). Negative health outcomes and adverse events in older people attending emergency departments: A systematic review. *Australasian Emergency Nursing Journal, 14*(3), 141–62.

Stanyon, M., Griffiths, A., Thomas, S. & Gordon, A. (2016). The facilitators of communication with people with dementia in a care setting: An interview study with healthcare workers. *Age and Ageing, 45*(1), 164–70.

Storlie, T. (2015). Person-centred communication: Ageism—the core problem. In T. Storlie, *Person-Centred Communication with Older Adults: The Professional Providers Guide* (pp. 73–86). London, UK: Academic Press, Elsevier.

Touhy, T. (2010). Communicating with elders. In T. Toughy & K. Jett (Eds), *Ebersole and Hess's Gerontological Nursing Healthy Aging* (pp. 25–47). St Louise, MO: Mosby Elsevier.

Travers, C., Byrne, J., Pachana, N., Klien, K. & Gray, L. (2013). Delirium in Australian Hospitals: A prospective study. *Current Gerontology and Geriatric Research*, Volume 2013 (Article ID 284780), 8 pages.

Traynor, V., Burns, P. & Britten, N. (2016). Developing the delirium care pathways. *Journal of Research in Nursing, 21*(8), 582–96. doi: 10.1177/1744987116661377

Wahr, J., Prager, R., Abernathy, J., Martinez, E., Salas, E., Seifert, P., … Nussmeier, N. A. (2013). Patient safety in the cardiac operating room: Human factors and teamwork. *Circulation, 128*(10), 1139–69.

Watkin, L., Blanchard, M., Tookman, A. & Sampson, E. (2012). Prospective cohort study of adverse events in older people admitted to the acute general hospital: Risk factors and the impact of dementia. *International Journal of Geriatric Psychiatry, 27*(1), 76–82.

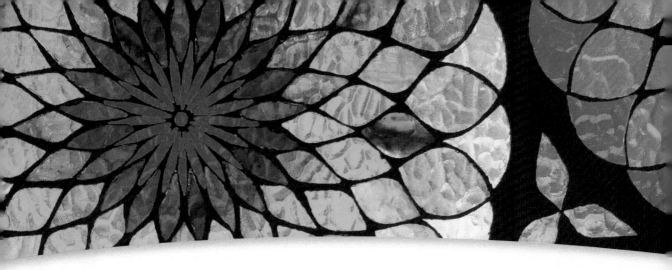

COMMUNICATING WITH CHILDREN AND FAMILIES

Jonathan Mould

LEARNING OUTCOMES

Chapter 13 will enable you to:

- discuss different communication techniques used with children and families
- explain why effective communication is paramount in meeting the healthcare needs of children and their families
- demonstrate an understanding of the relationship between effective communication and safety in paediatric settings
- outline the skills required to effectively communicate with children of all ages and stages of development
- identify different communication techniques needed at each developmental stage
- discuss the importance of families when communicating with children and young people.

KEY CONCEPTS

developmentally appropriate language | family-centred care

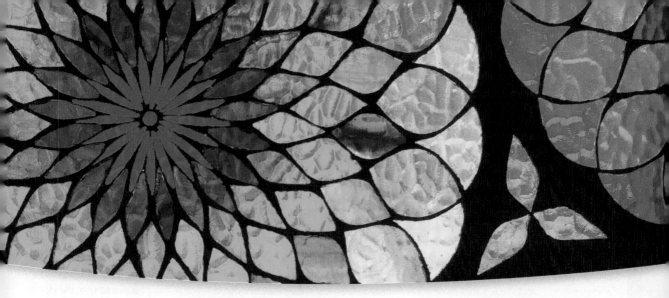

> Children are not little adults.
>
> (World Health Organization, 2008)

INTRODUCTION

There are many psychological and social differences between children and adults. It is essential to understand these differences in order to communicate with children and their families because, in paediatrics, effective communication is a fundamental element in safe and quality healthcare (Healy & Dugdale, 2009; Glasper, Coad & Richardson, 2015).

Because of the challenges presented when children require healthcare, paediatric experts argue that every conversation with children and their families is critical. Owens (2012) asserts that the emotional care of children is as important as their physical care. If children's emotional care is neglected, there is potential for them to experience long-term emotional harm (Kennardy, 2016).

When children are treated like small adults in healthcare settings, it results in the quality of care being compromised (Royal Australasian College of Physicians [RACP], 2008). Due to their immature emotions, their lack of understanding of concepts and their inability to communicate thoroughly, children cannot always verbalise their concerns if something seems incorrect. They cannot easily understand why they need healthcare and some preschool children may view a hospitalisation as punishment (Rokach, 2016). Hence, accurate communication with children and families is vitally important (Potts & Mandleco, 2012). If we fail to understand how children communicate and do not recognise parental[1] concerns, safety is compromised, and this can have serious outcomes.

---

1 Throughout this chapter the term 'parent' is used as the term for a child's main caregiver.

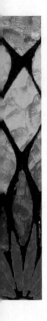

ROSIE'S STORY

Parents are similar to customers—they are usually right; thus, ignoring parental concerns can have grave consequences.

Three-year-old Rosie developed a high fever for four days following cold-like symptoms. Her mother, who is a healthcare professional, took her to the local hospital after Rosie vomited thick mucous. She was sent home with the instructions to give Rosie regular fluids and analgesia. Rosie's mother returned the next day as her daughter was no better and appeared to be in severe respiratory distress. Rosie was ordered a chest X-ray, which did not reveal anything abnormal. Consequently, she was sent home again and her mother was given the same instructions. Rosie's mother remembers the doctor and nurse being dismissive and saying that Rosie would be fine as it was 'just a cold'. As Rosie's mother was a healthcare professional, they made her feel as though she had overreacted.

Rosie's mother continued to be concerned, so she took her to the family doctor (GP) who referred them back to the hospital. Rosie was transferred to the paediatric intensive care unit (PICU) due to severe respiratory distress and she required mechanical ventilation following a diagnosis of influenza type A. Rosie recovered from the influenza and was discharged home. Her mother's perspective is that the initial hospital staff did not do any basic tests and that her concerns were ignored. Although Rosie's mother is unsure whether earlier interventions would have prevented the PICU admission, she felt extremely let down by all of the staff during her first two visits to hospital.

SOMETHING TO THINK ABOUT

Some illnesses do not fully manifest for several hours and therefore it is not unusual for children to be brought to hospital, examined and then sent home. Later, the symptoms may become much worse. For example, meningococcal septicaemia sometimes starts with a low-grade fever and a blanching rash. In some cases, by the time the telltale non-blanching rash has developed, a child may be near to death. Childhood diseases are not always easy to detect or treat, and listening to the child's parents is critical as they are best placed to report on changes from normal and impending clinical deterioration.

Listening to parents

Rosie's case highlights the importance of listening to parents, especially when they continue to be concerned. Rosie's mother felt that she was not listened to. The GP later told her that, in the discharge letter, the emergency department (ED) doctor had diagnosed Rosie with gastroenteritis, but this was never mentioned and nor were there any symptoms other than the mucous vomit. Ignoring parental concerns is perilous because in almost all cases parents know their child best, and children, especially young children, rely on parents to communicate their health needs. When adults need healthcare, they can usually tell healthcare professionals if they think something is amiss. Young children cannot do this as their perception of self and their language skills may not be developed enough to identify and/or acknowledge a change in their health status. We need to understand that children's physical and emotional development, and their limited communication skills, make them very vulnerable when needing healthcare. That is why parental presence is fundamental to children's wellbeing. This reliance on adults to interpret symptoms and feelings is particularly important for infants, toddlers and preschoolers.

SOMETHING TO THINK ABOUT

If parents have an increased level of anxiety, this increases the level of anxiety in children, and an increased level of anxiety in children increases parental anxiety. Therefore, effective communication with children's carers is as important as communicating with the children themselves (Adelaide Ear Nose and Throat Specialists, 2016).

Communication and child development

Children develop their language skills at various points, but usually by 18 months of age children can say simple sentences and make their basic needs known (Sheridan, 1985). Toddlers repeat words and they understand many more words than they can say (Devitt & Thain, 2011). Between the ages of three and four, the ability to understand language rapidly increases and children have a vocabulary of several thousand words (Berk, 2008). Thus, young children can understand some concepts as long as they are explained using age-appropriate language (Lloyd, Bor & Noble, 2018).

REFLECTIVE THINKING QUESTION

Children are often told that when they have a needle inserted it will feel like a mosquito sting. Do these misleading analogies help? How might you better convey to children concepts such as venepuncture/cannulation?

Parents need to be involved in procedures and these procedures need to be fully explained so that, if necessary, parents can explain them to their child (Van Horn et al., 2003). In addition, the explanations should be reframed to ensure that the parents have understood. Parents should be told how to contact staff for assistance and verbal information should be reinforced with written instructions (Glasper & Richardson, 2011). Parents can also be taught how to use distraction techniques to help with procedure and pain management (Tutelman et al., 2018).

Children should always be told what is being done and why (Hockenberry, Wilson & Winkelstien, 2007; Weller, 1986), and parents and children should not feel rushed as this prevents effective communication. If a child appears to be frightened or reluctant, healthcare professionals need to be sensitive to this. Using a toy, such as a doll or a teddy bear that the child is familiar with, can help children understand some procedures and help them feel more at ease (Association for the Wellbeing of Children in Healthcare [AWCH], 2008). In each step of any procedure in which the child cooperates, positive feedback should be used because children respond to being praised (Klossner & Hatfield, 2006). These techniques should be used whenever and wherever children and their families require healthcare, as they help to reduce anxiety and promote more effective engagement with the child and their parents. Parents can inform healthcare professionals if the child has special names for certain things, such as wanting the toilet or food (Kyle, 2008).

Another important fact regarding young children is that their understanding of explanations can be quite literal. Using phrases such as 'put to sleep' (used for being anaesthetised) may make them think of pets that have been euthanised, or using the word 'dye' for a diagnostic test may evoke fear that they are going to die (London et al., 2007). Even a relatively simple procedure, such as checking a child's vital signs, may evoke fear because, when they are told they are having their 'temperature taken', they may think that something is going to be removed. In addition, healthcare professionals often explain that they are 'putting the thermometer into the child's ear'. In research undertaken by Mould (2012), admitting nurses were observed asking parents to hold their child's head while they proceeded to check the temperature, without any explanation to either the child or the parents.

Using age-appropriate concepts such as asking children if they have seen a thermometer before and explaining what it does gains the cooperation of the child. If children do not know what a thermometer is, then a description such as 'it tells us how hot you are' and that it 'makes a beeping noise' can be used. This use of simple phrases is necessary when communicating with young children. Children enjoy games and asking a child to say when they hear a 'beeping noise' turns the assessment into a game and increases the child's cooperation.

The equipment used in healthcare can be scary for children, who may fantasise about what is going to happen to them. They need clear explanations about simple things that adults take for granted. For example, it is child-friendly to ask a child if they know what a blood pressure (BP) machine is. If a child asks if it will hurt, acknowledge that it may hurt a little but only for a short time, as this helps to reassure the child. Paramount when communicating with children of all ages is to be truthful. Saying that a procedure does not hurt, or saying that a medicine tastes nice when we either do not know whether it does or know for a fact that it has an unpleasant taste, will result in a lack of trust during future interactions. Using phrases such as the medicine tastes 'a bit yukky', or that the BP cuff squeezes the arm, is truthful and effective. Many adults testify that having their BP recorded is actually quite uncomfortable

This image depicts RN Sandra Rocha distracting four-year-old Lucas James by blowing bubbles (The Sydney Children's Hospital, Randwick, NSW).

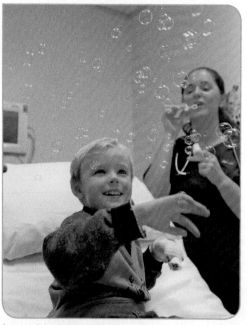

Source: © Rohan Kelly/News Corp Australia/Newspix

and children will almost certainly describe discomfort as hurt, especially if the pressure is set too high (Harman et al., 2005; Great Ormond Street Hospital for Children NHS Foundation Trust, 2015).

Another technique that helps healthcare professionals engage with children and their families is to sit near to the parents, but not so close as to frighten or overwhelm the child. Distraction also helps reduce discomfort and anxiety; for example, asking children who their favourite cartoon characters are will often engage the child. Mould observed a situation where a child could not be consoled, so bubble blowing was used (2012). This flexible approach to distraction helps the child become more settled. Having activities for children to do if they are not too unwell can also help children feel less anxious (Rezai et al., 2017; Klossner & Hatfield, 2006).

At the end of each procedure, thanking children when they cooperate, or telling them that they were 'a good boy/girl', is effective in helping them relax. Positive strategies such as these facilitate effective communication. They help prevent the emotional harm that can occur following healthcare interventions and reduce the fear of future healthcare encounters.

Still, it can be challenging when describing procedures to children, because of their aforementioned literal interpretation of things. Mould (2012) observed a child asking about the peripheral oxyhaemoglobin saturation (SpO2) probe that had been placed on his finger. The explanation involved the words 'blood haemoglobin', and as soon as the word 'blood' was mentioned the child immediately withdrew his finger and hid his hand behind his back, asking if it (the SpO2 probe) was going to make him bleed.

REFLECTIVE THINKING QUESTION

Telling a child that magic cream is going to make their skin numb so they won't feel the tiny straw going into their hand may be confusing, as children often associate straws with drinking. What might you think if you thought a cannula the size of a drinking straw was going to be inserted into your arm?

It is important to recognise that parents often become distressed when their child needs healthcare (Edwinson Månsson & Dykes, 2004). Mould (2012) reported on some families being left for up to an hour, in both emergency and non-emergency situations, without any explanation of the processes or procedures. Mould also observed some healthcare professionals starting procedures then leaving the family alone while they collected equipment or took telephone calls. These types of behaviour often increase the anxiety of families when their child needs healthcare, because they have longer periods of time to become fearful and concerned. A lack of information and direction has been reported as increasing parental anxieties (Coyne, 2013). Further, when parents observe busy healthcare professionals, it adds to their anxiety regarding the care their child may receive, as they fear the healthcare professionals may be too busy to deliver safe and appropriate care (Coyne, 2013). Timely, accurate information facilitates parents' trust (Potts & Mandleco, 2012) so, to alleviate parental anxiety, healthcare professionals should briefly explain the reasons for delays and inquire if they have any immediate needs (Coyne & Cowley, 2007). Sensitivity towards anxious parents is important because 'there is no such thing as minor surgery where your own child is concerned' (Fereday & Darbyshire, 2008, p. 4).

Family-centred care

Parental involvement in their child's care helps minimise any negative effects of hospitalisation on children; consequently, parents should be encouraged to participate in their child's care (Klossner & Hatfield, 2006; World Health Organization, 1955). This philosophy of a collaborative partnership is known as 'family-centred care' (or FCC) (Kyle, 2008; Shields, 2015). FCC boosts a family's confidence and capacity to care for their child's future health needs. However, Coyne (2013) described how FCC is sometimes interpreted by clinicians as parents providing nursing care to their child with minimal communication to the family. This is contrary to the philosophy of FCC, which includes involving and communicating with families and negotiating with them regarding what care they want to and can deliver. Shields (2015) states that FCC will only work if clinicians customise treatments to suit the child and their family's needs.

There is a great deal of evidence supporting the benefits of FCC (Coyne, 2013; Drew, Nathan & Hall, 2002; Young et al., 2006; Weller, 1986). For example, children's pain is managed more effectively when families are involved in the distraction of their child during the administration of medications (Bettle et al., 2018; Broome, 2000; Liossi, White & Hatira, 2006). Home cancer treatments are also more effective if families are supportive of their child's treatment, listen to their child's concerns about the disease and report the effects of medications to the oncology team (Bettle et al., 2018; Manne et al., 1990). Additionally, Kristensson-Hallström, Elander and Malmforss (1997) suggested that children recover more quickly from day surgery when families are fully involved in their post-operative care. In one study, children took fluids early, had less post-operative vomiting, reported less pain and were able to be discharged earlier as a result of the FCC provided. Chartrand, Tourigny and MacCormick (2017) also found there was less postoperative pain when parents were involved in the recovery room.

However, the extent and duration of parental involvement needs to be negotiated with the families so that they do not become overwhelmed with the demands of caring for their child (Coyne, 2013; Kelly, 2007). Communicating in a clear and concise manner, and checking that the parents have understood and are comfortable with the involvement, is essential. If parents do not understand something or are pressured into doing things that they are scared about, their levels of anxiety will be transmitted to their child and this can adversely affect the child's recovery (Potts & Mandleco, 2012).

Separation anxiety

Children who experience fear and anxiety in response to being parted from their parents are described as having separation anxiety (Bowlby & Robertson, 1952; Robertson, 1958). In the past, separation anxiety was observed in older infants and toddlers who were admitted to hospital without their parents and it may still be seen in hospitalised children in the 21st century. Children can become distressed when their parents are not with them (Kyle, 2008) and anxiety is observed when parents are advised not to accompany their child during an invasive procedure (AWCH, 2008). In addition, Ahmed et al. (2011) reported that separation anxiety is often seen in anaesthetic rooms prior to surgery if the clinician decides that a parent should not accompany their child prior to the induction of the anaesthetic, especially in younger children. The well-intentioned rationale for preventing parents being present seems to be that if the parents accompany them the child may blame them [their parent] for the distress experienced as a result of the procedure, and if parents are not present they can comfort their child when the procedure is completed. However, there is good evidence indicating that parental presence can reduce the amount of pain a child perceives; and anxiety caused by separation can heighten the pain sensation (Stafford, Boris & Dalton, 2007; Chartrand et al., 2017).

Quality care

Ensuring there is quality care for children requires knowledge of their physiological and psychological development, an ability to identify particular stages of development of every child encountered, age-appropriate interactions with children and families, and family-centred care (Coyne, Timmins & Neill, 2010; Hockenberry et al., 2017). Safe and quality healthcare does not focus solely on the prevention of adverse events, it also encompasses the experience of users of health services. Mould's (2012) research

---

BOX 13.1   Quality measures for admission of children

1   If the child can talk, endeavour to engage the child in social conversation, which may involve getting to the child's eye level to greet the child. If the child is a preverbal toddler, this social engagement may include making eye contact and saying simple repetitive phrases.

2   Endeavour to determine if the child has been in hospital before and, if so, establish whether the child remembers the experience. If the child can talk, ask the child what he or she knows about coming to the hospital.

3   Negotiate with parents about their level of participation in care giving.

4   When providing explanations to the child and parents, use age-appropriate language and/or concepts, and culturally appropriate language. Assess whether the child and parents have understood the explanations by reframing their responses.

5   If the child can talk, intentionally try to connect with them. This may include explaining to the child what you are going to do using words and phrases the child is able to understand and that are appropriate for the child's developmental age.

6   Help the child through the admission procedure, demonstrate sensitivity and use strategies to deal with a child who is reluctant to engage in any part of the admission procedure. Show patience and tolerance, and do not rush the child.

7   Be sensitive to cues indicating that the child is frightened or reluctant. Use a toy such as a doll or teddy bear to help the child feel more at ease with the admission procedure.

Source: Mould (2012).

---

emphasised the importance of the interaction between nurses and children and their families, and the effect of these encounters on the delivery of safe care. He developed a set of quality measures for admission of children based on a consensus of expert opinion (see Box 13.1). Although these quality measures were developed for nurses, they are relevant to all healthcare professionals.

Engaging with children and parents

When children and families arrive for a healthcare encounter, one of the first expectations is that there will be an attempt at social engagement from the professional. When parents are treated in a respectful manner and included in the admission procedure, it reduces their anxiety (Uhl, Fisher & Brandon, 2013). Healthcare professionals should use age-appropriate techniques such smiling and introducing themselves by name (Bowden & Greenberg, 2010; Mould, 2012; Schmidt et al., 2007), getting to the child's eye level and using simple phrases (Harding & Davis, 2015; Klossner & Hatfield, 2006; McKinney et al., 2018; Weller, 1986). There should also be an awareness of parental body language, because parents often feel a lack of control when their child is hospitalised (Kyle, 2008; Mould, 2012).

However, these techniques are not always used when children are admitted into hospital (Mould, 2012). At times there is a higher priority placed on administrative tasks such as ensuring that forms are completed. Even during emergency admissions, forms are sometimes completed before any assessments are conducted on the children.

Sometimes healthcare professionals can become so focused on the routine tasks they forget that children and parents are not at all familiar with these routines and need them to be explained (McKinney et al., 2018). For example, Mould (2012) witnessed a five-year-old boy being asked if he had a heart problem as a BP cuff was attached. This seemed to imply that the BP machine and the question may have been related, but no explanation was offered. Another child was asked if they had 'been here before' and if they knew where things were. Following these questions, no further engagement was observed with the child. Fear of the unknown will distract a child and cause unnecessary anxiety, which results in a less trusting relationship with the child and their family (Glasper et al., 2015). Effective

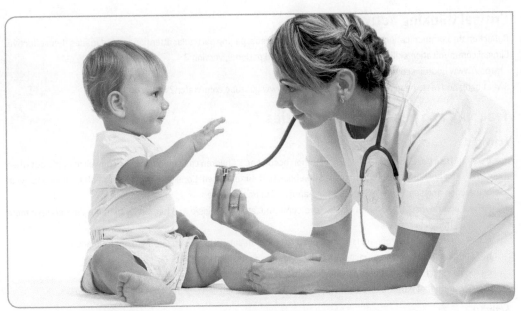

A nurse engaging with a child at eye level

Source: © Oksana Kuzmina/Shutterstock, Inc.

communication with children and parents establishes good relationships and contributes to positive and safer outcomes.

As described above, FCC involves negotiation with and respect for families. Mould (2012) observed an example of respect for a parent: a nurse intended to apply an SpO2 probe on a child but when the mother said, 'It would be better left until the child goes to sleep', the nurse immediately agreed to the suggestion.

Conclusion

Establishing age-appropriate communication with children is essential in order for therapeutic relationships to be created. An evidence-based approach to communication with children and their families is needed to ensure quality care for this population. Even the manner in which a child is spoken to or greeted when first met will determine the nature of the future relationship. If the relationship is therapeutic, it engages the child, leading to more effective clinical interventions. However, if language, body posture or actions are used that frighten a child, clinical interventions become more difficult and can cause long-term anxiety. This negative outcome can interfere with any future health encounters as the child will associate uniforms or equipment with previous negative experiences and become fearful regardless of the current circumstances.

Healthcare for children should integrate the universal principles listed below. Evidence indicates that when these principles are followed children's and family's emotional wellbeing and healthcare are positively affected, and safe and effective communication is optimised (Devitt & Thain, 2011; Potts & Mandleco, 2012):

- Healthcare professionals should be fully aware of the physical, psychological, emotional and social development of children at all ages.

- Healthcare professionals should be fully aware of the vital role that families play in children's lives.

- Healthcare professionals should engage with children and their families using appropriate verbal and non-verbal skills, which include age-appropriate language and concepts, establishing the family's previous experience of paediatric healthcare, and inquiring about whether the family members want to be or can be involved in the care of their child.

- Healthcare professionals should inform children and their families about the healthcare environment to reduce the level of anxiety experienced by both the children and their families.

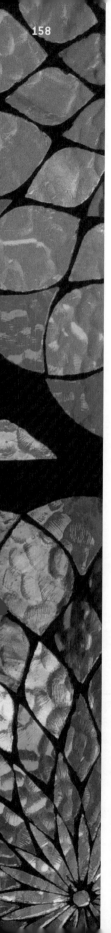

Critical thinking activities

Reflect on the communication strategies used in these videos, paying particular attention to what makes them effective:

Clinical communication skills—communication with child patients, version 2

<https://www.youtube.com/watch?v=I7QiPXqL9pY>

Sweet baby boy rests head on nurse's hand <https://www.youtube.com/watch?v=4SlcqOJj4RM>

Teaching and assessment activities

Activity 1

Rosie's story (see page 150) is a relatively common occurrence. Children can seem to be very unwell at home but when they arrive at a healthcare facility, they are often back to their usual self. Consequently, they are often diagnosed with a viral infection and sent home, which is what happened in Rosie's case.

1   Reflect on and discuss how you would have communicated with Rosie and her family to make their ED visit more positive. Things to consider:

   a.   The use of age-appropriate language used to communicate because 'children are not little adults'.

   b.   Toddlers cannot conceptualise time in the same way as adults can.

   c.   Ignoring parental concerns can be dangerous, even if we think they are overly anxious.

   d.   Ensuring that parents understand the situation so that they can explain it to their child.

Activity 2

Six-year-old David fell out of a tree resulting in a displaced fracture of his radius and ulna. The plan was to admit David for a manipulation under a general anaesthetic (MUA). He hadn't eaten for six hours and there was a space on the theatre list, so he was quickly transferred to the anaesthetic room so that the surgeon could complete the MUA prior to the afternoon theatre list. David is quite tall and looks older than his six years so his parents were advised that it would be better if David was on his own, as often children get more upset when their parents are with them. As a result, his parents agreed to comply. Due to the time constraints, there was not any time to apply local anaesthetic cream for the intravenous cannula insertion. David was told he wouldn't feel the needle anyway as it was just like a mosquito bite.

1   Identify and discuss the aspects of David's care that are likely to cause undue distress to David and his parents, both in the short and possibly longer term.

2   With consideration of the concept of family-centred care, discuss how David's care could have been improved?

3   Discuss the specific communication skills that could have been used in this situation.

Further reading

Hill, M. K., Pawsey, M., Cutler, A., Holt, J. L. & Goldfeld, S. R. (2011). Consensus standards for the care of children and adolescents in Australian health services. *Medical Journal of Australia, 194*(2), 78–82. Accessed January 2019 at

<https://www.mja.com.au/system/files/issues/194_02_170111/hil11049_fm.pdf>

NSW Health. (2010). *Policy directive: Children and Adolescents—Guidelines for Care in Acute Care Settings.* Accessed January 2019 at

<https://www1.health.nsw.gov.au/pds/ActivePDSDocuments/PD2010_034.pdf>

Queensland Government. (2018). *Children's Health Queensland Strategic Plan 2016–2020.* Accessed January 2019 at

<https://www.childrens.health.qld.gov.au/wp-content/uploads/PDF/chq-strat-plan-16-20.pdf>

World Health Organization, United Nations Children's Fund, World Bank Group. (2018). *Nurturing care for early childhood development: A framework for helping children survive and thrive to transform health and human potential.* Geneva:

World Health Organization. Accessed January 2019 at

<http://apps.who.int/iris/bitstream/handle/10665/272603/9789241514064-eng.pdf?ua=1>

Web resources

Sydney Children's Hospitals Network: This website focuses on the care of hospitalised children and family-centred care for all professionals and parents. The fact sheet link gives information about paediatric conditions but also about language development.

Talking Point: This UK website provides information for parents and professionals about helping children develop their communication skills. In addition, it provides fact sheets and information about the importance of play when communicating with children.

World Health Organization. (WHO). Maternal, newborn, child and adolescent health: This website focuses on WHO's initiatives for global child health and provides links to all aspects of child health.

<www.who.int/maternal_child_adolescent/en/index.html>

References

Adelaide Ear Nose and Throat Specialists. (2016). *Preparing Your Child for Surgery*. Accessed June 2018 at <http://www.adelaideentspecialists.com.au/preparing-your-child-for-surgery/>.

Ahmed, M., Farrell, M., Parrish, K. & Karla, A. (2011). Preoperative anxiety in children risk factors and non-pharmacological management. *Middle East Journal Anaesthesiology, 21*(2), 153–64.

Association for the Wellbeing of Children in Healthcare. (2008). *Standards for the Care of Children and Adolescents in Health Services*. Accessed June 2010 at <http://www.awch.org.au/pdfs/Standards_Care_Of_Children_And_Adolescents.pdf>.

Berk, L. (2008). *Child Development* (8th edn). New York: Pearson.

Bowden, V. & Greenberg, C. (2010). *Children and Their Families: The Continuum of Care* (2nd edn). Philadelphia, PA: Lippincott.

Bettle, A., Latimer, M., Fernandez, C. & Hughes, J. (2018). Supporting parents' pain care involvement with their children with acute lymphoblastic leukemia: A qualitative interpretive description. *Journal of Pediatric Oncology Nursing, 35*(1), 43–55.

Bowlby, J. & Robertson, J. (1952). A two-year-old goes to hospital. *Proceedings of the Royal Society of Medicine, 46*, 425–7.

Broome, M. (2000). Helping parents support their child in pain. *Pediatric Nursing, 26*(3), 315–17.

Chartrand, J., Tourigny, J. & MacCormick, J. (2017). The effect of an educational pre-operative DVD on parents' and children's outcomes after a same-day surgery: A randomized controlled trial. *Journal of Advanced Nursing*, 599–611.

Coyne, I. (2013). Families and health-care professionals' perspectives and expectations of family-centred care: Hidden expectations and unclear roles. *Health Expectations, 18*, 796–808.

Coyne, I. & Cowley, S. (2007). Challenging the philosophy of partnership with parents: A grounded theory study. *International Journal of Nursing Studies, 44*(6), 893–904.

Coyne, I., Timmins, F. & Neill, F. (2010). *Clinical Skills for Children's Nursing*. Oxford: Oxford University Press.

Devitt, P. & Thain, J. (2011). *Children and Young People's Nursing: Made Incredibly Easy* (1st UK edn). London: Lippincott, Williams & Wilkins.

Drew, J., Nathan, D. & Hall, D. (2002). Role of a paediatric nurse in primary care: Research issues. *British Journal of Nursing, 11*(22), 1452–9.

Edwinson Mansson, M. & Dykes, A. (2004). Practices for preparing children for clinical examinations and procedures in Swedish pediatric wards. *Pediatric Nursing, 30*(3), 182–7.

Fereday, J. & Darbyshire, P. (2008). Making the wait easier: Evaluating the role of supervised play in a surgical admission area. *Neonatal, Paediatric & Child Health Nursing, 11*(1), 4–9.

Glasper, A., Coad, J. & Richardson, J. (2015). *Children and Young People's Nursing at a Glance*. Oxford: Wiley.

Glasper, A. & Richardson, J. (2011). *A Textbook of Children's and Young Peoples' Nursing* (2nd edn). London: Elsevier.

Great Ormond Street Hospital for Children NHS Foundation Trust. (2015). *The Child First and Always*. Accessed June 2018 at <https://www.gosh.nhs.uk/health-professionals/clinical-guidelines/blood-pressure-monitoring#Rationale>.

Harding, J. & Davis, M. (2015). An observational study based on the interaction between the paediatric patient and radiographer. *Radiography, 21*(3), 258–63.

Harman, K., Lindsay, S., Adewami, A. & Smith, P. (2005). An investigation of language used by children to describe discomfort expected and experienced during dental treatment. *International Journal of Paediatric Dentistry, 15*(5), 319–26.

Healy, J. & Dugdale, P. (2009). *Patient Safety First: Responsive Regulation in Health Care*. Sydney: Allen & Unwin.

Hockenberry, M., Wilson, D. & Rodgers, C. (2017). *Wong's Essentials of Pediatric Nursing* (10th edn). St Louis, MO: Elsevier.

Hockenberry, M., Wilson, D. & Winkelstein, M. (2007). *Wong's Essentials of Pediatric Nursing* (8th edn). St Louis, MO: Mosby.

Kelly, M. (2007). Achieving family-centered care: Working on or working with stakeholders? *Neonatal, Paediatric, and Child Health Nursing, 10*(3), 4–11.

Kennardy, J. (2016). *Kids Can Be Traumatised by Hospital Stays, Research Shows*. Accessed July 2018 at <https://www.psychlopaedia.org/health/kids-can-be-traumatised-by-hospital-stays-research-shows/>.

Klossner, N. & Hatfield, N. (2006). *Introductory Maternity & Pediatric Nursing*. Philadelphia, PA: Lippincott.

Kristensson-Hallstrom, I., Elander, G. & Malmforss, G. (1997). Increased parental participation in a paediatric surgical day-care unit. *Journal of Clinical Nursing, 6*, 297–302.

Kyle, T. (2008). *Essentials of Pediatric Nursing*. Philadelphia, PA: Lippincott, Williams & Wilkins.

Liossi, C., White, P. & Hatira, P. (2006). A randomized clinical trial of a brief hypnosis intervention to control venepuncture-related pain of pediatric procedure related pain. *Health Psychology, 25*(3), 307–15.

London, M., Ladewig, P., Ball, J. & Bindler, R. (2007). *Maternal and Child Nursing Care* (2nd edn). New Jersey: Pearson.

Lloyd, M, Bor, R. & Noble, L. (2018). *Clinical Communication Skills for Medicine* (4th edn). Edinburgh: Elsevier.

Manne, S., Redd, W., Jacobsen, P., Gorfinkle, K., Schorr, O. & Rapkin, B. (1990). Behavioural intervention to reduce child and parent distress during venipuncture. *Journal of Consulting and Clinical Psychology, 58*, 565–72.

McKinney, E., James, S., Murray, S., Nelson, K. & Ashwill, J. (2018). *Maternal-Child Health Nursing*. St Louis, MO: Elsevier.

Mould, J. (2012). Paediatric nursing: An investigation of the effect of specialist paediatric nurse education on the quality of children's nursing care in Western Australia. Unpublished thesis, Edith Cowan University, WA.

Owens, A. (2012). Health, safety and wellbeing. *National Quality Standard Professional Learning Program e-Newsletter* 29.

Potts, N. & Mandleco, B. (2012). *Pediatric Nursing: Caring for Children and Their Families* (3rd edn). New York: Thomson Delmar.

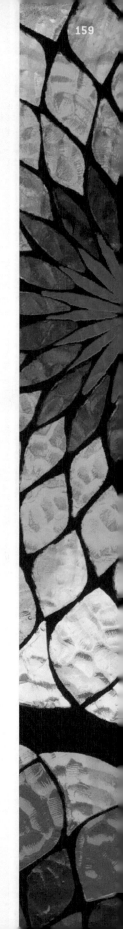

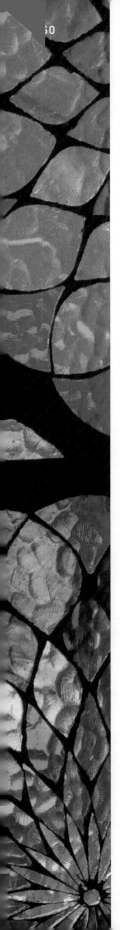

Rezai, M.S., Goudarzian, A.H., Jafari-Koulaee, A. & Bagheri-Nesami, M. (2017). The effect of distraction techniques on the pain of venipuncture in children: A systematic review. *Journal of Pediatric Review*, 5(1).

Robertson, J. (1958). *Young Children in Hospital*. New York: Basic Books Inc.

Rokach, A. (2016). Psychological, emotional and physical experiences of hospitalized children. *Clinical Case Reports and Reviews*, 2(4), 399–401.

Royal Australasian College of Physicians. (2008). *Standards for the Care of Children and Adolescents in Health Services*. Sydney: Australia Paediatrics & Child Health Division, RACP.

Schmidt, C., Bernaix, L., Koski, A., Weese, J., Chiappetta, M. & Sandrik, K. (2007). Hospitalized children's perceptions of nurses and nurses' behaviours. *MCN American Journal of Maternal Child Nursing*, 37(2), 336–42.

Sheridan, M. (1985). *From Birth to Five Years: Children's Developmental Progress*. Windsor: Nfer-Nelson.

Shields, L. (2015). What is family-centred care? *European Journal for Person Centered Healthcare*, 3(2), 139–44.

Stafford, B., Boris, N.W. & Dalton, R. (2007). Anxiety disorders. In R. Kliegman, R. Behrman, H. Jenson & B. Stanton (Eds), *Nelson's Textbook of Pediatrics* (18th edn, pp. 857–84). Philadelphia, PA: Saunders Elsevier.

Tutelman, P., Chambers, C., Stinson, J., Parker, J., Fernandez, C., Witteman, H., . . . Irwin, K. (2018). Pain in Children with Cancer. *The Clinical Journal of Pain*, 34(3), 198–206.

Uhl, T., Fisher, K., Docherty, S. L. & Brandon, D. H. (2013). Insights into patient and family-centered care through the hospital experiences of parents. *Journal of Obstetric, Gynecological and Neonatal Nursing*, 42, 121–31.

Van Horn, M., DeMaso, D., Lefkowitz, D. & Campis, L. (2003). Helping your child with medical experiences: A practical parent guide. *Center for Families*. Accessed at <http://www.experiencejournal.com/cardiac/clinic/parentguide.pdf>.

Weller, B. (Ed.) (1986). *The Lippincott Manual of Paediatric Nursing* (2nd edn). London: Harper & Row.

World Health Organization. (2008). Children are not little adults: Children's health and the environment. WHO training package for the health sector, July 2008 version. Accessed at <http://www.who.int/ceh/capacity/children_are_not_little_adults.pdf>.

World Health Organization. (1955). The child in hospital. *Chronicle of the World Health Organization*, 9, 6–10.

Young, J., McCann, D., Watson, K., Pitcher, A., Bundy, R. & Greathead, D. (2006). Negotiation of care for a hospitalised child: Parental perspectives. *Neonatal, Paediatric and Child Health Nursing*, 9(2), 4–13.

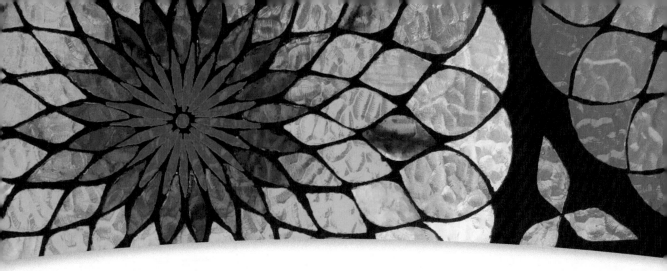

CHAPTER 14

COMMUNICATING WITH PEOPLE WHO HAVE A MENTAL HEALTH PROBLEM

Eimear Muir-Cochrane   Deb O'Kane   Lyza Helps

LEARNING OUTCOMES

Chapter 14 will enable you to:

◉ outline the prevalence of mental health problems in Australia

◉ define the terms 'stigma', 'co-morbidity' and 'diagnostic overshadowing'

◉ discuss the skills required to communicate safely with people experiencing mental health problems

◉ describe why effective communication with people experiencing mental health problems is essential

◉ outline some of the difficulties that can be encountered when communicating with a person with mental health problems.

KEY CONCEPTS

stigma | social exclusion | mental illness | co-morbidity | recovery

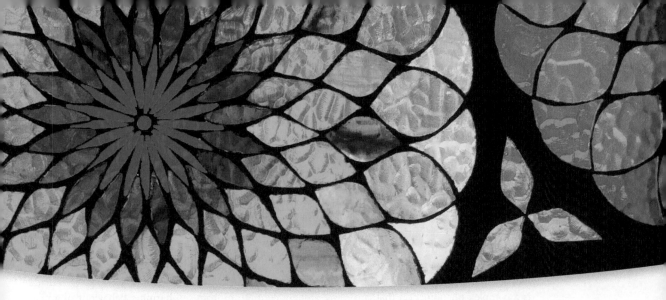

> It's not about us and them. It's about everyone. We know
> that people want to help but they don't know where to
> start ... They struggle to know how to talk about it and
> they worry that intervening will make things worse ... it
> used to be like this for other illnesses, for example cancer,
> but times have changed and attitudes and behaviour
> have moved on. It's now mental health's time.
>
> (Allan Fels AO)

INTRODUCTION

Mental health is everyone's business and communicating effectively with people who have mental health problems is vital to providing safe and effective healthcare. The prevalence of mental health problems is high, with one in five Australians experiencing a mental disorder at some point in their lives (Australian Bureau of Statistics [ABS], 2015b). Hence, people with mental health problems of varying severity will be seeking health services across the healthcare continuum, from primary healthcare settings to tertiary care, and across the life span.

Effective communication is not only fundamental to effective therapeutic relationships but is also essential to safe practice. This chapter explores the barriers and facilitators to effective communication with people who have a mental illness and outlines communication strategies that you can use to provide holistic person-centred care.

The prevalence of mental health problems in Australia

In March 2015, the Australian Bureau of Statistics (ABS) reported that some 4 million Australians had a mental health condition and 3.6 million also had a concurrent physical condition. Most common are anxiety disorders, which affect one in seven adults, followed by mood disorders (6.2%), depression (4.1%) and substance abuse disorders (5.1%, of which more than half is alcohol-related) (ABS, 2015b). Of note, the greatest numbers of people with a mental illness are between 18 and 24 years of age, a time when schizophrenia commonly emerges. Although schizophrenia is a low-prevalence disease, affecting approximately 1 per cent of the population worldwide, it nevertheless can be an extremely disabling and lifelong disease, so preventative and early intervention strategies are essential in the provision of mental healthcare to young people. Similarly, depression is one of the most common health conditions in young people and is exacerbated by substance abuse (ABS, 2015b).

Suicide is a serious act of self-harm where the person has acted with the intention of ending their life. It is the 17th leading cause of death worldwide (World Health Organization, 2017, p. 5). Suicide is a complex phenomenon that can move along a continuum from self-harming behaviour of a relatively minor nature through to having suicidal thoughts, making a formal plan and finally dying by suicide (Victoria Health, 2010). In Australia, people taking their own lives increased from 2300 in 2011 to 2800 in 2016, an increase of over 500 lives lost (ABS, 2017a). Intentional self-harm and suicide attempts leading to hospital admissions also continue to increase in Australia; in 2013–14 there were 33 956 hospital admissions for intentional self-harm, which increased in 2015–2016 to 39 579 admissions. Many more people self-harm but go unreported (ABS, 2017b).

It is essential to be able to communicate empathically and sensitively with people who have a mental health problem or may be suicidal, as well as communicating effectively with other healthcare professionals. The importance of effective communication for people with a mental illness is also emphasised in Standard 1.8 of the National Safety and Quality Health Service Standards (Australian Commission of Safety and Quality in Health Care [ACSQHC], 2017), where it is specified that 'processes' need to be in place to support the early identification, early intervention and appropriate management of patients at increased risk of harm.

JAMES' STORY

James was 19 when he experienced his first acute psychotic episode, leading to hospital admission. Until that point he had led what most would describe as a normal life. He was a high achiever and enrolled in a sports science degree at the local university. In his first year at university he smoked cannabis for the first time. Over a six-month period, his parents had become increasingly concerned about James' erratic behaviour and his tendency to spend long periods of time in his bedroom staring at his computer and saying odd things, such as he knew he was being followed.

In 2009, after returning home from a party in the early hours of the morning, James began to hear voices coming from the room next door. The voices were plotting ways to kill him, and he heard them say that they had installed cameras and microphones in his computer to monitor all his movements in preparation for the execution. James was too scared to sleep and remained awake all night. In the morning, his father found him hunched in the corner of his bedroom shaking uncontrollably but refusing to move. He finally agreed to go to the hospital with his parents. On arrival at the emergency department, as per hospital procedure, the triage nurse began to ask questions about the concerning health issue. As more questions were asked, James began to suspect that the triage nurse was an undercover CIA agent and refused to speak further. He remained in the waiting room for three hours, waiting to be seen by a doctor. During this time, he saw surveillance cameras watching him and he could hear the staff talking about him in a derogatory manner. James began pacing the floor of the waiting room, wringing his hands and clenching and unclenching his fists.

Paula, an experienced healthcare professional, was on duty in the emergency department that morning. She had 10 years of experience, facing the daily challenges of different presentations to the department, and on seeing James' agitation she approached him. She introduced herself and explained that she could see he was scared and how frightening it must be if he believed everybody was against him. She asked if she was safe and when James answered 'Yes', she asked if she could sit down and have a chat with him, so he could tell her what was happening. Paula sat on a chair and waited for James to begin. She did not ask questions, only interjected occasionally to clarify points or to reflect how James must have been feeling throughout the last 24 hours. James visibly relaxed. He described the past six months and the voices he had started to hear. He described being 'on edge' and smoking a cannabis joint in the hope it would relieve some of his tension before attending a party on the previous night. He went on to say how the voices appeared to get quieter until he returned home. They then returned ten times louder than on previous occasions. Paula suggested that cannabis, along with some physical or neurological disorders, can affect the way the mind works and asked if it might be a good idea to have a physical examination and bloods taken so that the team could help him in whatever way possible.

The impact of stigma

People with mental health problems remain one of the most stigmatised and discriminated groups in society today. Stigma is a social process whereby an individual or a group is defined by society as deviant, different or dangerous. Goffman (1963) defined the term 'spoiled identity' to describe how the stigma of having a mental illness disqualifies the person from full social acceptance. People with mental illness are often negatively stereotyped, grouped together and not viewed as individuals (Goffman; Scambler, 2011). The reactions of other individuals can preclude people with a mental illness from being fully allowed to take part in all aspects of the social world, through overt and covert exclusionary social processes.

Stigmatisation can be seen in acts of law, in that people with a mental illness are the only group with a health problem that, when acutely unwell, can be involuntarily held under legislation; this law is usually referred to as a Mental Health Act. The negative stereotyping of people with a mental illness as violent, unpredictable and dangerous led to the creation of laws to limit their freedom and compulsorily detain them in psychiatric hospitals. In this context, it is easy to understand why healthcare professionals, just like the public, can have reservations about working with people with mental health problems. A recent South American study found a correlation between self-perceived stigma and poor functioning in people with bipolar disorder, indicating the need for healthcare professionals to practise in ways that are respectful of people with a mental illness and that facilitate their recovery (Thome et al., 2012, p. 669).

People are largely influenced by the society and culture in which they live. This in turn contributes to the development of personal attitudes, values and beliefs. Developing and maintaining self-awareness (i.e. being aware of your own attitudes, values and beliefs) will help you to recognise how you communicate with others. Self-awareness is a necessary component of effective and safe communication, particularly in situations that are new or challenging (The Department of Health, 2013b). Standard 7 of the Standards of Practice in Mental Health Nursing states that, '… the mental health nurse demonstrates evidence-based practice and actively promotes practice innovation through lifelong education, research, professional development, clinical supervision and reflective practice' (Australian College of Mental Health Nurses, 2010).

REFLECTIVE THINKING QUESTIONS

Where and when might you meet a person with a mental illness?
How would you feel and why?
How would you behave?
What might you be thinking?
How would your own feelings, attitudes and perceptions of mental illness influence how you approach and communicate with the person?

Engaging in self-reflection and developing self-awareness allows healthcare professionals to examine their own values and beliefs and come to understand their actions better. By recognising the links between feelings, attitudes, thoughts and behaviours, healthcare professionals can also identify their strengths as well as any areas that require improvement. The development of self-awareness is not a static process; rather, it is one that is ongoing and continually explored throughout a professional career (Australian College of Mental Health Nurses, 2010).

Patient-safe communication with people experiencing mental health problems

Healthcare professionals can believe they are communicating in a therapeutic and helpful way with people with mental health problems, but this is often not the case. The healthcare professional's perception of doing 'right' can often be misplaced, with inappropriate communication resulting in adverse outcomes such as aggressive behaviour or suicidal gestures. Below are some clinical examples that illustrate these issues.

SYLVIA'S STORY

Part A

A team of paramedics attends an emergency call-out. A 34-year-old woman named Sylvia is found conscious and able to communicate. She contacted the service due to having taken an overdose to kill herself an hour ago. She states that she is now regretting the decision to call the ambulance and is reluctant to go with the team to the emergency department.

Source: This clinical practice example was adapted from L. Roberts (2012).

REFLECTIVE THINKING QUESTIONS

What would you say to encourage Sylvia to attend the emergency department?
When thinking about your response to Sylvia, what behaviours may hinder her cooperation with you?
What communication skills would you use and why do you think these may be effective?

There is evidence to suggest some healthcare professionals believe that people with mental health issues, in situations such as this, are 'game playing' and often label them as 'attention seekers'. Some paramedics have indicated that, though they initially start off the conversation by trying to engage with the person, if this isn't immediately effective other tactics may be employed, such as being direct and summoning them: 'Okay, we've tried being nice. We need you to get in the ambulance now and just come with us.'

While this type of communication may help the paramedics (or other healthcare professionals) believe they are taking control of the situation, it rarely helps the person feel supported and willing to cooperate. This type of communication implies a paternalistic or patronising approach and in some instances may antagonise the person further. Listening and validating Sylvia's fear, anxiety or thoughts about going to the emergency department demonstrates empathy and indicates that the healthcare professional is attempting to gain a sense of what she is experiencing. Thoughtful communication may take time and energy in the short term but it has positive and far-reaching consequences in the long term.

Part B

Sylvia attends the emergency department and, after various medical interventions to ensure her physical wellbeing, she is referred for a psychiatric consultation. She is on continual observation by a new graduate registered nurse after stating that she still wishes to end her life. The nurse attempts to engage Sylvia by asking questions about her family. Sylvia discloses that her long-time partner died six months ago and she has been struggling to pay the mortgage. The nurse also finds out that Sylvia has two young children and has recently been promoted in her current job. The nurse says, 'But you have so much to live for . . .'.

REFLECTIVE THINKING QUESTIONS

What do you think the nurse may be trying to achieve by making such a statement?
What impact may this type of comment have on Sylvia?

There is a fine line between providing reasons to live and sounding judgmental. The comment made by the nurse may be interpreted by a depressed person in a way that reinforces their guilt about contemplating leaving their family through suicide. It can also reinforce the negative thoughts they are experiencing about themselves and their lives (i.e. they are selfish and don't deserve to live). Offering hope to Sylvia should include acknowledging her concerns and communicating how her problems can improve with treatment. Such encouragement can provide reassurance and a sense of hope about the future.

A better example of this nurse–patient interaction would be: 'It sounds like it's been a tough year. But while it may be difficult at present to see how things can improve, I'm confident there are people who will help you feel better. Lots of people feel depressed and struggle to cope, but with the right treatment life can and does improve.'

Against this background, a brief look at the National Mental Health Strategy— launched in Australia in 1994—is warranted in order to gain an understanding of the vision for the future regarding the care of people with a mental health problem. The policies outlined in the Strategy are based on the concept of human rights and embracing access to services, equity in treatment and care, effectiveness and efficiency (World Health Organization, 2001). The Fifth National Mental Health and Suicide Prevention Plan (Council of Australian Governments Health Council, 2017) specifically targets the need for stigma reduction strategies to ensure the effective provision of care to people with mental health problems.

Over the last decade in Australia, the recovery philosophy model emerged from consumer advocates in mental health as a way of reducing stigma and raising consciousness among the public and healthcare professionals about person-centred care. Recovery, as a practical approach to care, emphasises the person's potential to lead their life as they wish. Thus, it is more than reducing symptoms; it is about supporting the individual's life journey and learning to live with mental health problems (Muir-Cochrane, Barkway & Nizette, 2018). As a part of this approach, the term 'patient' (in mental health services) has been replaced by 'consumer' to imply a partnership model between healthcare professionals and consumers. Recovery places the emphasis on the person's concerns as well as their perceived needs and goals. Being a strengths-based approach, emphasis is also placed on the person's abilities and motivations and how they can have more active control over their lives (agency) (The Department of Health, 2013a). In the recovery approach, engagement between healthcare professionals and consumers is at the core of the provision of care. For this to occur, healthcare professionals require open, honest and clear communication skills.

Communicating effectively in person-centred interactions has been demonstrated to improve care outcomes and remains central to the caring relationship (Hack et al., 2017, Davidson et al., 2015). However, unless experienced and trained in mental health, healthcare professionals may feel bewildered, puzzled or challenged when communicating with people experiencing mental health issues, particularly if the person is acutely unwell. Behaviour and speech patterns will vary from person to person but communicating with a mental health consumer may present complexities not previously encountered in other social or professional interactions. For example, conversing with someone who is acutely psychotic (i.e. hallucinating and/or delusional) may be very different from talking to someone who is morose, monosyllabic and diagnosed with depression.

Because of preconceived ideas and the stigma attached to mental illness, healthcare professionals may be scared of saying the 'wrong thing' and provoking aggressive or unpredictable behaviour; or concerned that saying the 'wrong thing' may make them responsible for the person's future behaviour, such as a suicide attempt. The truth is that all healthcare professionals should be willing to interact with people experiencing mental health problems. How you interact with each person will be different but empathic communication is key to his or her care and recovery.

Why is effective communication with people experiencing mental health problems essential?

Evidence indicates that both mental health professionals and healthcare professionals more broadly, too often give inadequate attention to the medical conditions of people with mental health problems (ABS, 2015a; Dornquast, et al., 2017). People with severe mental illness are at risk of several related and complex health problems, including obesity, diabetes and cardiovascular disease (Reisinger, 2017). Cigarette smoking, alcohol and substance abuse are also significant risks for people with mental health problems. Of note is the fact that a person with cancer, diabetes, stroke or coronary heart disease may stay up to four times longer in hospital if they have a pre-existing mental illness (Britt et al., 2016; ABS, 2015a). Communication between healthcare professionals about the complex needs of these individuals is therefore essential to ensure that a comprehensive and holistic plan is developed.

Mental health problems were the fourth most common reason for seeing a general practitioner (GP) in 2014–2015; and almost one in nine consultations involved a high-prevalence mental health problem such as depression or anxiety (Britt, et al., 2016). However, people with severe mental illness, including schizophrenia, are much less likely to present to a GP (Cameron et al., 2017). Further, this group of people is almost three times more likely to die of natural causes than the general population. Specifically, the conditions that commonly increase morbidity and mortality for people with mental health problems are ischaemic heart disease, cardiac arrhythmias and myocardial infarction (Cameron et al.). Unfortunately, taking medications to treat mental illness can have many side effects, many of which can be severe. These may include weight gain, sedation, hypotension, metabolic syndrome and lipid dysregulation, diabetes, and coronary vascular disease (Law et al.). So, while people with enduring mental illness are in dire need of appropriate healthcare, they typically receive less education, information and support related to medication management, and often experience a lack of continuity of care (Law et al.). For these reasons, mental illnesses such as schizophrenia and depression interconnect with a range of serious medical problems that need to be managed side by side. When healthcare professionals encounter people with mental health problems, clear communication and a thorough health assessment can identify health issues that may otherwise not be diagnosed.

Some of the barriers to people with mental health problems receiving prompt and appropriate physical healthcare include a lack of recognition by health professionals and the difficulties faced by consumers of mental health services in negotiating the healthcare system. Other barriers include, but are not limited to, those listed in Box 14.1.

BOX 14.1   Barriers to care for people with mental health problems

- A tendency by health professionals to focus on mental health issues while other health complaints are ignored.
- Reluctance of GPs to take comprehensive care of individuals with schizophrenia.
- Lack of continuity of care and follow-up due to itinerancy of patients.
- Screening for physical problems not carried out routinely.
- Physical symptoms diagnosed incorrectly as psychosomatic.
- Time and resources for general health check-ups not available in mental health service settings.
- Failure to receive primary health information; and available health information being inappropriate for consumer's needs.
- Fragmentation of the healthcare system, making it hard for people to negotiate it.
- Lack of sustained contact with GPs.

Source: Adapted from Jeste et al. (1996); Goldman (1999).

Difficulties in communication for people with mental health problems

People with mental health problems may avoid everyday social contact when their symptoms are severe. Severely unwell people may also have significant cognitive and psychosocial deficits, which can reduce accurate self-assessment of symptoms, and they may be unable to describe any medical problems they are experiencing. A lack of awareness of physical symptoms may also be due to a high pain tolerance associated with the use of antipsychotic medication.

PAUL'S STORY

Part A

Paul is 50 years old. He was diagnosed with paranoid schizophrenia at the age of 24. He has had several hospital admissions for his illness but has been able to successfully live independently with support from a local GP practice for the last five years. A community nurse visits him on a fortnightly basis to administer a depot injection and to check that his health is maintained, as Paul also has type 1 diabetes mellitus. It is the nurse's understanding, after speaking with the GP, that Paul can manage the diabetes himself via insulin and dietary management.

The community nurse has been visiting for three months and has noticed Paul's considerable weight gain, which is a common side effect of antipsychotic medications. Paul has also become lethargic. This is having an impact on his independence in managing activities of daily living and his personal hygiene. On the nurse's last few visits Paul appears unkempt; he walks very slowly and spends long periods of time in bed. There is also a distinct foul-smelling odor emanating from Paul.

REFLECTIVE THINKING QUESTIONS

What do you think might be happening with Paul's health?
How would you communicate with Paul in order to conduct a comprehensive health assessment?
What issues would you need to consider when talking with Paul?

Part B

After much questioning, Paul informs the nurse that, due to his weight gain, he is unable to reach his feet to untie his shoelaces. It quickly becomes apparent that Paul has been wearing the same canvas shoes for a few weeks. On removal of his shoes the community nurse identifies that the smell is from a chronic infected foot ulcer on his right foot that resulted from a minor injury Paul sustained after walking on a piece of broken glass a few weeks earlier.

REFLECTIVE THINKING QUESTIONS

What may have prevented Paul from telling the nurse about his foot on previous occasions?
Consider the impact and implications of having an untreated infected foot on Paul's social, mental and physical wellbeing.
How could this situation have been avoided?
How would you manage Paul's care in the future?

Paul's story highlights significant clinical and communication issues. For example, the inadequate physical assessment of Paul's health led to a failure to diagnose or treat his injured and infected foot, and to provide an opportunity for early intervention. The nurse may have focused predominantly on Paul's need for the depot injection, rather than also considering his physical health and the fact that behaviours such as lack of hygiene, lethargy and difficulties with activities of daily living can indicate both physical and mental ill-health. This resulted in diagnostic overshadowing, where healthcare professionals wrongly presume that physical symptoms are a consequence of a person's mental illness; and, as a result, the person receives inadequate diagnosis and/or treatment (Shefer et al., 2014).

A thorough history and comprehensive assessment would have allowed the nurse to identify both chronic illnesses, and provide appropriate treatment, education and management of Paul's health. There was also a clear need for the healthcare professionals involved to communicate about and coordinate Paul's care.

Table 14.1 provides suggestions for how healthcare professionals can develop communication strategies to enhance therapeutic engagement with people experiencing mental health problems.

	Intervention	Interaction
TABLE 14.1 Communication strategies for engaging with people experiencing mental health problems	**Observe the signs** The signs are what you can see and hear. **Observe and listen!**	• Detect the signs that the person is feeling angry, irritable, excitable, anxious, frightened or perplexed. • Observe for head shaking, fist clenching, pacing, facial expressions, hand wringing, tearful. • Listen for bizarre speech content, loud/quiet voice, rapid speech, profanities, suicidal ideation. • Detect early warning signs for agitated and aggressive behaviour. • Check the person's history for risk assessment and predictability of volatile behaviour.
	Be approachable. Being approachable refers to the way you initially engage the person that allows them to feel physically and psychologically safe in your presence.	• Adopt an open posture. • Remain calm and relaxed. • Use a soft voice. • Maintain eye contact (if culturally and socially appropriate). • Move slowly and be tentative as you approach, showing sensitivity to their needs. • Appear friendly by smiling (if appropriate to the context or situation).
	Establish a rapport. Starting a conversation with someone in the first instance can set the foundation for any following communication.	• Introduce yourself and explain your role. • Ask the consumer their name. • Use short clear sentences. • Ask how you can help. • Show an interest in the person. • Provide reassurance if required. • Answer any questions. • Use gentle persistence for those people difficult to engage.
	Respect and maintain personal space. It is important to be non-intrusive in your proximity to the person so that they can feel safe in your company. Different people have different personal boundaries; therefore, it is important to be respectful of culture and people's personal preferences.	• Acknowledge the person's boundaries. • Ask whether where you are sitting/standing is okay. • Provide information on any actions you and the team are doing so that the person has full awareness of what is happening. • Respect issues of consent and choice to ensure the person feels they have some control of events. If this is not possible, explain the reasons why and attempt to negotiate/compromise. • Listen to the person and respect their feelings. • Continually check to clarify that the person understands what is being said.

Intervention	Interaction	
Identify the problem/issue. Identifying the problem may be in the immediate situation or identifying problems that brought the person to the attention of the service in the first instance.	• Clarify the problem using active listening skills. • If there are several issues, try breaking the issues into smaller, more achievable areas to work on. • Make all your intentions clear to the person. • Avoid getting into arguments or disputes. • Empower the person to problem solve and discover their own answers rather than provide answers or advice.	**TABLE 14.1** Communication strategies for engaging with people experiencing mental health problems (Continued)
Maintain open dialogue. This involves the use of communication skills to encourage further conversation.	• Use open questions such as 'what, when, how, which'. • Provide opportunities for the person to ask questions. • Demonstrate empathy, acceptance and genuineness by being honest and thoughtful in your communication. • Respect times when silence or 'being with' the person is more helpful than talking. • Use touch, but only if appropriate and meaningful. • Listen and acknowledge the emotions the person is experiencing and use reflective skills to feed these back. • Clarify and summarise throughout the interaction, so that each party understands what is being said. • Clarify boundaries and expectations of the relationship and the service by being clear about what it is you want or need from the person. • Use assertiveness as necessary; however, be aware that there is a fine line between the right level of assertiveness and the wrong level of aggression. • Maintain a calm environment. • Be collaborative, using a person-centred approach throughout the interaction. • Utilise the techniques of reality and validation if the person is confused or acutely unwell.	
Ending the conversation. Finishing a conversation can be just as important as starting it and therefore needs time and effort from the healthcare professionals.	• Prepare the person from the onset by providing clear timeframes of your involvement. • Explain why the relationship is coming to an end. • Clarify that the person knows who they will see or what will happen next. • Ask how the person is feeling and constructively work with these feelings. • Offer reassurance as necessary.	

Conclusion

This chapter has provided the context in which people with mental health problems encounter care and the challenges they often face in communicating with healthcare professionals. Healthcare professionals require a sound understanding of the impact of stigma on how people with mental health problems interact with health services. A positive, reflective and non-judgmental approach can provide the opportunity for the establishment of rapport, leading to effective and patient-safe communication between consumers and health professionals. An understanding of the barriers to care for people with mental health problems, as well as knowledge of their associated physical health problems, will equip healthcare professionals to communicate more effectively and to provide comprehensive care to this disadvantaged and vulnerable group.

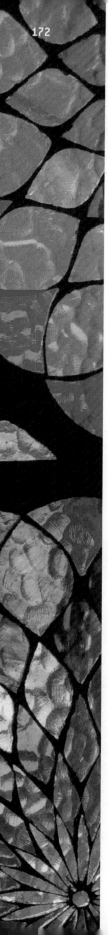

Critical thinking activities

Reflect on your personal and professional experiences. Can you recall any situations in which a person with a mental health problem encountered a lack of patient-safe communication? How did this influence their healthcare experience? How could the communication between the person and the healthcare professionals have been more therapeutic and person-centred?

How do the context, complexity and culture of mental health services influence communication between consumers and healthcare professionals and between the healthcare professionals themselves?

Teaching and assessment activities

The following list of questions can be used by educators to develop tutorial discussions and/or assessment items:

1   Discuss the ways in which healthcare professionals may use communication to develop partnerships with consumers and link them to community-based supports?

2   Discuss the term 'approachable' and identify what makes a healthcare professional *approachable*. How may using rapport-building skills enhance approachability?

3   What might be the key differences between communicating with someone who is profoundly depressed and someone who is experiencing psychosis?

4   Select one of the barriers outlined in Box 14.1 and discuss in more detail. Link your answers with the importance of effective communication.

5   Discuss the importance of both open and closed questions in communication with people with mental health issues. Explain how each type of question may be used to gain information and when each type may be used in an assessment interview?

6   Reflecting on the chapter, summarise the key learning you have achieved and how you will utilise this learning in your clinical practice?

Further reading

Bowers, L., Brennan, G., Winship, G. & Theodoridou, C. (2010). How expert nurses communicate with acutely psychotic patients. *Mental Health Practice, 13*(7), 24–6.

Muir-Cochrane, E., Barkway, P. & Nizette, D. (2018). *Mosby's Pocketbook of Mental Health (3rd edn)*, Sydney, Australia: Elsevier.

Web resources

Reshaping curricula: integrating culturally diverse/ mental health online content to prepare work ready health professionals
<http://flinders.edu.au/nursing/mental-health-and-culture/about.cfm>

ResearchGate. Talking with acutely psychotic people: Communication skills for nurses and others spending time with people who are very mentally ill
<https://www.researchgate.net/publication/257230982_%20>

Inky Smudge. Mental Health Liaison Nursing: An interactive eSimulation resource for generalist nurses.
<http://inkysmudge.com.au/eSimulation/>

Mental Health First Aid Australia
<www.mhfa.com.au/cms/mhfa-downloads/>

VinniesAustralia. Tips and Effective Communications— Understanding Mental Illness
<www.youtube.com/watch?v=is6v50LPqeg>

References

Australian Bureau of Statistics. (2015a). *National Health Survey: First Results, 2014–15* (Folio: 4364.0.55.001). Accesses February 2018 at <http://www.abs.gov.au/ausstats/abs@.nsf/Lookup/by%20Subject/4364.0.55.001~2014-15~Main%20Features~Key%20findings~1>.

Australian Bureau of Statistics. (2015b). *National Health Survey: Mental Health and Co-existing Physical Health Conditions, Australia, 2014–15* (Folio: 4329.0.00.004). Accessed February 2018 at <http://www.abs.gov.au/ausstats%5Cabs@.nsf/0/C0A4290EF1E7E7FDCA257F1E001C0B84>.

Australian Bureau of Statistics. (2017a). *Causes of Death, Australia, 2017* (Folio: 3303.0). Accessed January 2019 at <http://www.abs.gov.au/ausstats/abs@.nsf/0/47E19CA15036B04BCA2577570014668B?Opendocument>.

Australian Bureau of Statistics. (2017b, November). *Hospitalisations for Mental Health Conditions and Intentional Self-Harm in 2015–16.* Accessed April 2018 at <https://www.myhealthycommunities.gov.au/our-reports/mental-health-and-intentional-self-harm/november-2017>.

Australian College of Mental Health Nursing. (2010). *Standards of Practice in Mental Health Nursing.* Accessed April 2018 at <http://www.acmhn.org/publications/standards-of-practice>.

Australian Commission on Safety and Quality in Health Care. (2017). *National Safety and Quality Health Service Standards* (2nd edn). Sydney, Australia: ACSQHC.

Britt. H., Miller, G. C., Henderson, J., Bayram, C., Harrison, C., Valenti, L., . . . Gordon, J. (2016). *General Practice Activity in Australia 2015–16. General Practice Series no. 40*. Sydney, Australia: Sydney University Press.

Cameron, C., Cumsille-Nazar, J., Ehrlich, C., Kendall, E., Crompton, D., Liddy, A. & Kisely, S. (2017). General practitioner management of chronic diseases in adults with severe mental illness: A community intervention trial. *Australian Health Review, 41*(6), 665–71.

Council of Australian Governments Health Council. (2017). *The Fifth National Mental Health and Suicide Prevention Plan*. Accessed April 2018 at <http://www.health.gov.au/internet/main/publishing.nsf/content/mental-fifth-national-mental-health-plan>.

Davidson, L., Tondora, J., Miller, R. & O'Connell, M. J. (2015). Person-centered care, In P. W. Corrigan (Ed.), *Person-centered Care for Mental Illness: The Evolution of Adherence and Self-Determination* (pp. 81–102). Washington, DC: American Psychological Association.

Dornquast, C., Tomzik, J. & Reinhold, T. (2017). To what extent are psychiatrists aware of the comorbid somatic illnesses of their patients with serious mental illnesses? A cross-sectional secondary data analysis. *BMC Health Services Research, 17*, 162. doi: 10.1186/s12913-017-2106

Goffman, E. (1963). *Stigma: Notes on the Management of Spoiled Identity*. Englewood Cliffs, New York: Prentice Hall.

Goldman, K. (1999). Medical illness in patients with schizophrenia. *Journal of Clinical Psychiatry, 60*, 10–15.

Hack, S. M., Muralidharan, A., Brown, C., Lucksted, A. & Patterson, J. (2017). Provider behaviors or consumer participation: How should we measure person-centered care? *The International Journal of Person-Centered Medicine, 17*(1), 14–20.

Jeste, D., Gladsjo, J., Lindamer, L. & Lacro, J. (1996). Medical co-morbidity in schizophrenia. *Schizophrenia Bulletin, 22*, 413–30.

Muir-Cochrane, E., Barkway, P. & Nizette, D. (2018). *Mosby's Pocketbook of Mental Health (3rd edn)*. Sydney, Australia: Elsevier.

Reisinger, E. & Druss, B. (2017). Cumulative burden of comorbid mental disorders, substance use disorders, chronic medical conditions, and poverty on health among adults in the U.S.A. *Psychology, Health & Medicine, 22*(6), 727–35.

Roberts, L. (2012). Ethnography in the pre-hospital setting: An exploration of the culture of how paramedics identify, assess and manage psychiatric presentations in the community. Unpublished PhD thesis, Flinders University.

Scambler G. (2011). Stigma and Mental Disorder. In: D. Pilgrim, A. Rogers & B. A. Pescosolido (Eds), *The Sage Handbook of Mental Health and Illness* (pp. 218–38). London: Sage Ltd.

Shefer, G., Henderson, C., Howard, L. M., Murray, J. & Thornicroft, G. (2014). Diagnostic overshadowing and other challenges involved in the diagnostic process of patients with mental illness who present in emergency departments with physical symptoms—A qualitative study. *PLoS ONE, 9*(11).

The Department of Health. (2013a). *A National Framework for Recovery-Oriented Mental Health Services: Guide for Practitioners and Providers*. Commonwealth of Australia. Accessed January 2019 at <http://www.health.gov.au/internet/main/publishing.nsf/Content/mental-pubs-n-recovgde>

The Department of Health. (2013b). *A National Framework for Recovery-Oriented Mental Health Services: Guide for Practitioners and Providers—Capability 3C: Collaborative Relationships and Reflective Practice*. Commonwealth of Australia. Accessed April 2018 at <http://www.health.gov.au/internet/publications/publishing.nsf/Content/mental-pubs-n-recovgde-toc~mental-pubs-n-recovgde-app~mental-pubs-n-recovgde-app-3~mental-pubs-n-recovgde-app-3-c>.

Thome, E., Dargel, A., Migliavacca, F., Potter, W., Jaipur, D., Kapczinski, F. & Cereser, K. (2012). Stigma experiences in bipolar patients: the impact upon functioning. *Journal of Psychiatric and Mental Health Nursing, 19*(8), 665–71.

Victoria Health. (2010). *Suicide Risk Assessment and Management: A Systematic Evidence Review for the Clinical Practice Guidelines for Emergency Departments and Mental Health Services Project*. Mental Health, Drugs and Regions Division, Victorian Government, Department of Health, Melbourne, Victoria.

World Health Organization. (2001). *Mental Health Around the World: Stop Exclusion: Dare to Care*. Geneva: WHO.

World Health Organization. (2017). *Global Suicide Death Rates*. Accessed March 2018 at <http://www.who.int/mental_health/prevention/suicide/suicideprevent/en/>.

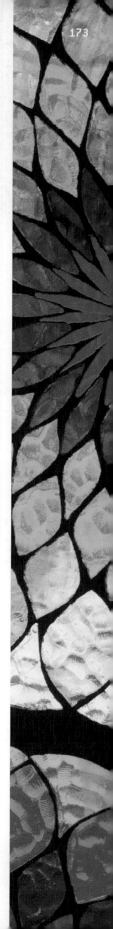

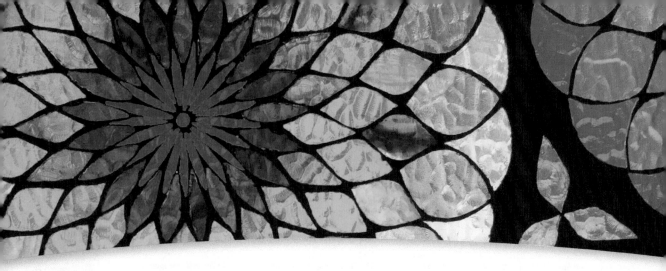

CHAPTER 15

COMMUNICATING WITH PEOPLE WHO HAVE COMMUNICATION IMPAIRMENT

Diane Tasker   Tania De Bortoli

LEARNING OUTCOMES

Chapter 15 will enable you to:

- demonstrate an understanding of different forms of communication impairment

- discuss how communication difficulties can affect patient safety

- outline strategies and approaches that healthcare professionals can use to enhance the safety of people with impaired communication when seeking healthcare.

KEY CONCEPTS

communication impairment | complex communication needs | augmentative and alternative communication (AAC) | communication partner | mindful dialogue framework

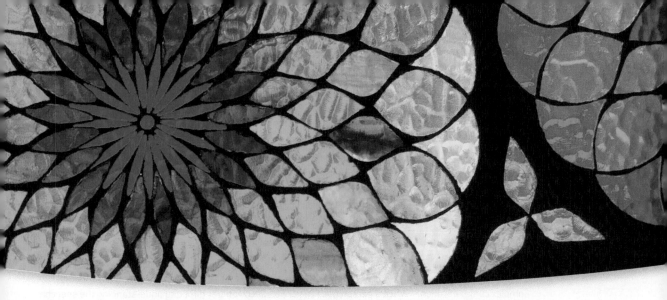

We are used to people saying we cannot communicate,
but of course they are wrong. In fact we have powerful
and effective ways of communicating and we usually have
many ways to let you know what it is we have in mind.

Yes we have communication difficulties and some of
those are linked with our impairments. But by far the
greater part of our difficulty is caused by 'speaking' people
not having the experience, time or commitment to try
and understand us or to include us in everyday life.

(Disabled People using Scope Services, 2002, pp. 1–2)

INTRODUCTION

As healthcare professionals, we encounter many people with communication impairments who require our care. Five to ten per cent of the population are estimated to have a communication impairment (Anderson, Ford & Thorpe, 2011, p. 44). People with such impairments are three times more likely than the general population to experience a negative healthcare outcome as a result of ineffective communication (Webber, Bowers & Bigby, 2012), and two to six times more likely to experience some form of abuse (including sexual abuse) while seeking healthcare (Collier et al., 2006).

Ineffective communication results not only from a person's communication impairment but also from the attitudes and assumptions of health professionals, who often have limited time, experience and knowledge about how to interact with people with communication impairments. See Table 15.1 for definitions associated with communication.

Impairment refers to 'loss or abnormality in body structure or physiological function' (WHO, 2007, p. 229)

but

Disability 'denotes the negative aspects of the interaction between an individual (with a health condition) and that individual's contextual factors (environmental and personal factors)' (WHO, 2007, p. 228).

TABLE 15.1

Definitions of 'communication' related terms

Term	Definition
Speech	Production of spoken words. Combines (a) knowledge of speech sounds and their combination to form words, and (b) the motor ability to produce these.
Language	A system for combining words into sentences to convey meaning. *Expressive language* is the construction and use of words and sentences to convey meaning. *Receptive language* is the understanding of the meaning of words and sentences.
Communication	The two-way process of conveying a message to a listener who understands the message and responds. It involves taking turns between communication partners.
Communication impairment	Difficulties in the use or understanding of speech and language that can impede communication processes.
Severe communication impairment (SCI)	Situations where people have little or no intelligible speech.
Complex communication need (CCN)	When a person has little or no speech and/or difficulty understanding the speech of others; they require additional support in order to be able to participate in the two-way process of communication.
Augmentative and alternative communication (AAC)	Strategies and systems that are used in combination with speech or in place of speech to enable a person to communicate.
Communication partner	Anyone who talks or interacts with another person; this means we can all be communication partners.

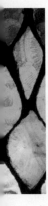

ERIC'S STORY

Taking time in a busy day to stop, look and listen can be difficult but, as this real story about Eric illustrates, it can help to keep a patient safe.

Eric was sitting trying to eat his dinner in the dining room of the rehabilitation unit. He was coughing. John, the medical resident, was passing by and thought how difficult it must be to feed yourself after having had a stroke. Eric was not able to speak, but he pointed to his throat and coughed. John noticed that Eric's neck looked swollen. On auscultation, John noted an unusual sound on expiration. *Something didn't seem right.*

John organised an X-ray. It identified that Eric had his partial denture stuck down his throat. The denture had gone missing about four days ago. No one had been able to find it, and no one had communicated with Eric about it.

As one medical educator told a researcher (V. Madigan, personal communication, 25 September 2012), 'Students read the patient notes and not the patient. We need to read our patients and act when something doesn't seem right.' Words may not be spoken, but messages are still being given.

Different forms of communication impairment

A communication impairment can be associated with a range of medical conditions, such as acquired head injury, autism spectrum disorder, stroke, cerebral palsy and a wide variety of other neuro-muscular conditions. Communication impairment may be temporary, permanent or deteriorating over time, or as a result of associated medical conditions. It often involves difficulty understanding the spoken language or body language of others.

People with communication impairments may also have *sensory impairments*, such as visual and/or hearing impairments. These present added challenges for communication. For example, people who have a *visual impairment* may have difficulty seeing the non-verbal behaviour of others and what is happening in their environment. So this information is not available to help them understand what others are saying. Instead, they may need to rely on their hearing only to understand what others are saying. People who have a *hearing impairment* may find it difficult to both hear and produce spoken words and, as a result, they may need to rely on their vision to help them understand what others are saying. They

Communication strategy	Elements of AAC strategies
Unaided	**Using the body to communicate:** • Auslan (the language used by the deaf community in Australia)[1]. • Key Word Signs (a simplified form of signs and gestures for use by people with intellectual disability). • Informal strategies such as gestures, facial expressions, body movements, eye gaze and vocalisations. These may be *idiosyncratic*; that is, gestures or body movements may be *particular to the individual* and have certain meanings.
Aided	**Using devices to assist communication:** • Computers and electronic devices, such as iPads, mobile phones and software applications (apps), e.g. Pictello. • Video clips, photos, pictures and text can also be uploaded into apps to be used for communication. Low-technology systems, such as communication books or boards. These may contain objects or parts of objects, photos, pictures, alphabet or words that allow people to communicate specific predetermined messages and may include strategies for responding, such as 'yes' and 'no'. These are some of the most commonly used forms of AAC (Finke, Light & Kitko, 2008).

TABLE 15.2
Augmentative and alternative communication (AAC)

1 Further information about Auslan, Key Word Signs and Pictello is provided in the *Further reading* section at the end of this chapter.

may use lip-reading, manual signing or other strategies (as outlined in Table 15.2). Some people may need to rely on their sense of touch, such as when reading Braille, because they have both vision and hearing impairments.

How people's communication difficulties can affect their safety in healthcare

Healthcare professionals frequently report difficulty communicating and, therefore, caring for people with complex communication needs (Campbell & Happ, 2010). Few healthcare professionals have the education or experience to prepare them to cope with such situations (Finke et al., 2008).

Augmentative and alternative communication

People with severe communication impairments (SCIs) use other ways to communicate than speech. Such strategies are known as 'augmentative and alternative communication' (AAC). AAC strategies can be difficult to use for both the person with an SCI and their communication partners. In healthcare interactions, this can result in ineffective communication between people with SCIs and their healthcare professionals. People with SCIs are therefore at greater risk of adverse health events (Webber et al., 2010).

Complex healthcare needs

When people have SCIs, they often also have complex healthcare needs. SCIs may be associated with (a) cognitive impairment, (b) multiple medical conditions, (c) polypharmacy (the prescription of multiple medications), (d) a limited support system and income, and (e) a narrow margin of good health due to the impact of neurological disease on the body (Cristian, 2009, p. 229). There may also be situations when people are unconscious and therefore unable to communicate.

It may be difficult for a person with an SCI to convey the necessary information or communicate their needs to healthcare professionals. They may be unable to tell the healthcare professional their history or report presenting conditions, such as allergies or subjective symptoms (e.g. areas of pain).

It is important to keep in mind that, when speaking to a person with communication impairments, it is helpful to keep sentences short, use simple words and ask questions that only require a yes/no response; e.g. 'Are you feeling okay today?' is better than asking 'How are you feeling today?'.

Speaking more loudly to a person with a disability is not necessary unless that person has a hearing impairment.

It may also be difficult for people with SCIs to understand and remember advice; for example, about medications or discharge instructions.

Ineffective communication

Researchers have identified a number of potential barriers to communication between healthcare professionals in hospital settings and patients who have SCIs (Balandin et al., 2007; Finke et al., 2008). Such barriers include:

- difficulty gaining the attention of staff when needed
- few opportunities for communication because staff tend to focus on healthcare procedures and do not take the time to interact
- limited knowledge and education of staff in the use of AAC
- lack of access to AAC systems or devices
- healthcare professionals' lack of recognition and/or understanding of patients' attempts to communicate
- lack of response to patients' communicative attempts from healthcare professionals
- lack of continuity in staff assigned to a patient's care
- healthcare professionals taking the attitude that it is 'not their problem'.

In the United Kingdom, MENCAP (2007) reported that doctors often made personal judgments about patients' quality of life if those patients had a learning disability[1], despite evidence of poor correlation between a doctor's opinion of a person's quality of life and that person's own opinion. Healthcare professionals may also assume that people with SCIs experience less pain or emotional distress than other people. In a classic study, Baer, Davitz and Lieb (1970) found that healthcare professionals attributed lower pain levels to non-verbal patients than to verbal patients.

Consequences of ineffective communication

People's SCIs, coupled with barriers to effective communication, can place them at risk of 'inadequate care' or 'harmful situations' (Hemsley & Balandin, 2004, p. 250). Limited communication between nurses and patients has resulted in increased risk of patients being neglected, ignored, isolated and injured (Finke et al., 2008). People with SCIs may also not have the means to report abuse (Collier et al., 2006). Participants in a study by Collier et al. used AAC to tell of their experiences of physical, verbal, sexual and financial abuse; threats of abuse; neglect; their equipment being destroyed; inappropriate administration of medications; inappropriate exertion of control; and not being allowed to communicate.

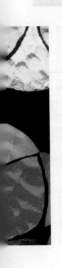

Access Helen Ross' story to learn more about empathic and effective communication with a person with a communication impairment at <https://www.virtualempathymuseum.com.au/wp-content/uploads/2018/10/PERSON-WITH-CEREBRAL-PALSY-TOOLKIT-IN-TEMPLATE.pdf>.

ROBERT'S STORY

Robert is a young adult with cerebral palsy who is not able to use his arms or hands to feed himself. He depends on carers to do this for him.

Robert was moaning and refusing to eat. He pressed his lips together and turned his head away when his carer tried to feed him and he sometimes cried after meals. A modified barium swallow showed that he had severe gastro-oesophageal reflux disease.

Robert had no speech and instead used his body to communicate what he wanted and needed. Turning his head away and pressing his lips together were communication strategies that he used. With his moaning/crying, he was trying to communicate that he did not want to eat because this caused him pain.

Robert's carer appeared to be aware that Robert was communicating refusal, but she did not know how to respond. The resulting breakdown in communication exposed Robert to untreated pain and risk of further harm if his underlying condition was not treated.

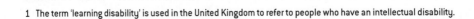

1 The term 'learning disability' is used in the United Kingdom to refer to people who have an intellectual disability.

Ensuring safety in healthcare processes for people with impaired communication

Person-centred care can assist to keep people with SCIs safer within healthcare settings because it provides more opportunities to source the necessary information to achieve positive health outcomes. For example, a framework of *Mindful Dialogues* can be used to enhance person-centred relationships between healthcare professionals, patients and families, and when people have complex care needs and communication impairment (Tasker, Loftus & Higgs, 2012).

> Being mindful
> Staying engaged
> Becoming responsive

Being mindful: Acknowledging a person's humanity and individuality

Mindful practitioners use a variety of means to enhance their ability to engage in moment-to-moment self-monitoring, bring to consciousness their tacit personal knowledge and deeply held values, use peripheral vision and subsidiary awareness to become aware of new information and perspectives, and adopt curiosity in both ordinary and novel situations.

(Epstein, 1999, p. 2)

You can be a mindful healthcare professional by:

- *constantly observing your patient and their environment;*
- *including your patient in all communication exchanges;*
- *individualising your approach to communication with each person;*
- *finding out how your patient can communicate*—Always read the person's own profile information and ask carers and family members to explain how the person with SCI communicates. However, be aware that communication situations may be assisted but also complicated by the efforts of staff, family or friends as they try to explain how they see the situation. In the United Kingdom, work has been done to introduce and use *patient passports* about peoples' needs and preferences (Broderick et al., 2011);
- *ensuring that AAC systems are available* and that you know how they work—If no communication system is available, make a referral to a speech pathologist to ensure that some form of communication system is established (Finke et al., 2008);
- *ensuring that the person has the vocabulary or other means to communicate symptoms or concerns* (Campbell & Happ, 2010)—Encourage the use of *gesture* and *pointing* to indicate symptom location. Use *communication boards* to communicate about symptom location, intensity and quality. Include vocabulary for communication of all forms of abuse. Picture Communication Symbols (PCS) in Boardmaker software have been developed to provide a way of communicating abuse (Collier et al., 2006, p. 70);
- *being a communication partner with and for people*—The success of communication is as reliant on the healthcare professional's skills as a communication partner as it is on the person's ability to use their AAC strategies (State of Queensland [Department of Communities], 2009);
- *actively involving people with SCIs in supported decision making about their care* (see Web resources at the end of this chapter);
- *communicating and collaborating with other healthcare professionals*—Communication breakdown between care providers can cause errors to occur. Staff need to be aware of how a person is currently communicating and that this can quickly change. Such information needs to be part of the handover process.

> Some people may require a support person to provide medical information and a legally designated person to give consent for medical procedures (Lip Chew, Iacono & Tracy, 2009). For example, if a person is unconscious, healthcare professionals must include a legally designated person in any decision-making processes. Legally designated guardians should be contacted immediately to avoid any delay in the initiation of treatment.

> Get on the same level (face to face) to communicate with your patient, especially if they are lying down or sitting in a chair or wheelchair.

Dr Diane Tasker and Dr Tania de Bortoli were given permission by Melissa and her family to use this photo in teaching healthcare students about patient safety from the perspective of patients and their families.

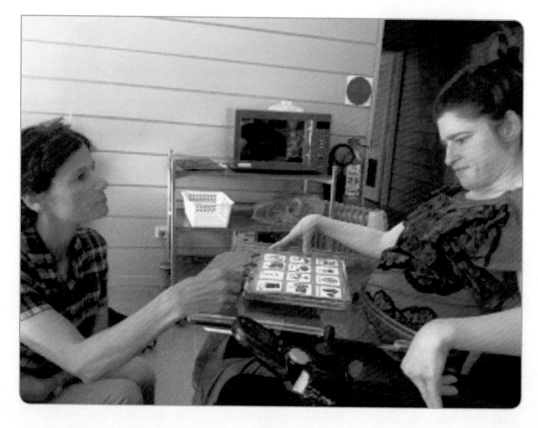

Staying engaged: Maintaining connection with your patient

Be quiet

Listen to me.

I need you to listen to me.

I can't communicate as well as you.

So I need you to listen to me and hear me!

Stay with me and be quiet.

Be with me.

Lack of confidence and experience can make healthcare professionals reluctant to interact with people with whom they have difficulty communicating (Hemsley & Balandin, 2004). The following strategies may assist in interacting with people who have SCIs.

- ■ *Take time to observe,* looking for cues and non-verbal signs of pain or discomfort (V. Madigan, personal communication, 25 September 2012). The *'OBSERVE': Non-verbal assessment tool for clinical evaluation* (Figure 15.1) and the *Non-verbal and behavioural pain indicators using the acronym 'PAINFUL'* (Figure 15.2) provide some further guidance for this process (Madigan, 2013a and b).

- ■ *Speak directly and use reassuring non-verbal communication,* such as eye contact, smiling and shaking hands.

- ■ *Establish a system for the person to indicate 'yes' and 'no'.*

- ■ *Use the person's communication system consistently in all interactions with them.*

- ■ *Ensure that safety information (e.g. taking of medication) is presented to people in a way that they can understand or remember.* If this is not possible, ensure that carers are clear about this information.

- ■ *Emphasise those parts of their communication system that deal with pain, comfort and emotions* and encourage people to use them.

- ■ *Allow time for people to respond.* Some people with SCIs may need 15–20 seconds to process information and then respond to a question. You can encourage communication by avoiding the appearance of being hurried. Also be aware that some people can be overwhelmed by interpersonal interactions (e.g. people with autism).

FIGURE 15.1
OBSERVE: *Non-verbal patient assessment tool for clinical evaluation*

Overall physical assessment

Body language

Behaviour

Safety/**S**urroundings

Emotions/moods/demeanour

Relationship with others

Vocalisation

Eyes/re-**E**xamine, **E**valuate

FIGURE 15.2 *Non-verbal and behavioural pain indicators using the acronym* **'PAINFUL'**

Posture abnormal/pupils dilated

Appearance

Increased heart rate/respirations/blood pressure

Nausea and vomiting

Noise/vocalisations

Facial grimacing

Favouring gestures

Unstable mobility/gait impairment

Lassitude

Loss of appetite

JOEL'S STORY

This is a quote from Joel Smith, who lives with autism and wrote online to try to inform people about how someone with a communication impairment related to autism can feel when trying to communicate.

> Sometimes autistics need to be left alone, so that we can calm our minds and bodies. We'll often retreat when we're experiencing sensory overload or when we are under a lot of stress.

> If you see me push you away in a stressful time, please realise that I'm not doing it because you did something wrong. I sometimes push my friends away when I need quiet and solitude to regain my senses. Let me know you are available, and that you care, but please don't push the issue if I am unable to interact at that moment.

(Smith, 2001, Solitude)

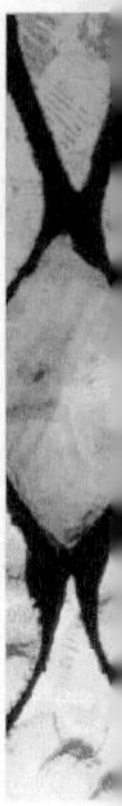

Becoming responsive: Enhancing perception of people's individuality in light of knowledge gained with and about them

Responsiveness does not refer only to *responding to issues*; it also refers to *responding to people and their concerns*. Conversations that occur between healthcare professionals and their patients, families and carers can assist the process of becoming responsive, but this requires healthcare professionals to have an open attitude.

■ *Use language appropriate to a person's age and cognitive ability* to help them to better understand you. If the person has an intellectual disability and/or hearing impairment, use materials (e.g. pictures) to support their understanding of explanations. Be careful not to speak to people in a childish manner.

- *Check your interpretations of a person's message* by repeating back key points or words and ask for feedback, or watch for relief or recognition.
- *Continuously observe and assess people* (Gibson-Mee, 2011). People who have little or no intelligible speech and other physical impairments may not be able to signal for attention.
- *Assess people's health and wellbeing so that behaviour changes that may signify illness or changes in condition are not misinterpreted as signs of their disability* (Blair, 2011, p. 24).
- *Delineate care roles* being undertaken by carers and hospital staff so that mistakes or omissions of care do not occur.
- *Encourage patients, carers and families to be involved* as much as they want to be. Importantly, there may be some situations when people will *not* want their attending carer to be present. Ensure that you make time to be alone with them, in case they are trying to disclose instances of concern or abuse. Bear in mind that anyone may be a perpetrator of abuse or hold attitudes that discourage patients from disclosing that abuse (Collier et al., 2006).
- *Document family and carer contributions and support needs* in the person's care plan and notes (e.g. need for respite, transportation).

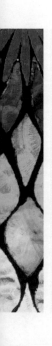

JENNY'S STORY

Jenny was a young woman with an intellectual disability. Her general practitioner, Gwen, had cared for her for many years. Although Jenny's communication was impaired, she always said 'Good' when she visited her doctor. She had very few other words.

Jenny had started repeatedly hitting her head. Her carers reported that she was increasingly moody, less active and had a decreased appetite. They thought that her self-abusive behaviour had increased after an altercation with another resident in her group home.

Gwen sought an opinion from a consultant doctor who specialised in the care of people with developmental disability. On her advice, a range of medical tests was ordered, including brain CT scans, and it was thought that her problem could be depression. Jenny was started on medication but she continued to be agitated and self-harming.

On the following appointment, she was still self-harming but now she was also vomiting, had lost weight and constantly wanted to go to bed. Gwen arranged an urgent gastroscopy, which revealed a helicobacter stomach infection. This condition was treated with a combination course of medication.

Gwen's notes written two months later read: 'Jenny appears to be a lot better ... She said to me, 'Good, good'

In 'Jenny's story' we can see how frustrating health problems can be when people are unable to communicate clearly about their symptoms. Collaboration is important; information may need to be gained from many different sources and combined with careful observation to solve health-related problems. Persistence by carers and healthcare professionals is necessary to achieve successful outcomes.

Conclusion

Communicating with people who have a severe communication impairment can be challenging for healthcare professionals, but 'people with CCNs (complex communication needs) have a right to expect the same quality of care as the rest of the community' (Hemsley & Balindin, 2004, p. 244). We need to persist in our efforts to communicate and challenge our underlying assumptions about the subjective experiences of people with severe communication impairments.

Critical thinking activities

Annie had an acquired brain injury and was unable to speak, but she was able to nod or shake her head to provide yes/ no responses. She was waiting to have some tests done to identify why she had been experiencing abdominal pain. Lying in her hospital bed facing the window, Annie could see out of the window, but she was unable to use the call button because she had insufficient movement to do that activity. Her face was not visible from the door of her room.

1 How might you feel if you were Annie and admitted to hospital without the ability to speak?
2 If you were lying in a hospital bed unable to move or talk, what sort of physical and emotional attention would you like to receive?
3 What position would you prefer to be placed in to be able to communicate with people coming into your room?
4 Where would you like healthcare professionals to sit or stand when they speak to you?
5 How could you modify your approach to the next patient you meet who has impaired communication?

Teaching and assessment activities

The following activities may help students to more deeply consider how to interact with people with SCI's.

1 *Lip reading.* Students form into pairs and position themselves to carry out a lip reading activity. One student will take the role of a patient and the other student will take the role of a healthcare professional. Have a conversation! The roles can then be reversed. Educators and students should then discuss the experience to highlight any factors that contributed to a successful or unsuccessful interaction.
2 *Asking 'Yes/No' questions.* Students form into groups of three or four. Refer to the *Critical thinking activity* above to provide some context for this activity. As a group of healthcare professionals, determine what information you would like to gain from your interaction with Annie and build some appropriate 'Yes/No' questions to achieve this outcome. Students can then discuss the challenges associated with this communication activity.
3 Arrange a visit by a person who uses an AAC device so that students can gain skills and insights about this communication approach.
4 Refer students to the *Critical thinking activity* above and instruct them to devise a communication board of pictures that Annie could use to communicate. They should be guided to thoughtfully consider what Annie might need or want to communicate while in a hospital setting.

Further reading

Blair, J. (2011). Care adjustments for people with learning disabilities in hospitals. *Nursing Management, 18*(8), 21–4.

Broderick, D., Lewis, D., Worth, A. & Marland, A. (2011). One-page passport for people with learning disabilities. *Nursing Standard, 25*(47), 35–40. Accessed May 2018 at <http://nursingstandard.rcnpublishing.co.uk/archive/article-one-page-patient-passport-for-people-with-learning-disabilities>

Disabled People Using Scope Services. (2002). *The Good Practice Guide for Support Workers and Personal Assistants Working with Disabled People with Communication Impairments.* London: Scope. Accessed May 2018 at <http://www.scope.org.uk/Scope/media/Documents/Support/The-Good-Practice-Guide.pdf>

Tasker, D., Croker, A., McAllister, L. & Sefton, A. (2012). Talking with colleagues, patients, clients and carers. In J. Higgs, R. Ajjawi, L. McAllister, F. Trede & S. Loftus (Eds), *Communicating in the Health and Social Sciences.* *Melbourne, Australia:* Oxford University Press. (This chapter provides some more detailed advice about how to communicate with people with disability and the use of AAC devices.)

Web resources

Helen's story: These two videos below depict different aspects of Helen Ross' experiences of hospitalisation. They were designed to enhance empathy and raise awareness of the challenges that can be experienced by people with cerebral palsy, and complex communication needs when interacting with healthcare professionals.
Acknowledging the person:
<https://bournemouth.cloud.panopto.eu/Panopto/Pages/Viewer.aspx?id=1f4078dd-20be-46e6-b4db-a96500ac6d52>

Finding alternative ways:
<https://bournemouth.cloud.panopto.eu/Panopto/Pages/Viewer.aspx?id=55edc654-3557-4cde-9106-a96500acd885>

Auslan Signbank, a resource site for Auslan (Australian Sign Language).
<http://www.auslan.org.au>

Communication is Key. Communicating with deaf and hearing impaired patients: This resource was designed by Molly Sullivan, a former nursing student from the University of Newcastle to help healthcare professionals communicate with deaf and hearing-impaired patients. The website provides information on the deaf culture, links to interpreter services and videos demonstrating some AUSLAN signs.
<http://msullivan72.wixsite.com/communicationiskey>

ISAAC (International Society for Augmentative and Alternative Communication): ISAAC is a non-government organisation in consultative status with the United Nations

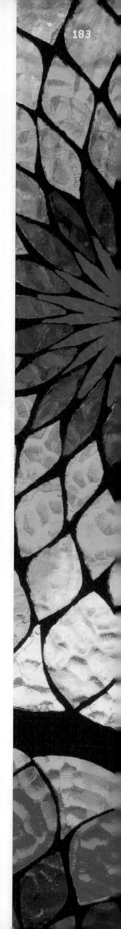

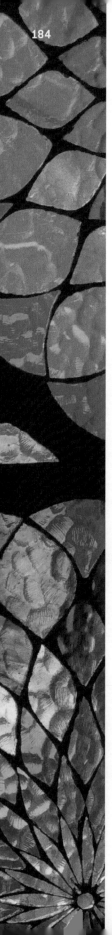

Economic and Social Council (ECOSOC). Its website provides information and resources about the use of AAC for adults and children.
<www.isaac-online.org/english/home/>

Key Word Sign Australia (Scope Australia)
<www.scopeaust.org.au/key-word-sign-australia>.

Pictello (AssistiveWare 2017; software application)
<www.assistiveware.com/product/pictello>.

Also available on Apple App Store at
<https://itunes.apple.com/au/app/pictello>

Speak Up Project (Safeguarding People who use Augmentative and Alternative Communication (AAC) from Sexual Abuse/Victimization): This website is maintained by Augmentative Communication Community Partnerships, Canada (ACCPC). It has a wide variety of resources that explore AAC use, and its use to protect people with communication impairment from harm related to sexual abuse.
<http://www.speakupandbesafe.com.au/>

New South Wales Government Family and Community Services: A useful website with information about supported decision-making.
<https://www.adhc.nsw.gov.au/individuals/inclusion_and_participation/supported-decision-making>

References

Anderson, E., Ford, F. & Thorpe, L. (2011). Learning to listen: Improving student communication with disabled people. *Medical Teacher, 3*(3), 44–52.

Baer, E., Davitz, L. & Lieb, R. (1970). Inferences of physical pain and psychological distress in relation to verbal and nonverbal patient communication. *Nursing Research, 19*(5), 388–92.

Balandin, S., Hemsley, B., Sigafoos, J. & Green, V. (2007). Communicating with nurses: The experience of 10 adults with cerebral palsy and complex communication needs. *Applied Nursing Research, 20*(2), 56–62.

Blair, J. (2011). Care adjustments for people with learning disabilities in hospitals. *Nursing Management, 18*(8), 21–4.

Broderick, D., Lewis, D., Worth, A. & Marland, A. (2011). One-page passport for people with learning disabilities. *Nursing Standard, 25*(47), 35–40.

Campbell, G. & Happ, M. (2010). Symptom identification in the chronically ill. *AACN Journal of Advanced Critical Care, 21*(1), 64–79.

Cristian, A. (2009). Patient safety. In A. Cristian (Ed.), *Medical Management of Adults with Neurologic Disabilities* (pp. 229–38). New York, NY: Demos Medical Publishing.

Collier, B., McGhie-Richmond, D., Odette, F. & Pyne, J. (2006). Reducing the risk of sexual abuse for people who use augmentative and alternative communication. *Augmentative and Alternative Communication, 22*(1), 62–75.

Disabled People Using Scope Services (2002). *The Good Practice Guide for Support Workers and Personal Assistants Working with Disabled People with Communication*

Impairments. London: Scope. Accessed May 2018 at <http://www.scope.org.uk/Scope/media/Documents/Support/The-Good-Practice-Guide.pdf>.

Epstein, R. (1999). Mindful practice. *Journal of the American Medical Association, 282*(9), 833–9.

Finke, E., Light, J. & Kitko, L. (2008). A systematic review of the effectiveness of nurse communication with patients with complex communication needs with a focus on the use of augmentative and alternative communication. *Journal of Clinical Nursing, 17*(16), 2102–15.

Gibson-Mee, S. (2011). Communication skills to improve experiences of hospital. *Learning Disability Practice, 14*(9), 28–30.

Hemsley, B. & Balandin, S. (2004). Without ACC: The stories of unpaid carers of adults with cerebral palsy and complex communication needs in hospital. *Augmentative and Alternative Communication, 20*(4), 243–58.

Lip Chew, K., Iacono, T. & Tracy, J. (2008). Overcoming communication barriers: Working with patients with intellectual disabilities. *Australian Family Physician, 30*(1-2), 10–14.

Madigan, V. (2013a). *'OBSERVE': Non-verbal Assessment Tool for Clinical Evaluation.* Contact Veronica Madigan: VMadigan@csu.edu.au.

Madigan, V. (2013b). *Non-verbal and Behavioural Pain Indicators Using the Acronym 'PAINFUL'.* Contact Veronica Madigan: VMadigan@csu.edu.au.

MENCAP: Understanding Learning Disability. (2007). *Death by Indifference: Following Up the Treat Me Right! Report.* London: MENCAP Accessed January 2018 at <https://www.mencap.org.uk/sites/default/files/2016-06/DBIreport.pdf>.

Smith, J. (2001). *Solitude. This Way of Life: Living with Autism* [website]. Accessed February 2013 at <http://www.geocities.com/growingjoel/whatisitlike.html> (website no longer being updated). New website: <http://thiswayoflife.org/contact.html>.

State of Queensland [Department of Communities, Child Safety and Disability Services]. (2009). *Complex Communication Needs.* Accessed December 2012 at <http://www.communities.qld.gov.au/resources/disability/community-involvement/communication/documents/complex-communitaction-needs.pdf>.

Tasker, D., Loftus, S. & Higgs, J. (2012). Fusing interpersonal horizons in community-based physiotherapy. Paper presented at the Physiotherapy New Zealand 2012 Conference 'Expanding Horizons', 4–6 May, Wellington, New Zealand.

Webber, R., Bowers, B. & Bigby, C. (2012). Hospital experiences of older people with intellectual disability: Responses of group home staff and family members. *Journal of Intellectual and Developmental Disabilities, 35*(3), 155–164.

World Health Organization. (2007). *International Classification of Functioning, Disability and Health: Children and Youth Version.* Geneva: WHO.

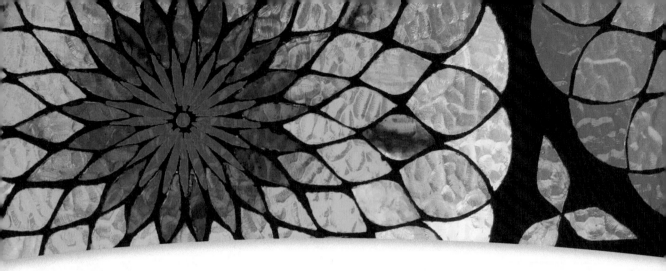

CHAPTER 16

COMMUNICATING WITH ABORIGINAL AND TORRES STRAIT ISLANDER PEOPLES

Natalie Strobel   Dan McAullay   Moira Sim
Colleen Hayward   Cobie Rudd

LEARNING OUTCOMES

Chapter 16 will enable you to:

- outline the impact of communication on Aboriginal and Torres Strait Islander peoples' health outcomes

- demonstrate an understanding of how conscious and unconscious bias influences healthcare professionals' attitudes, communication behaviours and clinical decision making

- discuss the importance of cultural empathy

- outline the importance of effective listening and demonstrating respect for Aboriginal and Torres Strait Islander peoples

- discuss strategies for addressing miscommunication in healthcare.

KEY CONCEPTS

cultural empathy | assumptions | conscious bias | unconscious bias

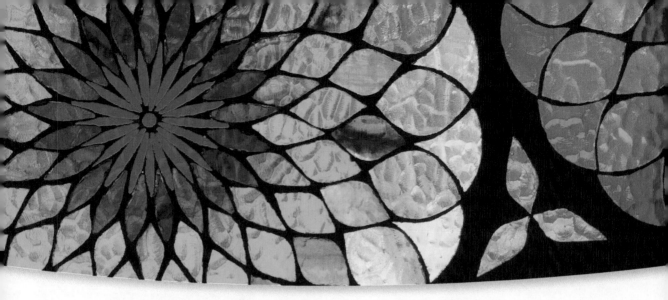

INTRODUCTION

Previous chapters have emphasised how effective communication is fundamental for quality healthcare and safe patient outcomes (Jha et al., 2010). Communication also has a significant impact on the quality of care provided to Aboriginal and Torres Strait Islander peoples (Lowell et al., 2012), with stigmatism and bias having an ongoing impact on interactions between patients and healthcare providers. A body of evidence has identified that Aboriginal and Torres Strait Islander peoples have poorer health outcomes than non-Indigenous Australians, and that there is a significant gap in life expectancy between Indigenous and non-Indigenous Australians (Anderson et al., 2016). These factors are exacerbated by poor communication, as a number of studies have reported that Aboriginal and Torres Strait Islander peoples often feel intimidated, belittled, annoyed, dissatisfied and alienated when accessing healthcare services (Kendall & Barnett, 2015).

This chapter discusses how to communicate effectively and empathically with Aboriginal and Torres Strait Islander peoples in culturally appropriate ways that have a positive impact on safety and wellbeing. The communication strategies included are based on the personal and professional experiences of the five authors, two of whom are Aboriginal—Associate Professor Dan McAullay (Noongar man) and Professor Colleen Hayward (senior Noongar woman).

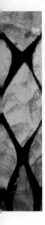

THE WILUNA SCHOOL PRINCIPAL'S STORY

The moment I tell them I'm of Aboriginal descent they speak to me like I'm not worth talking to or I'm too stupid to know (Kendall & Barnett, 2015).

When my dad was teaching at Wiluna, he had a series of heart attacks that were misdiagnosed by the Flying Doctor as indigestion. One day, when his level of discomfort was unbearable, he was taken to Meekatharra hospital by my brother and brother-in-law. The car journey was 180 kilometres along a gravel road. When he arrived the hospital staff assumed he was 'just another Aboriginal person' and said 'he's probably putting it on'. He was left untreated for several hours on a gurney in the corridor before someone went past him and said, 'You should look after him, he's the principal of Wiluna school'.

Source: Professor Colleen Hayward, Pro-Vice-Chancellor Equity and Indigenous, and Head of the Centre for Indigenous Australian Education and Research (Kurongkurl Katitjin), Edith Cowan University, personal interview, 3 October 2012.

The impact of communication on Aboriginal and Torres Strait Islander peoples' health outcomes

Communication is a highly complex process that is influenced by many factors. Figure 16.1 illustrates the factors that can influence communication with Aboriginal and Torres Strait Islander peoples.

Communication is critical for building trusting relationships, strengthening engagement and producing positive health outcomes for Aboriginal and Torres Strait Islander peoples (Jennings, Bond, & Hill, 2018). However, a recent systematic review identified that poor communication, such as the use of medical jargon, talking down to people or judgmental language reinforces power differentials between Aboriginal clients and healthcare professionals (Jennings et al., 2018). Alternatively, culturally appropriate and person-centred communication can enhance positive healthcare experiences and improve health outcomes (Jennings et al., 2018).

> When a blackfella goes to the health centre, he's looking around nervous . . . while he's in with the doctor he's looking around and trying to get out of the place. About a quarter of what the doctor's saying will sink in (Kendall & Barnett, 2015).

Communication also plays a significant role in determining the actual services that are provided, or in some cases not provided, to Aboriginal and Torres Strait Islander peoples. For example, in Australia, Aboriginal and Torres Strait Islander peoples with cardiovascular conditions have been reported to have 40 per cent less coronary procedures performed and twice the in-hospital mortality rate compared to non-Indigenous Australians. This has been attributed to poor communication between healthcare professionals and clients, including the withholding of information or the provision of limited explanations about healthcare options (Lopez et al., 2014; Tavella et al., 2016).

How conscious and unconscious bias influences healthcare professionals' attitudes, communication behaviours and decision making

Assumptions, biases, stereotypes and stigmatism can negatively influence how healthcare professionals communicate and respond to other people (Croskerry, 2003). Cognitive biases can arise from the tendency to group people, prefer people who are similar to ourselves, and try to make a complex world simple (Glaser, Spencer & Charbonneau, 2014). As a result of these biases, our judgments and communication behaviours can be influenced in a negative way.

We are often unaware of the biases and prejudices that we hold as they are deeply imbedded and long standing. However, these biases can have a significant impact on the way healthcare is provided to (or withheld from) Aboriginal and Torres Strait Islander peoples. In Western Australia, for example, 52 per cent of urban residents and 69 per cent of regional residents admitted that they are prejudiced against Aboriginal Australians (Pedersen et al., 2000). These racist attitudes have been identified as a

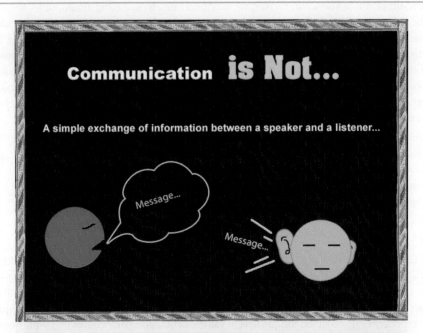

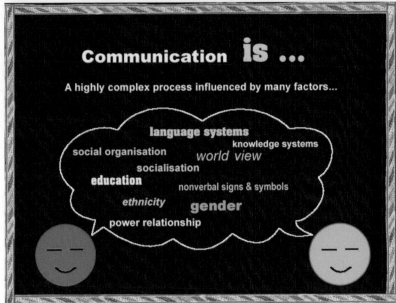

FIGURE 16.1
The context of communicating with Aboriginal and Torres Strait Islander peoples
Source: Reproduced with permission of Charles Darwin University <http://www.cdu.edu.au/centres/stts/home.html>.

significant cause of the socioeconomic and health disadvantage of Indigenous Australians (Artuso et al., 2013; Worrall-Carter et al., 2016). One of our authors expressed their thoughts on racism and how it may influence our thinking:

> *We all have blinkers on whether we like it or not. We can think that we are not racist but we are. Racism originates from a survival instinct in which human beings favour their own tribe over others. We identify with people who are similar to ourselves and we have less understanding of people who seem different to us. If everyone recognised their own tendency to racism things would be different.*

As a result of this tendency to racism, we may find ourselves making assumptions about how we treat patients (as shown in the story about the principal of Wiluna School). There is also evidence that healthcare professionals' attitudes and prejudices influence their clinical decision making and their interpretation of patient's symptoms (Cooper & Roter, 2003). Healthcare professionals must seek to develop emotional intelligence and self-awareness by deliberate reflection on their biases, assumptions and preconceptions, as failure to do so can undermine the accuracy of their communication, clinical decision making and, consequently, patient safety. One of our authors explained how biases and assumptions could influence our practice:

> If we make assumptions about people not having intelligence, we may not explain certain things. If we make assumptions about what may be important to patients, we might not tell them certain things, we might not offer certain options and we might not ask certain things. And if we don't ask, we don't listen, then we probably advise things that are not necessarily appropriate and which might not be followed through because they are not appropriate.

The importance of cultural empathy

As Reid (2012, p. 216) describes, at the heart of racist attitudes and shortfalls in the healthcare system lies a 'lack of respect, lack of compassion and failure to uphold the dignity of patients'. However, cultural empathy can help to break down some of the communication barriers that currently exist in healthcare (Kendall & Barnett, 2015). Cultural empathy is defined as the learned ability to appreciate or imagine experiences through the unique lens of values, beliefs and perspectives of people from cultural backgrounds different to one's own (Wang et al., 2003). Cultural empathy is a precursor to cultural competence (Sales et al., 2013).

Developing self-awareness and empathy through cultural training programs can help to improve communication between Aboriginal and Torres Strait Islander peoples and healthcare professionals (Bainbridge et al., 2015; Freeman et al., 2014). Training programs can also enhance cultural awareness; that is, knowledge and understanding of Aboriginal people's histories, values, belief systems, experience and lifestyles. Being culturally aware refers to having an appreciation and acceptance of cultural differences (Weetra, 2001).

> To understand what some of your own implicit biases are go to *Project Implicit*® and take the implicit association test: <https://implicit.harvard.edu/implicit/>.

> Biases and assumptions need to be discussed in cultural training. This needs to include reflection about self. We need to understand ourselves before we can consider how we act and react to others.

Could cultural training have helped in this situation?
In the Pilbara, a male Aboriginal patient was asked whether he'd passed water, and his reply was 'No, I haven't'. The conversation went on and on to the point where hospital staff were contemplating the use of a catheter. The patient thought that passing water referred to passing a creek on his way to the hospital. The healthcare professionals did not know that in this man's language the word for urine was 'koomp'.

BOX 16.1   Matching verbal and non-verbal signals

Communication involves both verbal and non-verbal behaviours. How you listen, look and react helps your patient to determine whether or not you care, whether you are being truthful, and how well you are listening. When verbal and non-verbal signals align, there is increased engagement, trust and building of rapport (Kelly & Brown, 2002; Vicary & Westerman, 2004). However, when verbal and non-verbal signals do not match, anger, mistrust and a lack of engagement with the healthcare professionals and healthcare services can result.

Therapeutic interactions with Aboriginal and Torres Strait Islander peoples require healthcare professionals to be mindful of the various ways that culture affects clinical encounters. Indeed, inherent in cultural awareness is a recognition that culture is much more than country of origin, but it is a complex reflection of each individual's 'sense-making' schemas. Effective cultural practice and respectful relationships are also a core element of professional practice (Cusack et al., 2018).

Listening to Aboriginal and Torres Strait Islander peoples

As healthcare professionals, listening to patients is essential to building trust and developing therapeutic relationships. However, Aboriginal and Torres Strait Islander peoples sometimes tell healthcare professionals what they think they want to hear rather than what is truly happening. This occurs for a range of reasons, including a lack of trust and a perceived power differential between healthcare professionals and patients. Further, a 'yes' response is often used as an indication that an Aboriginal person has heard the question, not that they have understood it or are actually answering it. Many Aboriginal and Torres Strait Islander peoples relay stories about how previous negative communication interactions with healthcare professionals often discourage them from responding to potential medical emergencies, for example:

> I said 'I need to see a doctor'. At the end of the line was an arrogant white lady who had no patience. She said 'Speak up I can't understand you' ... and then she put the phone down. I won't ring up again (Kendall & Barnett, 2015).

Healthcare professionals need to reflect on their communication approaches in order to become more self-aware and attuned to the needs of individual patients. They also need to check their understanding of what other people have said. For example, one of our authors said:

> I often find myself testing that I've heard what someone is telling me. I say 'I think what you've said to me is this ...' or 'I'm trying to understand and what I've heard is ...'.

The next time you have a conversation with a patient, reflect and ask whether you listened and really heard what the person was saying, instead of what you thought they were saying.

Demonstrating respect

Effective communication with Aboriginal and Torres Strait Islander peoples is not always easy, and in healthcare contexts, when personal space and a range of intimate factors are at play, it is even more challenging. Effective communication requires much more than information provision, courtesy and kindness. It is also about conveying messages in a respectful way that is easily understood, unlikely to be misinterpreted or cause offence, and not threatening or intimidating.

In a hospital setting, a nurse might say to a patient, 'We have had two new patients admitted to the ward, so it might be some time before I can get back to you.' While this may seem to be courteous and thoughtful, the long history of systemic racism in healthcare can lead to Aboriginal and Torres Strait Islander patients feeling as if they have no control in the hospital environment, and this message can be misinterpreted as 'I'm in control and you'll have to fit in with me'.

If you wanted to explain to an Aboriginal patient that you are busy while at the same time reassuring them that their care is important, what words could you use to ensure the message has been received as intended, and at the same time give the person control over their care?

When miscommunication occurs ...

We don't always get it right the first time. In healthcare, sometimes we are rushed and say or do the wrong thing. But there are usually opportunities to go back and try again. This can be as simple as stopping at the next opportunity and picking up the conversation again. Where appropriate, it is always good to apologise: 'I'm sorry I was in a rush yesterday. I didn't get a chance to ... Can we start again?'

SOMETHING TO THINK ABOUT

At the end of the day, even sincere and well-meaning attempts to communicate can go awry. There will be many times when you won't know the impact of your communication, but there will also be times when you become aware that you have communicated poorly with Aboriginal and Torres Strait Islander peoples and, as a result, you will need to re-engage your patient. Box 16.2 summarises a number of strategies to address miscommunication.

BOX 16.2   Repairing miscommunication when it occurs

- If you recognise that a communication problem has occurred reflect on the part you played in the interaction and how you can approach the situation more appropriately.

- If you need advice about how to address miscommunication, seek guidance from Aboriginal Liaison Officers, Indigenous Outreach Workers or people who have experience working with the patient's specific language/cultural group (see Box 16.3).

- If you are discussing a topic with your patient and they become agitated, distressed or non-responsive, leave the topic and come back to it later. Don't keep pushing but wait until the person regains composure.

- Encourage the person to explain concepts/issues that are not clear to you.

- Consider whether the concepts or ideas that you need to communicate might be specific to your own cultural/professional experience. If so, take the time to explain them in detail and check that the person understands what you are saying. Drawings can also be used to help convey the message.

Source: Reproduced with permission of Charles Darwin University <http://www.cdu.edu.au/centres/stts/home.html>.

BOX 16.3   People who can help facilitate communication and cultural empathy with Aboriginal and Torres Strait Islander peoples

Aboriginal Liaison Officers *(ALOs) are* employed in hospitals to ensure that Aboriginal and Torres Strait Islander peoples have equitable access to mainstream healthcare services. ALOs can be found in all states and territories in Australia and can assist in:

- emotional, social and cultural support to patients and their families

- liaison services for patients and their families

- information about hospital services and the linkage between the hospital and other Indigenous community resources.

Indigenous Outreach Workers *can* help local Indigenous Australians make better use of the available healthcare services through:

- establishing links with local Indigenous communities to encourage and support the increased use of healthcare services

- assisting to identify barriers that may impact on access to healthcare services by Indigenous Australians

- providing practical assistance to Indigenous Australians to attend appointments for recommended health checks and follow-up care

- providing feedback to the healthcare organisation and healthcare professionals regarding issues that may be restricting Indigenous Australians' access to healthcare or related services, and working collaboratively to resolve these problems.

Sources: Reproduced with permission of ACT Government Health Directorate; and from <http://www.health.gov.au/internet/ctg/publishing.nsf/Content/prog-guidelines-ihpo-toc~outreach>, used by permission of the Australian Government.

Conclusion

The Aboriginal approach to health is 'holistic, steeped in history, religion, interconnectedness with the land, and obligatory requirements in relation to kin' (Kendall & Barnett, 2015). However, these factors are poorly understood by most non-Aboriginal healthcare professionals. Because of this, Aboriginal and Torres Strait Islander peoples often choose not to access the mainstream healthcare services, even though their general health is much worse than that of non-Aboriginal Australians. Factors such as poor communication, systemic racism and a lack of cultural competence have had a negative and ongoing impact on the engagement of Indigenous Australians with the healthcare system. However, it is evident from a wide body of literature, that when healthcare professionals practice in a culturally empathic manner, communication with and attitudes towards Aboriginal and Torres Strait Islander peoples improve.

This chapter has also emphasised the importance of trust, respect and emotional intelligence to the development of therapeutic relationships; and although the focus has been on communicating with Aboriginal and Torres Strait Islander peoples, the communication skills outlined will be relevant to all patients.

Watch 'I just want to go home' to gain further insights into how to address miscommunication and enhance cultural empathy: <http://www.ecu.edu.au/schools/medical-and-health-sciences/our-facilities/interprofessional-learning-resources/resources/i-just-want-to-go-home>

Critical thinking activities

I had been backwards and forwards from the family planning clinic for a good 12 months before my surgery. And my line was consistent: I don't know what's wrong . . . but something is wrong, and it doesn't feel right. I'd had two clear pap smears in the nine months before. And when doctors couldn't find any diagnoses, then it had to be all in my head. 'Are you alright? How's your relationship? Are there any problems at home?' Now that doesn't actually endear you to going back, but I persisted. When I was referred to the gynaecological oncologist, I didn't know what an oncologist was. Nobody in my realm at that time had ever had cancer. It's a very different story now. But in those days . . .

So, I had miscarried, and I went to the gynaecological oncologist. I fully expected to go in and find a little bit more about why I had miscarried and what my chances were of falling pregnant soon. That bit made sense. So I was going along to that appointment for something entirely different to why I'd been referred.

I went along to the gynaecological oncologist and after waiting three or four hours I left—clearly it wasn't important, I wasn't a priority. I'd miscarried now anyway. And then the doctor intervened and said I had to go back. When I went back the following day, he was fantastic but it was very much 'I think when we do surgery that I will find this but I won't find that'. He ran through a list of about 17 things, all of which ended up being absolutely on the money. In my head still I'm thinking two clear pap smears in nine months and the second one was only three months earlier. So, I'm asking questions like 'What are the chances of my falling pregnant and carrying a baby to term before we have to do anything about this?' And his response was, if we don't operate in the next fortnight I won't be able to save your life. I will meet you at the hospital in the morning.

1 Write down your initial thoughts and feelings about this Aboriginal woman's experience.
2 Consider what the instances of miscommunication were and what you could have done to repair them.
3 How would you have ensured that there was a safe space for the patient to ask questions about the situation?
4 How would you have asked whether the person understood what was happening and why?

Teaching and assessment activities

Access the stories at the 'Creating cultural empathy and challenging attitudes through Indigenous narratives' website: <https://altc.betterhealth.ecu.edu.au/>. The narratives profile authentic stories of Aboriginal and Torres Strait Islander peoples' experience of healthcare, both positive and negative, to enhance the development of cultural empathy (Edith Cowan University, 2012). They were collected to facilitate discussion and highlight communication styles, stereotypes and cultural issues. These narratives can be used in tutorial discussions and assignments about topics such as cardiovascular disease, diabetes, infection, palliative care and mental health. The aim is to use these narratives to encourage students to recognise their unconscious biases in a non-threatening environment. Ultimately it is hoped that the use of the narratives will positively influence the health and wellbeing of Australian Aboriginal and Torres Strait Islander peoples by improving the education of healthcare professionals.

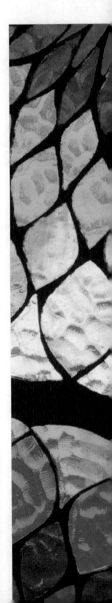

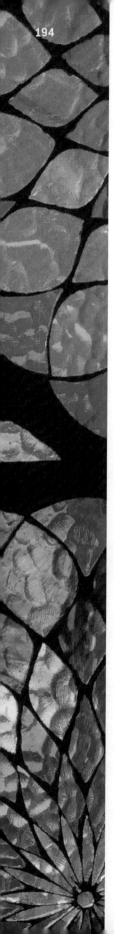

The 41 Indigenous narratives include themes such as paying respects to dying relatives, drunken stereotypes and the forced removal of children from their families. The narratives provide experiences of individuals within health systems and supporting materials for teaching, such as facilitator's guides and reflective thinking questions.

After watching particular narratives, students can discuss some of the points below:

1   What is important to this Indigenous person?
2   What are their values and beliefs?
3   How are these values and beliefs similar or different from your own?
4   What examples of good or poor care were illustrated in this narrative?
5   What are the facilitators or barriers to developing trust with Indigenous people? How can you develop trust with Indigenous Australians in your care?
6   How can you show respect to Indigenous Australians in your care?
7   Indigenous people (as most people) understand disease and medical terms when they are explained using simple language and diagrams.
8   How can healthcare professionals improve their communication with Indigenous Australians?

Further reading

'Closing the Gap' is a commitment by all Australian governments to improve the lives of Indigenous Australians, and in particular provide a better future for Indigenous children. For more information, go to the Department of the Prime Minister and Cabinet <https://www.pmc.gov.au/indigenous-affairs/closing-gap>.

Taylor, K. & Guerin, P. (2010). *Health Care and Indigenous Australians: Cultural Safety in Practice*. Victoria: Palgrave Macmillan.

Trudgen, R. (2000). *Why Warriors Lie Down and Die*. Aboriginal Resource and Development Services Inc., Darwin.

Web resources

Creating cultural empathy and challenging attitudes through Indigenous narratives
<https://altc-betterhealth.ecu.edu.au/index.php>

Sharing the True Stories: Improving communication between health staff and their Indigenous patients. This website aims to develop a more informed understanding of intercultural communication in Aboriginal healthcare, identify strategies to improve communication, and provide resources on communicating with Aboriginal and Torres Strait Islander peoples.
<www.cdu.edu.au/centres/stts/home.html>

Mungabareena Aboriginal Corporation & Women's Health Goulburn North East (2008). Working with Aboriginal people and communities: Health and community services audit tool. This tool is part of the 'Making Two Worlds Work' project. It enables agencies to audit their practices and make small changes, which can lead to big differences in providing better care.
<www.whealth.com.au/mtww/documents/MTWW_Audit_Tool.pdf>

The Lowitja Institute: Australia's National Institute for Aboriginal and Torres Strait Islander Health Research—a source of information about how to communicate research to Aboriginal and Torres Strait Islander peoples and communities.

References

Anderson, I., Robson, B., Connolly, M., Al-Yaman, F., Bjertness, E., King, A., . . . Yap, L. (2016). Indigenous and tribal peoples' health (The Lancet-Lowitja Institute Global Collaboration): A population study. *Lancet, 388*(10040), 131–57. doi:10.1016/S0140-6736(16)00345-7

Artuso, S., Cargo, M., Brown, A. & Daniel, M. (2013). Factors influencing health care utilisation among Aboriginal cardiac patients in central Australia: A qualitative study. *BMC Health Serv Res, 13*, 83. doi:10.1186/1472-6963-13-83

Bainbridge, R., McCalman, J., Clifford, A. & Tsey, K. (2015). *Cultural Competency in the Delivery of Health Services for Indigenous People. Issues paper no. 13.* Produced for the Closing the Gap Clearinghouse. Retrieved from Canberra: Australian Institute of Health and Welfare; Melbourne: Australian Institute of Family Studies.

Cooper, L. A. & Roter, D. L. (2003). Patient-provider communication: The effect of race and ethnicity on process and outcomes of healthcare. In B. D. Smedley, A. Y. Stith, & A. R. Nelson (Eds), *Unequal Treatment: Confronting Racial and Ethnic Disparities in Health Care* (pp. 552–93). Washington, DC: National Academy Press.

Croskerry, P. (2003). The importance of cognitive errors in diagnosis and strategies to minimize them. *Academic Medicine, 78*(8), 1–6.

Cusack, L., Kinnear, A., Ward, K., Mohammad, J. & Butler, A. (2018). *Cultural Safety: Nurses and Midwives Leading the Way for Safer Healthcare.* Accessed January 2019 at <https://www.acn.edu.au/wp-content/uploads/2018/03/Nursing-and-Midwifery-Board-Statement-Nurses-and-midwives-leading-the-way-for-safer-healthcare.pdf>

Edith Cowan University. (2012). Creating cultural empathy and challenging attitudes through Indigenous narratives. Accessed January 2019 at <https://altc.betterhealth.ecu.edu.au/index.php>.

Freeman, T., Edwards, T., Baum, F., Lawless, A., Jolley, G., Javanparast, S. & Francis, T. (2014). Cultural respect strategies in Australian Aboriginal primary health care services: Beyond education and training of practitioners. *Aust N Z J Public Health, 38*(4), 355–61. doi:10.1111/1753-6405.12231

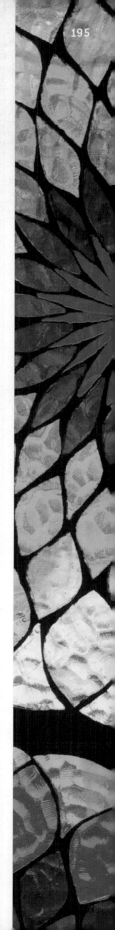

Glaser, J., Spencer, K. & Charbonneau, A. (2014). Racial bias and public policy. *Policy Insights from Behavioral and Brain Sciences, 1*, 88–94.

Jennings, W., Bond, C. & Hill, P. S. (2018). The power of talk and power in talk: A systematic review of Indigenous narratives of culturally safe healthcare communication. *Aust J Prim Health*. doi:10.1071/PY17082

Jha, A. K., Prasopa-Plaizier, N., Larizgoitia, I. & Bates, D. W. (2010). Patient safety research: An overview of the global evidence. *Qual Saf Health Care, 19*(1), 42–7. doi:19/1/42 [pii] 10.1136/qshc.2008.029165

Kelly, L. & Brown, J. B. (2002). Listening to native patients. Changes in physicians' understanding and behaviour. *Can Fam Physician, 48*, 1645–52.

Kendall, E. & Barnett, L. (2015). Principles for the development of Aboriginal health interventions: Culturally appropriate methods through systemic empathy. *Ethnicity & Health, 20*(5), 437–52. doi: 10.1080/13557858.2014.921897

Lopez, D., Katzenellenbogen, J. M., Sanfilippo, F. M., Woods, J. A., Hobbs, M. S., Knuiman, M. W., . . . Thompson, S. C. (2014). Disparities experienced by Aboriginal compared to non-Aboriginal metropolitan Western Australians in receiving coronary angiography following acute ischaemic heart disease: The impact of age and comorbidities. *Int J Equity Health, 13*(1), 93. doi:10.1186/s12939-014-0093-3

Lowell, A., Maypilama, E., Yikaniwuy, S., Rrapa, E., Williams, R. & Dunn, S. (2012). 'Hiding the story': Indigenous consumer concerns about communication related to chronic disease in one remote region of Australia. *Int J Speech Lang Pathol, 14*(3). 200-208. doi:10.3109/17549507.2012.663791

NSW Department of Community Services. (2009). *Working with Aboriginal People and Communities—A Practice Resource*. Accessed January 2019 at <http://www.carersaustralia.com.au/storage/2011Working%20with%20Aboriginal%20People%20and%20Communities.pdf>.

Pedersen, A., Griffiths, B., Contos, N., Bishop, B. & Walker, I. (2000). Attitudes toward Aboriginal Australians in city and country settings. *Australian Psychologist, 35*(2), 109–17.

Reid, J. (2012). Respect, compassion and dignity: The foundations of ethical and professional caring. *The Journal of Perioperative Practice, 22*(7), 216–19.

Sales, I., Jonkman, L., Connor, S. & Hall, D. (2013). A comparison of educational interventions to enhance cultural competency in pharmacy students. *American Journal of Pharmaceutical Education, 77*, 76.

Tavella, R., McBride, K., Keech, W., Kelly, J., Rischbieth, A., Zeitz, C., . . . Brown, A. (2016). Disparities in acute in-hospital cardiovascular care for Aboriginal and non-Aboriginal South Australians. *Med J Aust, 205*(5), 222–27.

Vicary, D. & Westerman, T. (2004). 'That's just the way he is': Some implications of Aboriginal mental health beliefs. *Australian e-Journal for the Advancement of Mental Health 3*(3), 103–12.

Wang, Y.-W., Davidson, M. M., Yakushko, O. F., Savoy, H. B., Tan, J. A. & Bleier, J. K. (2003). The scale of ethnocultural empathy: Development, validation, and reliability. *Journal of Counseling Psychology, 50*, 221–34.

Worrall-Carter, L., Daws, K., Rahman, M. A., MacLean, S., Rowley, K., Andrews, S., . . . Arabena, K. (2016). Exploring Aboriginal patients' experiences of cardiac care at a major metropolitan hospital in Melbourne. *Aust Health Rev, 40*(6), 696–704. doi:10.1071/AH15175

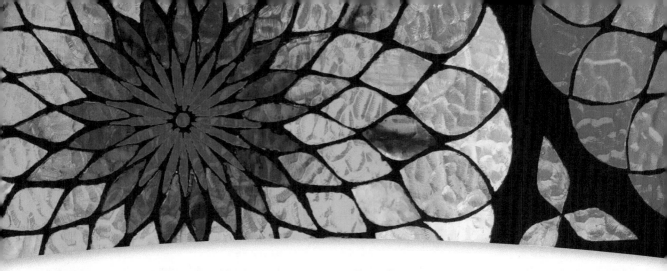

COMMUNICATING WITH PEOPLE FROM CULTURALLY AND LINGUISTICALLY DIVERSE BACKGROUNDS

Conor Gilligan   Sue Outram   Helen Buchanan

LEARNING OUTCOMES

Chapter 17 will enable you to:

- discuss the factors that influence migrant and refugee health

- describe the meaning of the term 'culture' and the complexities of cultural diversity

- outline the attributes of culturally competent healthcare professionals

- discuss when interpreters may be needed, and how to appropriately access and use interpreters

- describe effective strategies for communicating with people from culturally and linguistically diverse backgrounds

- identify barriers to culturally appropriate healthcare communication

- reflect on your own personal attitudes to cultural diversity, and your experience of the healthcare environment in delivering safe care to culturally and linguistically diverse backgrounds.

KEY CONCEPTS

culture | linguistic diversity | cultural competence

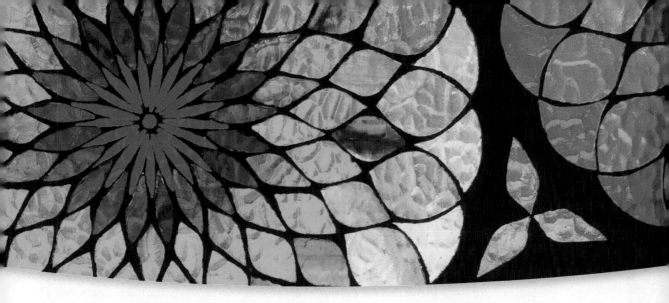

Cultural competence is much more than awareness of cultural differences, as it focuses on the capacity of the health system to improve health and wellbeing by integrating culture into the delivery of health services.

(Eisenbruch, 2004)

INTRODUCTION

Australia is one of the most culturally and linguistically diverse nations in the world. The 2016 Census shows that nearly half (49%) of the Australian population had either been born overseas (first-generation Australian) or one or both parents had been born overseas (second-generation Australian) (Australian Bureau of Statistics [ABS], 2016). The fact that there are 5.3 million first-generation Australians puts the need for culturally appropriate healthcare into focus. There have been many terms used to encompass this culturally diverse population. This chapter uses the term 'CALD' to refer to people from culturally and linguistically diverse backgrounds.

Communication can be particularly challenging when barriers such as language and cultural difference are encountered. Australia's increasing cultural diversity has placed pressure on the healthcare system to ensure that all people, including migrants and refugees, have access to culturally appropriate and safe healthcare. Quality healthcare is a basic human right and the absence of patient-safe communication can have life-threatening consequences resulting in long-term harm. Despite ongoing efforts in Australia, reports frequently describe misunderstandings, miscommunication and inappropriate cultural assumptions in the care of patients from CALD backgrounds. For example, experiences of having no interpreter to explain blood test results (Brough, 2006), having the need for an emergency caesarean and being misdiagnosed with a mental illness have been recounted (Manderson & Allotey, 2003).

This chapter addresses the meaning and impact of culture and the impact of culturally competent communication on patient safety. It emphasises that communication is not primarily about language but awareness that the complexities of an individual's relationship with their culture, and the capacity to respond appropriately to these differences, are central to cultural competence.

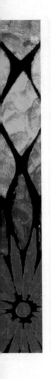

SUSAN'S STORY

Susan is a 25-year-old woman who fled the Congo after her village was attacked by rebels. She witnessed the brutal deaths of her husband and father, and she, her mother and her sisters were raped repeatedly by rebel militia in front of her children. Susan fled to Kenya with her three children where she sought refuge in Kakuma refugee camp.

As a single woman, Susan was often ostracised during her time in Kakuma. Many people called her names and abused her, and it became increasingly difficult for her and her children to survive. Her case came to the attention of protection officers within Kakuma and she was eventually resettled in Australia.

Susan arrived severely traumatised and with complex physical and psychological health needs. Because she spoke some English, her case worker assumed she would need only limited support. Subsequently, Susan only saw her case worker three times before being referred to a new service provider who had no information on her history. Susan was forced to retell all aspects of her story. Susan refused to return to the service and subsequently tried to seek assistance through a number of other services, without success. At one stage Susan was referred to a torture and trauma counselling service but she was terrified this would be seen as confirmation that she was mentally ill.

Susan had limited community support as she found it very difficult to trust people. She felt isolated and often only left her house to take her children to school. As a single mother Susan worked hard to care for her children but continued to struggle. Three years after arriving in Australia, Susan was reviewed by a mental health nurse practitioner who was experienced in working with women at risk. The nurse practitioner communicated empathically and over many months she provided the individualised and person-centred support that Susan needed. Susan and her family are now doing well.

Migrant and refugee health

In Australia, people who were born overseas generally enjoy good health, and in fact even better health than many Australian-born individuals according to mortality data, hospitalisation rates and rates of lifestyle-related risk factors. Most migrants enter Australia under the skilled worker scheme and they (and their dependents) undergo rigorous medical screening before being approved. However, the health of migrants appears to decline with their length of stay in Australia (Smith, 2015).

This decline in health status may be explained, in part, by an uptake of behaviours associated with health risk, but it is also likely to be associated with a lack of access to culturally appropriate healthcare. There is also evidence that disparities in the incidence of disease and health outcomes exist for people from CALD backgrounds. It seems there is less participation in healthcare and less involvement in decision making for many patients from CALD backgrounds (Harun, Harrison & Young, 2012). The exclusion of CALD patients from many intervention trials to improve the quality of care, as well as from many clinical trials, highlights some of the challenges faced in providing equitable care to CALD patients, as well as the treatment gap that exists for these patients.

In 2016, Australia resettled 34 193 refugees (1.43% of the global total), which was an increase from 2015 due to a one-off commitment of 12 000 places for Syrian and Iraqi refugees (Refugee Council of Australia, 2017). In contrast to the good health among migrants in Australia, humanitarian refugees arrive from different backgrounds, and in many cases have been forced to flee to save their lives or preserve their freedom. A significant proportion of refugees come with a history of severe trauma. Some have been tortured and have spent years (for some, up to 15 years) in refugee camps that provided limited protection and healthcare. Refugees living in pre-settlement countries have often experienced serious threats such as arbitrary arrest, detention and severe discrimination. Educational opportunities are often very limited with schooling frequently interrupted.

Differences in language, culture and health practices represent substantial challenges for refugees arriving in Australia. Physical as well as social and emotional health issues often lead to contact with the healthcare system but the care available is not always culturally appropriate and may not give adequate consideration to peoples' social history and cultural needs.

In one study, a large group of refugee women from the Middle East and the Horn of Africa were interviewed to identify problems that affected their reproductive health in Australia (Manderson &

Allotey, 2003). These women experienced strong feelings of discrimination, miscommunication and poor-quality provision of health and social services. One-fifth spoke about specific communication problems: lack of interpreters, being given information by healthcare professionals that they judged as inappropriate, and the inability of the doctors to 'hear' or understand the meaning of what the women told them.

Communication challenges are also regularly experienced in caring for older refugees and migrants, many of whom are now facing chronic illnesses, dementia and the need to access aged care with associated end-of-life issues. English language learnt after migration often fades under these circumstances and older people may revert to their original language. Older migrant women who have been socially isolated are particularly vulnerable.

The meaning of culture

While language barriers can be quite readily identified, cultural barriers are more difficult to recognise. 'Culture' refers to ways of thinking and behaving that are socially accepted among a particular group or society. Thus, every individual has a culture that is influenced by the social norms and the context in which they live. It is often only when cultural differences become apparent that we are conscious of culture. The aspects of culture we can easily see in others (e.g. food, dress and language) can be likened to the tip of an iceberg—the majority is hidden from view and largely unknown. Culture can exist at many levels: the culture of a country or region, the culture associated with a sport or leisure activity, or the culture associated with a profession.

Different age groups within the population can also be seen as cultural entities in themselves. Adolescents have a language and culture that often seems quite foreign to adults. Similarly, our ageing population represents a cultural group who grew up in a different time in society, with different approaches and attitudes about social issues. Cultural differences can be encountered not only with people from other countries and within a mainstream culture but also with colleagues from different 'subcultures' in the healthcare professions. Different behavioural norms, expectations and even language are passed on from one generation to the next in medicine, nursing, physiotherapy, social work, etc. (see Chapter 5).

Culture and language are strongly connected, not only in the primary language spoken but also in the use of slang and jargon, and in the different meanings attached to some common words. The English language provides many examples of confusing double meanings. For example, in Australian culture the word 'tea' is sometimes used to describe an evening meal or dinner, but in other contexts can be misunderstood to mean the hot beverage or an afternoon snack. These subtleties of language are not of the type that requires an interpreter but they can sometimes cause embarrassing miscommunication.

While we acknowledge the breadth of different cultures and subcultures in a society, this chapter focuses primarily on ethnic cultures, and safe communication with migrants and refugees from CALD backgrounds.

A framework for thinking about culture

Culture has been described as a framework people use to solve human problems (Orque, 1983). While healthcare professionals are taught to use scientific evidence and technical knowledge to explain and understand illness and treatment approaches, lay people often use spiritual and cultural world views to explain life events. Within the context of healthcare, cultural backgrounds can influence people's views on health, wellbeing and illness, which in turn impact their perceptions of healthcare and healthcare outcomes (Leininger, 1991).

Figure 17.1 presents a framework for thinking about individual identity and culture based on Orque's (1983) ethnic/cultural system. This framework recognises the complexity of culture and the components that influence the culture of an individual or a society. The model illustrates how our culture is intrinsic to our identity and influences our world views—our ways of thinking about, and experiences of, social interaction, language, healing practices, family life, history and politics, food, and religion.

All of the eight domains shown in Figure 17.1 are interdependent. As healthcare professionals, we often concentrate on knowing about healing beliefs and practices; however, it may be impossible to

Person-centred communication

'I kept telling them I am a Muslim woman, I want a female nurse' (Arabic woman) (Garrett et al., 2008).

FIGURE 17.1

A framework for thinking about culture.

Source: Based on Orque, M. (1983). Orque's ethnic/cultural system: A framework for ethnic nursing care. In M. Orque, B. Bloch & L. Monrroy (Eds), *Ethnic Nursing Care: A Multicultural Approach* (pp. 5–48). St Louis, MO: Mosby.

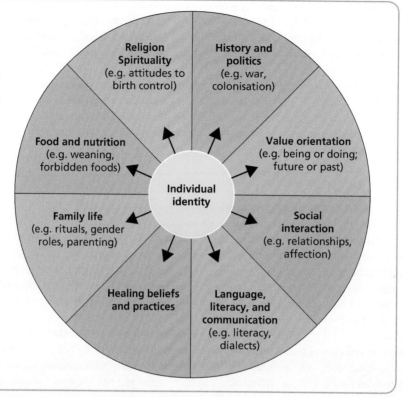

make sense of these without an understanding of family dynamics—for example, gender roles and the expectations of extended family.

Culture is not static. It is influenced by political and economic conditions and varies with factors such as age, gender, class, education and personality. Culture changes over time, both in the country of origin and in the host country. Healthcare professionals often ask for factual documents to guide them in understanding the illness beliefs and practices of an unfamiliar ethnic group. While this desire comes from good intentions, a prescriptive list can be misguided and can result in stereotyping, cultural assumptions, diagnostic blindness and cognitive error. (See the 'Example from clinical practice' in Box 17.1.)

BOX 17.1   Example from clinical practice

When facilitating prenatal classes with newly arrived Vietnamese migrants, the midwife told the women about the diet necessary to ensure a healthy baby. This advice emphasised the importance of dairy (cheese, milk, yoghurt). However, dairy foods are not part of a normal Vietnamese diet and would not be physically tolerated by these women. Of course they ate other foods rich in calcium (soy products, small fish bones) but, in Vietnam, many foods are prescribed depending on the stage of pregnancy. Early in pregnancy, a woman is considered to be 'cold' and needs foods with 'hotter' properties. Later in pregnancy, the woman becomes 'hot' and requires foods with 'cold' properties to bring her into balance. In the period after childbirth, the woman is considered particularly vulnerable, thus needing 'warm-up' foods (not salads) and she may wear many layers of clothing, even in hot weather.

This example highlights the need to acknowledge the positive practices that have maintained health among a particular cultural group, rather than assuming that practices which differ greatly from our Western ways are in fact deficits (Sidelinger et al., 2005).

However, having a framework can provide a broad set of possible behaviours and ideas that *may* be applicable to a particular situation and person. The use of a framework can increase the likelihood that a healthcare professional will be equipped to work with patients to effectively 'see' and 'hear' their meaning and understand their needs.

Kleinman describes being asked by staff to provide a medical anthropology consult where a Mexican-American man—a widower caring for his four-year-old son who has HIV—had not been attending the clinic for care. Contrary to staff assumptions, the father had a near perfect understanding of the disease but, as a low paid bus driver on shift work, he could not afford time off to attend (Kleinman & Benson, 2006).

Chapter 3 emphasised the importance of person-centred care in healthcare. Silverman, Kurtz and Draper (2005) also argue for a person-centred approach to clinical communication, where the patient's perspective (concerns, ideas and expectations) about their illness is as important as their physical examination and past medical history. The skills required to carry out this conversation are no less important in a consultation with a person from a CALD background. However much we know, or think we know, about the practices and beliefs of the cultural group they belong to, the perspective of *each* patient must be sought.

Use the **'Ask–Tell–Ask'** model. *Ask* the patient to describe their current understanding of the issue, so you can take into account their level of knowledge and emotional state. *Tell* the patient briefly and clearly what you need to communicate. *Ask* if the patient understood what you just said.

Complex and interwoven sets of beliefs and practices are often part of a world view and are hard to articulate as 'cultural' beliefs. Asking a woman who is pregnant with her second child, 'What foods do you usually eat when you are pregnant? Are there any that you avoid?', may be preferable to asking, 'What do women in your culture eat when they are pregnant?'

Cultural competence

Cultural competence is a set of congruent behaviours, attitudes and policies that come together in a system, agency or among professionals and enable that system, agency or those professionals to work effectively in cross-cultural situations.

(Cross et al., 1989)

The healthcare system in Australia and other developed countries is aimed at literate people. This is the same with our legal and educational systems. To ensure that simple messages and essential information get to vulnerable CALD individuals, healthcare professionals need to adapt information to the needs of the client groups.

- What are some ways that you can openly invite discussion and dialogue about a person's beliefs in regards to special remedies and foods?
- How might you manage to convey evidence-based practice to replace myths or beliefs that may present risk or danger to a person, child or infant from another culture?
- Reflect upon health remedies that you believe have been passed down through your family or culture. How would you feel if someone explained that these were not good for your health or your families' health?

Culturally competent healthcare professionals have the ability to deliver safe and high-quality care to all people regardless of their race, ethnicity, culture or language proficiency (Kramer, Ivey & Ying, 1998). Increasingly, healthcare professionals—including students, clinicians and administrators—are offered cultural competency training to improve their understanding of the healthcare experiences of CALD patients, as well as their skills in working effectively in cross-cultural situations. A healthcare professional who is culturally competent engages in assistive, supportive, facilitative or enabling acts that are tailored to fit with individual, group or cultural values, beliefs and world views to provide safe and quality healthcare (Lehman, Fenza & Hollinger-Smith, n.d.).

The perceived cultural competence of healthcare professionals is linked to improved patient care (Paez et al., 2009). There are direct links with patient outcomes (Fernández et al., 2012) and the emotional burden associated with illness (Slean et al., 2012), particularly in chronic diseases. Culturally competent healthcare leads to increases in health-seeking behaviours, more appropriate screening and testing, fewer diagnostic errors, greater adherence to healthcare advice, and reduced medication errors (Lehman et al., n.d.). The example in Box 17.2 illustrates another assumption error based on cultural differences and how it was remedied with cultural competence.

Garrett et al. (2008) explored the experiences of 59 patients and carers of patients with limited English in a large Australian tertiary hospital. They generated six competencies that were derived from the patients' own perspectives:

1   Facilitating language (using interpreters or bilingual health staff)
2   Negotiating the nature and extent of family involvement
3   Understanding patient beliefs, expectations, experiences and constructions (introducing name and role to the patient and family, responding to cues regarding the frequency and appropriateness of eye contact, etc.)
4   Being empathic and respecting patient and human rights (hold regular open conversations directly with patients and their families in order to demonstrate kindness and respect)
5   Negotiating a care partnership (requires an open exploration of the patient and family's view of the cause of the illness, when, how and why it started, its severity, the expected treatment and results, and what they call the problem)
6   Providing systems so healthcare services and professionals can be competent (multilingual signage, relationships with religious leaders, ensuring the availability of a range of food options, providing cultural competency training, ensuring that data collections include a field about English proficiency).

In addition, we suggest that language comprehension be facilitated by using translated literature and computer-based translation or interpreting as bedside tools.

Attributes of culturally competent healthcare professionals

Awareness

■   Understanding that people have different frameworks, and that one can't possibly know everything about every culture
■   Knowledge of self and awareness of own culture

Attitudes

■   Willingness to learn, curiosity about others
■   Humility
■   Perseverance (bounce back, don't take it personally)

Knowledge

■   Knowing your organisation's policies, protocols, resources (e.g. is there a multicultural liaison officer?)
■   Knowing your patients and their history
■   Knowing the social and political environment from which the patient has come
■   Understanding non-verbal cues, and that cues are not universal (e.g. smiling and silence can mean different things to different people)

BOX 17.2   Example from clinical practice: The dangers of assumption-based communication

Part A

A woman came to give birth at a large public hospital. She spoke minimal English and had not been in Australia for very long. The woman had migrated from an area of the Middle East where it is not the norm for the father of the baby to be present during birth. In fact, it is seen as wrong for men to enter the hospital until the birth is over, and the baby is washed and dressed. The father is then allowed a short visit but has minimal involvement in the daily care and hygiene of the infant. It is also expected that women will immediately resume their duties as a mother and wife within hours of the birth.

During the admission, staff discussed how things would unfold and the role of the father during the birth. The woman had explained that her husband would go home and wait until the baby is born. However, the hospital policy encouraged fathers to be present for the birth, spend time supporting his wife/partner, hold the newborn baby and assist with its care.

Should the husband be invited or even encouraged to stay, or should he be sent home?

The interpreter being used in this interaction was male, a member of the minority community and known to the couple. How might the family feel about the male interpreter being present with or without the husband's presence?

REFLECTIVE THINKING QUESTIONS

- What is the difference between knowledge and assumption in clinical practice?
- What impact might this encounter have had for the woman, her husband and other female relatives?
- What strategies can you implement in your daily clinical practice to reduce the dangers of assumptions and unsafe care?

Part B

Reflecting the principles of open and honest communication, staff decided to discuss the differences in cultural expectations with the couple. They began by talking openly about the Australian custom of the father being present during the birth of their child and how research has shown that this is not only beneficial for a strong and healthy relationship with their child, it can also be a strong support for mothers. Strategies were also offered for the male interpreter to work behind a screen, or to instead use a female phone interpreter.

The family talked intensely for a time and discussed at length with the interpreter. They became very animated and excited. Speaking through the interpreter, they told staff that this new way of being together is very scary for them but they want to experience it, and they asked for assistance in navigating through the experience.

REFLECTIVE THINKING QUESTIONS

- Consider the way in which open and honest communication may lead a person or family to trust healthcare professionals to support them through their healthcare experiences.
- How did the clinicians work with the various cultural assumptions in this example—the woman's, the families and their own?
- Can you think of times when more open and honest communication might have assisted you in your clinical practice?

Practice tips for communicating with people from CALD backgrounds

- Develop a trusting relationship.
- Be honest and admit to mistakes.
- Pay attention to your body language.
- Be explicit and speak slowly and clearly.
- Avoid metaphors, jargon, irony, slang or local sayings.
- Invite an exchange of cross-cultural information; ask people to tell you about their culture, country and healthcare.
- Explore the patient's perspective of their illness.
- Have patience—each healthcare encounter may take 2–3 times as long.
- Identify specific ethnicity, country of origin and spoken language (e.g. a person of Chinese ethnicity from Malaysia who speaks Cantonese).
- Use computer-based translation and telephone interpreter services as appropriate.
- Use Ask–Tell–Ask.

Using interpreters in healthcare

I went to have some blood tests. The person doing the test was asking me questions but I couldn't understand anything. There was no interpreter. I couldn't ask for one because I don't speak any English. Some days later they called me on the mobile. He was talking in English. I tried to get someone off the street to listen and translate but the doctor just kept talking, talking and then hung up the phone. I don't know how to get the results of my tests.

(Brough, 2006, p. 14)

However conscientious health professionals are, cultural awareness and sensitivity will always be inadequate to ensure patient safety and quality healthcare if the health professional is not able to communicate with a patient who is not proficient in English. A large proportion of people from CALD backgrounds who do not have English proficiency live in urban areas of Australian cities. For example, 71 per cent of people in Fairfield, NSW, speak a language other than English at home (the most common being Vietnamese, Assyrian, Arabic, Cantonese), and a large proportion are not proficient in English (ABS, 2016).

'I know you're not supposed to use family but you still do. If they are there at the moment you're not going to get an interpreter' (Cioffi, 2003).

The use of qualified healthcare interpreters is an important strategy to reduce healthcare barriers for people who are not proficient in English. There is an improvement in the quality of healthcare when qualified interpreters are used (Flores, 2005; Karlinger et al., 2007): client safety is improved, access to healthcare is promoted, unnecessary health expenditure is avoided, stress on families is reduced, and the risk of healthcare professionals incurring legal liability for adverse outcomes is minimised (Thomas, Beckmann & Gibbons, 2010).

For many years the person closest to the encounter who spoke the language of the patient was used to translate the clinical communication between a patient and healthcare workers. This might be a member of the administrative staff or support staff such as cleaners, or a member of the family, including young children. Not only were these encounters potentially dangerous when the person interpreting did not have the technically correct language, but they could cause emotional harm to children when they were used to break bad news to parents (e.g. a diagnosis of cancer) or to speak about a sensitive area such as sexuality or mental illness. Despite the best efforts of proponents of cultural competency, this informal translation of illness symptoms, history and treatment still occurs in many healthcare encounters. It has been estimated that only 1 in 100 general practice consultations use qualified interpreters (Phillips & Travaglia, 2011). Review the barriers to the use of interpreters in Box 17.3.

BOX 17.3   Barriers to the use of interpreters

Organisational/health professional barriers

- Lack of protocols in organisations to identify patients with poor English proficiency
- Poor facilities and equipment (private space, access to three-way telephones)
- Cost (allied health and private practice not always free)
- Increased length of consultation
- Lack of awareness, knowledge and skills relating to the use of interpreters among health professionals

Patient related factors

- Refusal by the patient or by members of the patient's family due to lack of knowledge about services
- Fear of confidentiality breaches, especially within one's community
- The private and sensitive nature of some issues such as reproduction and sexuality (the belief that this should be contained within the family)
- The family wanting to shield the patient from a life-limiting diagnosis (see Mr Lee's Story)

Access to interpreter services for healthcare is a human rights issue and as such is reflected in the Australian Charter of Health Care Rights, from the Australian Commission on Safety and Quality in Health Care, and adopted by federal and state health ministers in July 2008. The use of qualified healthcare interpreters is now mandated in many national, state and local health systems and often backed by legislation. While the situation varies across states and territories in Australia, we will use New South Wales as one example. In New South Wales, public sector agencies and services are required by legislation to provide equitable access to people from non-English-speaking backgrounds and to people who are deaf. The relevant laws include the *Anti-Discrimination Act 1977*, the *Mental Health Act 1990*, and the *Community Relations Commission and Principles of Multiculturalism Act 2000*.

The NSW Department of Health, Standard Procedures for Working with Health Care Interpreters (NSW Ministry for Health, 2006) states:

> *Healthcare interpreters are to be used in all healthcare situations where communication is essential including admission, consent, assessment, counselling, discharge, explanation of treatment, associated risks and side-effects, health education and medical research, and day only surgery.*

Compliance with this directive is *mandatory* for NSW Health and is a condition of subsidy for associated public health organisations. The specific use of services to address communication barriers caused by poor English proficiency in CALD patients can be confusing. Interpreting and translating services vary between states, healthcare professions and the site of the service. Most people (patients and staff) prefer to meet face to face with the interpreter and the patient; however, there are situations where telephone or video interpreting is preferable (e.g. when there is short notice, a medical emergency, when the patient prefers an interpreter outside the community) or in situations when there is no other option (e.g. rural and remote contexts, after hours).

The Health Care Interpreter Service is a free service operating across New South Wales—24 hours a day, 7 days a week—to ensure that non-English-speaking patients/clients are able to communicate effectively with any health provider of the New South Wales health system. Since the year 2000, a Commonwealth government service (Telephone Interpreter Service or TIS) has

'You take it for granted that exactly what you're saying is being interpreted. Some patients feel if they tell too much it will get back to the community. So they may not want to tell you. It has happened with a particular ethnic group who wasn't happy with their particular interpreter because they thought it was getting back to their community' (Cioffi, 2003).

provided medical practitioners (and nurses working with them) free access to interpreters for Medicare rebatable services. TIS is also available for some private sector healthcare consultations. Despite this, many general practitioners are still not aware of the service and a majority have not used an interpreter (Bird, 2010).

MR LEE'S STORY

Mr Lee, a 76-year-old man who migrated from China 20 years ago, was admitted to the cardiology ward of a tertiary referral hospital, accompanied by his wife and adult daughter. On admission, the family declined the use of an interpreter when asked. Nursing and medical staff on the ward became increasingly concerned over the next few days about what seemed to be the patient's lack of knowledge of the seriousness of his condition, and his apparent history of non-compliance with medication and other treatment recommendations such as fluid restriction. The nurse unit manager (NUM) told the patient, his wife and his daughter that the doctor would like the assistance of an interpreter. The family was adamant that this was not necessary, and they did not want an interpreter. The daughter told the nurses that her father was not aware of the seriousness of his illness and they did not want him told. While initially the staff were guided by the family, they felt they had a duty of care to the patient that outweighed the family's desire, and an appointment with a qualified healthcare interpreter (Cantonese-speaking) was made so that the doctor could communicate directly with the patient. Through the use of the interpreter, the extent of the patient's ignorance about his condition became apparent. The history that had previously been taken, including medication use and fluid restriction, upon which the current treatment was based, were all called into doubt. This situation was complicated by the father having lost some of his English language skills during ageing and illness. His wife had poor English literacy, and the adult daughter, although fluent in English, did not have the medical language in her first language to interpret for her mother and father.

Mr Lee's story illustrates the following:

■ Assessing the need for interpreters can be complex.

■ Barriers to safe healthcare can originate from patients and families rather than healthcare professionals.

■ It is the right of the healthcare professional to ask for an interpreter even if the patient or family decline.

■ The duty of care towards the patient requires diagnosis and treatment to be based on the correct history and involvement of the patient in the treatment plan.

■ Persistence on the part of healthcare professionals may be required to achieve quality healthcare.

■ Fluency in English and other languages within a family group may not extend to a technical level and may be insufficient to understand instructions for treatment, thus not facilitate safe healthcare.

REFLECTIVE THINKING QUESTIONS

• List three reasons why a patient or family (such as in the scenario above) may refuse an interpreter.

• List three reasons why a healthcare professional may not use a trained interpreter in a situation such as the pregnant woman from Box 17.2.

In complex clinical interactions where there is, at minimum, a three-way communication (often many more with the inclusion of family members), it is not only the interpreters who need training. Healthcare workers need to learn how to effectively use interpreters in clinical encounters. This includes a pre-consultation briefing, the way in which they will communicate during a consultation (e.g. seating arrangements, consecutive or simultaneous interpreting) and a debriefing.

Healthcare students should understand the rationale for using qualified interpreters and the problems that occur in using family and other non-professional interpreters (native speakers), in the context of equity of healthcare, patient safety, and improved patient satisfaction. However, as in learning any new skill, knowledge is not enough and the required skills need to be practised, ideally in a simulated environment with the opportunity for feedback and rehearsal. Training in the use of interpreters has been associated with increased use of professional interpreters and increased satisfaction with the healthcare provided (Karlinger et al., 2007). See the links provided in Box 17.4, Guidelines for the use of interpreters, and Box 17.5, Working with interpreters: A summary.

BOX 17.4　　　Guidelines for the use of interpreters

- Guidelines for working effectively with interpreters in mental health settings <http://framework.mhima.org.au/pdfs/VTPU_interpreter_guidelines_book.pdf >

- Speaking with clients who have low English proficiency <https://www.ceh.org.au/speaking-clients-low-english-proficiency/>

- Assessing the need for an interpreter <file:///C:/Users/118130/Downloads/interpreters.pdf>

BOX 17.5　　　Working with interpreters: A summary

Preparation

- Book the interpreter with as much advance notice as possible and allocate sufficient time (sometimes double what you would normally need) for the session.

- Brief the interpreter before the session, especially if it is a complex or sensitive issue.

- Arrange a private space with adequate seating or a three-way phone.

The session

- Always remember that you are the person leading the session, not the interpreter.

- Address the patient directly, introducing yourself, the interpreter and setting up the agenda.

- Look at the person and address them in the first person: 'How can I help you today?'

- Speak for two or three sentences and then wait for the interpreter to finish.

- Do not talk with the interpreter and exclude the client.

- Clarify understanding, summarise the discussion and allow for questions.

Follow-up

- Debrief the interpreter if necessary.

- Arrange any further appointments while the interpreter is present.

Cultural competence training

Cultural competence training typically covers cultural awareness as well as communication skills. These types of programs help learners to gain:

■ skills to communicate effectively across cultures and deliver culturally appropriate care

■ skills for interpreting and responding appropriately to verbal and non-verbal communication cues

■ an appreciation of variations in the understanding of core concepts, such as time, personal space, group dynamics and relationships, authority, and task sharing

■ an appreciation of differences in communication styles

■ skills in decoding facial expressions and vocal tones that may have different meanings in different cultures and contexts

■ an understanding of an assets approach rather than deficits to assessing communities and different cultures.

The evidence base for long-term change as a result of one-off cultural competency training, or a course of study as part of a healthcare professional training program, is mixed. A systematic review of health workforce cultural competency interventions in the US, Canada, Australia and New Zealand identified 16 studies that aimed to improved cultural competency through health workforce development (Jongen et al., 2018). Eleven of these studies provided cultural competence training as the primary intervention. The training programs delivered across all of these studies appeared to be quite generic, with common strategies and outcomes reported. In general, the studies reported positive effects on practitioner attitudes/beliefs, skills and confidence. However, there remains a dearth of evidence regarding impact on actual clinical practice and patient health outcomes.

Training approaches are usually described as either categorical, or cross-cultural. Categorical approaches provide information about particular cultural, ethnic or racial groups and offer advice on working with patients from such groups in clinical practice (Betancourt et al., 2003a). In contrast, cross-cultural approaches focus on teaching knowledge, attitudes and skills that can be applied to any cross-cultural encounter (Betancourt, 2003b). This approach aligns with Kleinman and Benson's (2006) explanatory model and offers a more generalised approach to teaching the skills necessary for culturally safe healthcare. The successful integration of cultural competence training into healthcare education is important but an ongoing challenge.

Medical students at a Canadian university were surveyed after a new course in social and cultural issues was introduced. While they enjoyed the course, once in the wards the students did not recognise, or denied, the effects of race, class, gender and culture, and felt that what they had learnt had little to do with clinical practice (Beagan, 2003). The authors concluded that greater attention needs to be given to enabling students to recognise and challenge their own biases and privilege. In this study, it was apparent that the medical students were taught to be neutral and almost blind to differences in gender, skin colour, sexuality, etc. (Beagan, 2003). Cultural competence education should challenge this approach and make students more aware of their own social factors and influences, and to consider how these might influence their practice. Much of the bias that healthcare professionals have towards certain patient groups is unconscious, so making those assumptions conscious is a beginning goal (Teal et al., 2012).

Challenges

Definitions of cultural competence tend to be based on provider and academic representations; yet a great many aspects of culturally competent care are contextually and temporally based—in effect, a social construction of the care process. Indeed, the same behaviour might be considered 'culturally competent' in one situation and quite incompetent in another (Manderson & Allotey, 2003).

Because of the complexity of culture, it is unlikely that cultural competence can be reduced to a technical skill measured reliably with a checklist, as is common in other competency-based healthcare skills. Poor care can result from stereotyping and assumptions (as discussed above) but, in addition, some patients can become distressed and concerned that they are being singled out and stigmatised when asked directly about their cultural background (Kleinman & Benson, 2006). Dean (2001) believes that if healthcare professionals know that cultural competence is challenging to achieve, greater awareness of the need to gain an understanding of the patient's circumstances will result and this will impact positively on safety.

Not getting it perfect every time

It is important to remember that no individual can be expected to know and understand the complexities of every cultural group with which they come into contact. When we travel to a foreign country we respect the culture and values of that country and people (e.g. by dressing appropriately, removing our shoes to enter a sacred place or home, respecting rules about separate men's and women's bathing areas), but we do so without actually assimilating into the associated culture or religious beliefs. Similarly, we can respect the needs and considerations of patients without needing to know every detail of their culture. For example, in some cultures it is a sign of disrespect to make eye contact with a person who is considered more senior than oneself, or an elder in the community. A healthcare professional who does not belong to such a culture and who unknowingly makes eye contact with a patient from that culture should not feel ashamed or worry that they have broken a cultural rule. Rather, it is important that healthcare professionals respect the fact that some patients may not feel comfortable making eye contact with them and find other ways of engaging and connecting with the patient. This level of competency is based on being sensitive and patient, taking time to get to know the person, and giving them an opportunity to share their concerns and express their needs.

Conclusion

Individuals can attend cultural diversity training, learn many skills and enjoy the experience, but it is only by their personal commitment that cultural competence will be evidenced by behaviour change. Communication in healthcare is not primarily about the shared language or the use or non-use of interpreters. Awareness of the diversity of cultures, the complexities of an individual's relationship with their culture, and the capacity to respond appropriately to these differences are central to cultural competence. Acknowledgment of the inadequacies of knowledge, humility to learn from our mistakes, and a focus on putting the patients at the centre of the health encounter so that their perspective is sought and considered, are the ingredients that allow culturally effective conversations in healthcare to be realised.

Critical thinking activities

1   What are some of your own personal barriers to effective cross-cultural healthcare delivery?
2   Have you identified any unconscious biases in yourself as a result of reading this chapter?
3   Reflect on what you have been taught about cultural awareness in your university program. Are there any differences between what you have been taught and what you have observed in the clinical environment? How will you reconcile these differences?
4   What are the challenges to practicing in a culturally competent manner?

Teaching and assessment activities

1   Invite students to define their own cultural identity by listing their cultural identity elements (the way they identify themselves and the groups they belong to). Then ask them to create a pie chart reflecting the importance of each element to their sense of self. This activity is a helpful self-reflection to enhance students' openness to learning about other cultures and having empathy for people from other cultures.
2   While there is no single way to address culturally competent communication in teaching and assessment, some opportunities include:
     •   using culturally diverse patient cases in role-plays during teaching and assessment
     •   training students in the use of interpreters

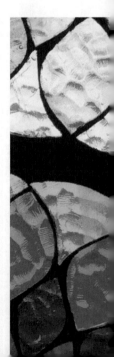

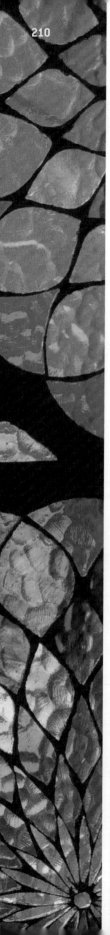

- inviting people from culturally diverse backgrounds to share their stories and experiences with students (this can be done with larger groups)
- inviting students to reflect on their cultural empathy using some of the available assessment scales
- setting assignments for students to engage with culturally diverse patients and write or present these cases with reflection on the patients' cultural needs and safety.

Further reading

Fadiman, A. (2012). *The Spirit Catches You and You Fall down: A Hmong Child, Her American Doctors, and the Collision of Two Cultures*. New York: Farrar, Straus & Giroux.

El Masri, A. (2000). *Tea with Arwa: One Woman's Story of Faith, Family and Finding a Home in Australia*. Sydney: Hachette Australia.

Kagawa-Singer, M. & Backhall, L. (2001). Negotiating cross-cultural issues at end of life. *Journal of American Medical Association*, 286(3001), 2993. <https://www.ecald.com/assets/Resources/ABCD-Cultural-Assessment-Model.pdf>

Web resources

Centre for Culture, Ethnicity and Health.
<www.ceh.org.au>

NSW Government Multicultural Health Communication Service.
<www.mhcs.health.nsw.gov.au>

Promoting Refugee Health: A guide for doctors, nurses and other healthcare providers caring for people from refugee backgrounds.
<http://refugeehealthnetwork.org.au/wp-content/uploads/PRH-online-edition_July2012.pdf>

Migrant and refugee resilience and wellbeing.
<http://flinders.edu.au/nursing/mental-health-and-culture/migrant-mh/mental-health.cfm>

References

Australian Bureau of Statistics (2016). *Cultural Diversity in Australia: 2016 Census Data Summary* (no. 2071.0). Accessed January 2019 at: <http://www.abs.gov.au/ausstats/abs@.nsf/Lookup/by%20Subject/2071.0~2016~Main%20Features~Cultural%20Diversity%20Data%20Summary~30>.

Beagan, B. (2003). Teaching social and cultural awareness to medical students: 'It's all very nice to talk about it in theory, but ultimately it makes no difference'. *Academic Medicine, 78*(6), 605–14.

Betancourt, J. R., Green, A.R., Carrillo, J. E. & Ananeh-Firempong, O. (2003a) Defining cultural competence: A practical framework for addressing racial/ethnic disparities in health and health care. *Public Health Reports, 118*(4), 293–302.

Betancourt, J. R. (2003b) Cross-cultural medical education: Conceptual approaches and frameworks for evaluation. *Academic Medicine, 78*(6), 560–9.

Bird, S. (2010). Failure to use an interpreter. *Australian Family Physician, 39*(4), 241–2.

Brough, C. (2006). Language Services in Victoria's Health System: Perspectives of Culturally and Linguistically Diverse Consumers. State Government, Victoria. Published by the Centre for Culture, Ethnicity and Health, Melbourne. Accessed at <www.ceh.org. au/resources/resbyceh.html>.

Cioffi, R. (2003). Communicating with culturally and linguistically diverse patients in an acute care setting: Nurses' experiences. *International Journal of Nursing Studies, 40*(3), 299–306.

Cross, T., Basron, B., Dennis, K. & Isaacs, M. (1989). *Towards a Culturally Competent System of Care* (Report). Georgetown University Child Development Center, Washington DC.

Dean, R. (2001). The myth of cross-cultural competence. *Families in Society: The Journal of Contemporary Human Services, 82*(6), 623–30.

Eisenbruch, M. (2004). *The Lens of Culture, the Lens of Health: Toward a Framework and Toolkit for Cultural Competence*. University of New South Wales. Cited in Cultural Responsiveness Framework, published by Rural and Regional Health and Aged Care Services (2009), Department of Health, Victorian Government, Melbourne. Accessed at <http://www.health.vic.gov.au/cald>.

Fernández, A., Seligman, H., Quan, J., Stern, R. & Jacobs, E. (2012). Associations between aspects of culturally competent care and clinical outcomes among patients with diabetes. *Medical Care, 50*(9) (Suppl 2), S74–S79.

Flores, G. (2005). The impact of medical interpreter services on the quality of health care: A systematic review. *Medical Care Research and Review, 62*(3), 255–99.

Garrett, P., Dickson, H., Young, L., Whelan, A. & Forero, R. (2008). What do non-English-speaking patients value in acute care? Cultural competency from the patient's perspective: A qualitative study. *Ethnicity and Health, 13*(5), 479–96.

Harun, A., Harrison, J. & Young, J. (2012). Interventions to improve patient participation in the treatment process for culturally and linguistically diverse people with cancer: A systematic review. *Asia-Pacific Journal of Clinical Oncology*.

Jongen, C., McCalman, J. & Bainbridge, R. (2018). Health workforce cultural competency interventions: A systematic scoping review. *BMC Health Service Research, 18*(232), 1–15. Accessed January 2019 at <https://www.ncbi.nlm.nih.gov/pmc/articles/PMC5879833/>.

Karlinger, L., Jacobs, E., Chen, A. & Mutha, S. (2007). Do professional interpreters improve clinical care for patients with limited English proficiency? A systematic review of the literature. *Health Services Research, 42*(2), 727–54.

Kleinman, A. & Benson, P. (2006). Anthropology in the clinic: The problem of cultural competency and how to fix it. *PLoS Medicine, 3*(10), 1673–6.

Kramer, E., Ivey, S. & Ying, Y.-W. (Eds) (1998). *Immigrant Women's Health: Problems and Solutions*. San Francisco: Jossey-Bass.

Lehman, D., Fenza, P. & Hollinger-Smith, L. (n.d.). *Diversity and Cultural Competency in Health Care Settings*. Mather LifeWays.

Leininger, M. (1991). *Culture Care Diversity and Universality: A Theory of Nursing*. New York: National League for Nursing Press (redistributed by Jones & Bartlett Publishers, Inc., New York, 2001).

Manderson, L. & Allotey, P. (2003). Cultural politics and clinical competence in Australian health services. *Anthropology & Medicine, 10*(1), 71–85.

NSW Ministry for Health (2006). *Interpreters—Standard Procedures for Working with Health Care Interpreters*. Accessed at <www.health.nsw.gov.au/policies/pd/2006/pdf/PD2006_053.pdf>.

Orque, M. (1983). Orque's ethnic/cultural system: A framework for ethnic nursing care. In M. Orque, B. Bloch & L. Monrroy (Eds), *Ethnic Nursing Care: A Multicultural Approach* (pp. 5–48). St Louis, MO: Mosby.

Paez, K., Allen, J., Beach, M., Carson, K. & Cooper, L. (2009). Physician cultural competence and patient ratings of the patient–physician relationship. *Journal of General Internal Medicine, 24*(2), 494–8.

Phillips, C. & Travaglia, J. (2011). Low levels of uptake of free interpreters by Australian doctors in private practice: Secondary analysis of national data. *Australian Health Review, 35*(4), 475–9.

Refugee Council of Australia. (2017). *UNHCR Global Trends 2016—How Australia Compares with the World*. Accessed April 2018 at <http://www.refugeecouncil.org.au/>.

Sidelinger, D., Meyer, D., Blaschke, G., Hametz, P., Batista, M., Salguero, R. & Reznik, V. (2005). Communities as teachers: Learning to deliver culturally effective care in pediatrics. *Paediatrics, 115*, 1160–4.

Silverman, J., Kurtz, S. & Draper, J. (2005). *Skills for Communicating with Patients*. Oxford: Radcliffe Publishing Ltd.

Singh, M. & de Looper, M. (2002). *Australian Health Inequalities: 1 Birthplace*. Bulletin No. 2, AIHW Cat No. AUS 27. Canberra: AIHW.

Slean, G., Jacobs, E., Lahiff, M., Fisher, L. & Fernández, A. (2012). Aspects of culturally competent care are associated with less emotional burden among patients with diabetes. *Medical Care, 50*(9) (Suppl 2), S69–S73.

Smith, L. (2015). *The Health Outcomes of Migrants: A Literature Review*. Canberra: Migration Council Australia. Accessed January 2019 at <http://migrationcouncil.org.au/wp-content/uploads/2016/06/2015_Smith.pdf>.

Teal, C., Gill, A., Green, A. & Crandall, S. (2012). Helping medical learners recognise and manage unconscious bias toward certain patient groups. *Medical Education, 46*, 80–8.

Thomas, P., Beckmann, M. & Gibbons, K. (2010). The effect of cultural and linguistic diversity on pregnancy outcome. *Australian and New Zealand Journal of Obstetrics and Gynaecology, 50*(5), 419–22.

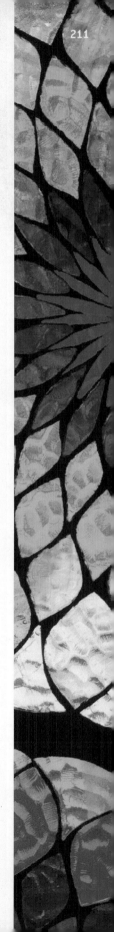

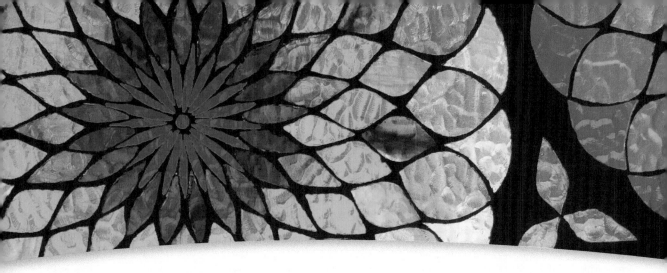

COMMUNICATING WITH PEOPLE ABOUT THEIR SPIRITUAL NEEDS

Pamela van der Riet   Victoria Pitt

LEARNING OUTCOMES

Chapter 18 will enable you to:

- discuss the meaning and importance of spirituality
- clarify the difference between spirituality and religiosity
- describe how to communicate with people about their spiritual needs
- identify the barriers to the provision of spiritual care.

KEY CONCEPTS

spirituality | spiritual care | spiritual distress | therapeutic communication | holistic care

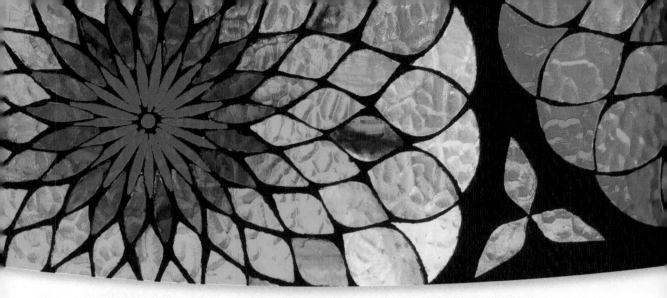

Attitudes toward spirituality in healthcare appear to be changing ... a transition to a deeper calling is becoming apparent. Research suggests that patients desire and feel more comfortable with healthcare professionals who are not only open to their own humanity, but who also are willing to allow patients to discuss their spiritual needs.

(Morrison, 2009, p. 322)

INTRODUCTION

Effective communication about a person's spiritual needs requires healthcare professionals to recognise that spiritual care is an essential element of person-centred holistic practice (Phelps et al., 2012; Ronaldson et al., 2012; Attard, Baldacchino & Camilleri, 2014). However, our own under- standings and personal experiences of spirituality can influence our ability and willingness to com- municate with others about their spiritual needs (Noble & Jones, 2010; Smyth & Allen, 2011). Too often, healthcare professionals feel reluctant or uncomfortable when communicating with people about their spiritual needs, and as a result, these important interactions can be overlooked or fraught with difficulty (Ford et al., 2012; Phelps et al., 2012). This reluctance may stem from a lack of understanding of spirituality and spiritual needs (Hodge & Horvath, 2011). This chapter explores the importance of spirituality to health and wellbeing and provides practical strategies that can be used when communicating with people about their spiritual needs.

The meaning and importance of spirituality

'Prayer, ritual, meditation, and music have the power to heal, and yet we don't use them seriously and widely in healthcare practice because they lie outside the paradigm, the myth, and the accepted story of modern medicine' (Moore, 2010, p. xxi).

While typically recognised as important to end-of-life care, spirituality is also important to people who are confronted with life-changing events, such as pregnancy, miscarriage, still birth, traumatic injury or illness. In addition, spirituality can have a positive affect on recovery and healing. For these reasons, patients and families often want to be able to discuss their spiritual needs (Phelps et al., 2012; Smyth & Allen, 2011) with healthcare professionals. Conversations about spiritual needs can strengthen therapeutic relationships and allow people to find emotional comfort (Hodge & Horvath, 2011; Puchalski, 2006), and evidence suggests that attending to a person's spiritual care can improve health outcomes and quality of life (Phelps et al., 2012; Vlasblom et al., 2011; Barton et al., 2018).

Spirituality, in its many interpretations, is a core dimension of the human experience (Ronaldson, 2012) and is often about a search for meaning or inner peace. It is an elusive, individual and subjective term without a clear and consistent definition. Stevenson and Berry (2015), suggest that the essence of spirituality is 'beliefs connecting transcendence and value'. Spirituality also refers to the mind–body–spirit connection.

Spirituality is an inner resource that helps people face illness and life-threatening events. People who have had their spiritual needs addressed have noted a reduction in depression, anxiety and sense of hopelessness (Chochinov et al., 2005), as well as improved recovery (Ford et al., 2012) and ability to cope with grief (Lovgren et al., 2017). Omitting spiritual care from our conversations with patients can cause spiritual distress and negatively impact their perception of emotional safety and wellbeing.

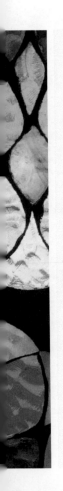

MAI'S STORY: A STORY OF SPIRITUAL DISTRESS

Mai is 98 years old and has lived by her Buddhist beliefs all her life. She immigrated to Australia from Thailand many years ago and now lives with her daughter. In the Thai culture it is common for older relatives to live with family. Mai, like many Thai people, doesn't like to be away from home, even for a night, and is reluctant to go to hospital if unwell.

Recently, Mai collapsed at home and was brought to the emergency department. She was observed for two hours and then discharged. The family decided that she should stay with her granddaughter Achara, a 36-year-old first-generation Australian, whose home was only five minutes from the hospital.

Mai was not happy about this arrangement. Two days later Mai became quite ill again and was taken back to the hospital. She became agitated, pale and restless. She pleaded with her family and the nurses to be taken back to her home, as she felt she was dying. When this was ineffective, she pleaded with the doctor. He stated, 'The hospital is the best place for you right now.'

Over the next two days, Mai refused to talk or to acknowledge any of the nurses or doctors that attended her. Her family noted that she ate little and had very little to say to them except, 'I need to go home. That is where I need to be!' The healthcare professionals met with Achara and explained that, although Mai was in heart failure, her condition was stable and she was well enough to be discharged. However, they were concerned about Mai's emotional distress and reluctance to stay with her granddaughter. Achara explained that she wanted her grand-mother to live with her so that she was close to the hospital in case she collapsed again. She said, 'What do I do, let her go home and die? I need her to be close to hospital to save her life.'

This story illustrates the intergenerational tension that can exist within families, particularly when spiritual and religious beliefs appear to conflict with healthcare needs. In this scenario, Achara and the healthcare professionals involved needed to understand that for many Thai Buddhist people it is important to die in a place of comfort and familiarity, as this contributes to a sense of peace and serenity. This state of peace and calmness at the time of death is essential to move on after death to a better afterlife (Tang, 2002).

The difference between spirituality and religiosity

To aid in communicating with people about their spiritual needs, we first need to understand the difference between religiosity and spirituality. Religiosity, in its broadest sense, is a comprehensive sociological term used to refer to an organised system of beliefs and the numerous aspects of religious activity. It often includes certain rituals, retelling stories, prayer, worship, revering certain symbols, or accepting particular doctrines about deities and the afterlife (Cooper et al., 2012). In Australia, the largest religious affiliation is Christianity (61%) (Australian Bureau of Statistics (ABS), 2012). This number has been steadily decreasing over the last decade, while at the same time there has been an increase in non-Christian religions (ABS).

Some suggest that the concept of spirituality has changed over time from a religious view to a more secular one (Tiew, Creedy & Chan, 2013). Ronaldson suggests that 'spirituality has been viewed more from a secular stance in order to fit it into a holistic framework for health care' (2012, p. 56). Spirituality can involve the search for meaning, hope, forgiveness and a sense of emotional healing (Ronaldson, 2012). It has also been referred to as 'an existential mode of human functioning' (Vlasblom et al., 2011, p. 791). Spirituality has been defined as an 'aspect of humanity that relates to the way individuals seek and express meaning and purpose, and the way they experience connectedness to the moment, to self, to others, to nature and to the significant or sacred' (Puchalski et al., 2009).

In van der Riet's (1999) research involving cancer patients' experience of massage and visualisation, patients did not use the term 'spirituality'; however, they used metaphors of spirituality to mean peace, comfort, healing, wellbeing, intimacy and reconnection with their bodies. For them, spirituality involved an awareness of their bodies as new and no longer as diseased, and it assisted them to deal with the loss experienced by illness. The building of a therapeutic partnership enabled these patients to communicate their feelings to the clinician providing the massage, and to recognise their experience of spirituality.

Awareness of the connectedness between spirituality and safety is integral in communications concerning spirituality. Potentially the person might be left feeling psychologically unsafe and experience spiritual distress if communications concerning spirituality are not adequately or appropriately addressed (Sinclair & Chochinov, 2012). Unrecognised spiritual distress may lead to depression, anger and confusion (Helming, 2009). This distress can be avoided by supporting individuals to express their spiritual needs as part of a holistic health assessment (Amoah, 2011). Empathic interactions and therapeutic communication allows patients to express their perspectives, views, needs and feelings. (Levett-Jones et al., 2017).

JACKSON'S STORY

A mother sat beside her son's hospital bed, her head bowed. Although the room was quiet, anguish and fear seemed to pulsate in the room. Jackson was 12 years old but seemed so much younger. A week before, Jackson had been playing with his friends at school. He had slid down a handrail, overbalanced and fallen six metres down onto a concrete quadrangle. Since his admission to intensive care, Jackson had been stabilised but had not regained consciousness. His prognosis was poor. His mother remained at his side.

Jackson's admission notes stated that he was a Catholic. A priest who had been visiting another patient was asked by one of the nurses to see if Jackson's mother needed his support. As he entered the room, he introduced himself saying 'I am Father Colin. Would you …' He never finished the sentence. Jackson's mother stood to face him, never letting go of her son's hand. Her face red, she hissed vehemently, 'Get out … get out!' She turned back to her son and quietly sobbed. When the nurse came into the room the mother asked, 'Why would God let this happen to my son?'

How would you respond to the question?

Communicating with people about their spiritual needs

Spiritual care is an important component of holistic healthcare, and failure to initiate conversations about spiritual needs can contribute to a sense of spiritual suffering (abandonment, feeling ill at ease) or discomfort (Ford et al., 2012; Vlasblom et al., 2011). Communicating with people about their spiritual needs can strengthen trust and facilitate the development of a therapeutic relationship. It can also improve quality of life and reduce pain (Brady et al., 1999) and depression (Nelson et al., 2002).

As spirituality is such an elusive concept, talking to people about their spiritual needs can be challenging. Although there is no clear format or approach, there are some important points to consider. These include understanding your own views about spirituality, establishing trust, having basic communication skills, understanding the importance of language and presence, encouraging the person to communicate their needs, and understanding your own limitations and professional boundaries.

Self-awareness

Having a degree of self-awareness is important when conversing with patients about their spiritual needs. In particular, it is important for healthcare professionals to understand their own perceptions and prejudices about spirituality. People who see themselves as spiritual or religious are more likely to discuss spiritual issues with their patients (Olson et al., 2006). However, these healthcare professionals may sometimes experience moral distress when confronted with decisions and behaviours that conflict with their own spiritual or religious beliefs.

Developing trust and rapport

Creating an environment of trust so that people feel safe to share their concerns is an essential aspect of communicating about spiritual needs (Ford et al., 2012). In order to develop trust, healthcare professionals must acknowledge a patient's vulnerability, be non-judgmental, and allow brief periods of silence for the person to collect their thoughts or handle their emotions (Helming, 2009). The use of silence can also allow the healthcare professional to do the same and to reflect on the most appropriate response to the patient's disclosure. It is important to acknowledge that healthcare professionals are not expected to have the answers to an individual's questions concerning spirituality but are expected to create a therapeutic relationship that enables a person to express their needs and concerns.

Terminology or language

The terminology or language used in communications regarding spirituality is extremely important. We have already noted the complexity and ambiguity that exists in defining spirituality. For people who have strong religious beliefs, the use of the term 'spirituality' may be offensive and hinder further trust. On the other hand, using terms that relate to religion may stifle the confidence of the person with more secular beliefs. Attentive listening will ensure that your language reflects the language familiar to the patient (Sinclair & Chochinov, 2012).

What questions to ask?

The acronym SMACC (Spirituality, Meaning, Activities, Connection and Care) can be used to guide your assessment of your patient's spiritual needs (Cacciatore, 2011; Sinclair & Chochinov, 2012). The questions below are provided as examples; however, your questions should be tailored to each person's needs.

Spirituality

The initial assessment of a patient's beliefs establishes the language you will use in further communications, including words such as 'religion', 'God', 'spirituality', 'belief' and 'faith':

- Do you consider yourself a religious or spiritual person?
- What gives you a sense of inner peace?

Meaning

These questions assess the meaning or importance that spirituality plays in the person's life:

■ How important is faith/religion/spirituality in your life?

■ How much meaning does your faith/beliefs have in decisions related to your illness?

Activities

Assess the spiritual or religious behaviours that the patient engages in. For some, these may include prayer, church or meditation.

■ Do you ever pray?

■ What do you do to reduce stress in your life?

■ When you are angry or distressed, what helps calm you?

Connection

To establish the role that spirituality plays in dealing with the loss or the experience of illness try these questions:

■ How has your relationship with the important things in your life changed since your illness/grief?

■ How has your loss/illness changed your relationship with God/faith/beliefs?

Care

This question elicits how the healthcare professionals may provide ongoing care or support to assist with the patient's spiritual journey or discovery:

■ How can we help you to continue or develop your faith/spirituality during this time in your life?

Barriers to the provision of spiritual care

In order to communicate with patients concerning their spiritual needs, health professionals must reflect, recognise and work to overcome the personal and situational barriers that exist. Perceived barriers to communicating with patients concerning spirituality may include:

■ insufficient time

■ attitudes of healthcare professionals

■ lack of privacy

■ lack of education or confidence.

Insufficient time

Insufficient time and a heavy workload can be a barrier to communicating with people about their spiritual needs (Casarez & Engebretson, 2012; Edwards et al., 2010; Helming, 2009). Patients sometimes feel that healthcare professionals are too busy dealing with their physical needs to be concerned about their spiritual needs (Phelps et al., 2012; Noble & Jones, 2010).

Attitudes of healthcare professionals

Negative attitudes about spirituality and a lack of understanding of one's own spiritual beliefs can act as a deterrent to meeting patients' spiritual needs. Healthcare professionals sometimes feel that spiritual care is not their responsibility (Vermandere et al., 2016) and is less important than other clinical needs (Ford et al., 2012). Avoiding conversations about spiritual needs can be linked to a healthcare professional's fear of being overwhelmed by the perceived emotional demands of patients, especially when caring for oncology patients. For example, participants in Noble and Jones' (2010) study stated that attending to patients' spiritual needs 'can be quite draining' and 'giving all this support is lonely' (p. 568). Healthcare professionals may also have a fear of imposing their own views of spirituality

(Sinclair & Chochinov, 2012; Casarez & Engebretson, 2012), or may feel that they do not have the skills needed to engage in conversations about spirituality with their patients (Phelps et al., 2012). Two strategies that can be used to overcome these barriers are self-awareness and education (refer to 'Communicating with people about their spiritual needs' earlier in this chapter).

Lack of privacy

A lack of privacy in clinical contexts often prevents healthcare professionals from discussing personal issues with patients (Ronaldson et al., 2012; Sinclair & Chochinov, 2012). This is a particular issue when communicating about spirituality with patients who are dying (Smyth & Allen, 2011). When considering conversations about spiritual needs, the setting should be private, quiet and peaceful. In hospitals, such places include the hospital chapel or garden. Other areas to consider are vacant teaching rooms or a private lounge area.

Lack of education or confidence

A lack of education and confidence concerning spiritual care has been identified as the most significant constraint to conversations about spiritual needs (Edwards et al., 2010; Ross, 2006; Vermandere, et al., 2016). Despite spiritual care being incorporated into many healthcare curricula, most programs do not spend enough time on this important area (Puchalski, 2006; Tiew et al., 2013; Vlasblom et al., 2011; Attard et al., 2014). This has been reported across all healthcare disciplines (Hodge & Horvath, 2011; Phelps et al., 2012; Ronaldson et al., 2012). However, when spiritual care training is provided, healthcare professionals report that they feel better equipped to recognise the spiritual needs of their patients, have improved confidence, and are more receptive to questions regarding the meaning of life and death (Ford et al., 2012; Vlasblom et al., 2011).

Conclusion

Spirituality is at the core of human existence, integrating and transcending the physical, emotional, intellectual and social dimensions (Reed, 1996). It involves a person's beliefs and values and cannot be viewed in isolation from the person's culture and background (Abbas & Panjwani, 2008). Failure to provide spiritual care means failure to provide holistic care. Spirituality can serve to provide a framework for patients and their families to reflect and find meaning, hope and purpose when experiencing illness and other issues related to the fragility of mortal existence. Spirituality and religious beliefs support personal coping in the event of sickness and suffering. They can be a means of gaining hope in the face of inevitable pain and suffering, chronic illness, and even life-threatening or terminal illnesses. Spiritual care leads to enhanced wellbeing and emotional and psychological safety. More positive and significant life events, such as childbirth, can also be a time for people to explore and celebrate the spiritual dimensions of their lives.

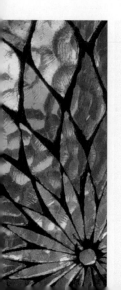

Critical thinking activity

The following scenario reflects on interactions between clinicians and a woman who has experienced a miscarriage. Remember that spiritual care is premised on the ability of the healthcare professional to build a therapeutic relationship with the patient that is both supportive and empathic. As you read this scenario, reflect on how your attitudes and values can impact on your ability to understand the experiences and responses of others.

> The walls seem to be closing in, the weight is oppressive, the noises around me seem muffled. The doctor states blankly, 'You have had a miscarriage ... you will be okay to go home as soon as the paper work is complete.'
>
> I sit on a bed in the emergency department. The pain has gone from my abdomen but the pain and heaviness in my heart remains. The doctor asks, 'I notice that you have noted a religion on your admission. Do you want me to get the pastoral care worker or the social worker?'
>
> It seems so superficial, I don't respond. The doctor leaves ... I stare blankly at the curtains that surround the bed. At least with the pain there was hope ... but now there is nothing.

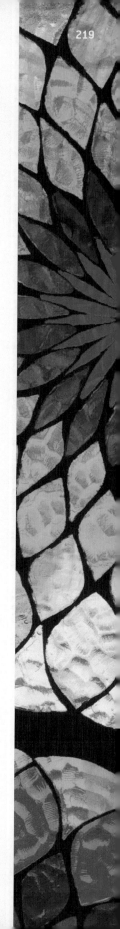

The nurse comes in, his face full of concern; it is hard to look at him. He quietly sits beside me and rests his hand gently on my forearm. It should feel wrong, a stranger being there, but it doesn't ... I don't feel like I am being rushed out for the next patient. I feel like I matter, like my baby matters ... I feel the pain ... the agony of my body not being able to protect my child ... I feel the tears begin to slip down my face.

'The doctor asked if I wanted pastoral care,' I whisper. 'I am not religious even though I have a religion ... if that makes sense ... I am from the country, a small town with open spaces. It just feels so heavy and closed in here ... like I can't breathe ... How can I begin to heal from this if I can't even breathe.'

The nurse asks, 'Where do you go when you are at home and life is tough?' I reply, 'I walk outside and smell the bush and feel the peace and quiet.' He asks, 'Would you like to take a walk outside and sit in the garden?' He adds, 'It is not like the bush, but you will be able to smell the earth and see the sky.'

As we sit out in the small courtyard, I look up to the perfectly blue sky and close my eyes. I block out the busy noises of the hospital and smell the rich smells of the earth and the flowers. I think of home. It does not stop the pain of the loss, but I feel a little freer so I can think. I feel the nurse's presence next to me. I turn to him and say, 'Thank you.'

1   Reflect on what spirituality means to you. How could your beliefs and experiences influence your practice and assist in communicating with your patients about their spiritual needs?

2   How might your own perceptions of spirituality influence how you would provide spiritual care to the woman in this scenario?

Teaching and assessment activity

Students may well be faced with situations that require empathic communication for people requiring end-of-life care. The scenario in Box 18.1 can be used as a stimulus for discussions about spiritual-care needs.

BOX 18.1   Scenario

Michael is a 55-year-old man. Three months ago he was told that he had inoperable colorectal cancer and liver metastasis. Michael lives in a small coastal town with his wife Teresa and two daughters, Charlie and Anthea aged 14 and 16 years.

Michael was initially treated with an extensive chemotherapy regime that resulted in severe nausea, vomiting and weight loss of 15 kg. During this time Michael sought the support of a naturopath who encouraged him to commence a vegan diet to cleanse his body. His wife Teresa, a yoga teacher encouraged him to learn to meditate.

Recently, Michael has lost another 5 kg in weight and he was admitted to a metropolitan hospital for treatment. An endoscopic stent was inserted to relieve symptoms of jaundice and itchiness. However, this procedure was unsuccessful and Michael developed the complications of pancreatitis and a pulmonary embolus. Michael's overall condition continued to deteriorate. Michael and Teresa, with the support of the treating oncologist, decided against any further active treatment and for Michael to be transferred to the palliative care team for support at home.

This scenario introduces a particularly stressful family situation as for many people the transfer to palliative care services can mean 'no hope' of cure. Provide an opportunity for students to reflect on the scenario and discuss the following questions:

1   If you were the healthcare professional visiting Michael and his family at home, what assistance might you provide during this time?

2   What communication skills/approaches would you need in this situation?

3   What spiritual care may be needed to support Michael and his family as they come to terms with Michael's prognosis and imminent death?

4   Working in groups, allocate roles and simulate the use of these communication strategies in providing spiritual care to Michael and his family.

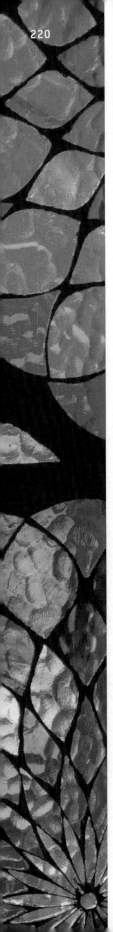

Further reading

Puchalski, C. (2006). Spiritual assessment in clinical practice. *Psychiatric Annals, 36*(3), 150–5.

Roy, D. (2011). Editorial. Does 'spiritual' indicate a limit to palliative care? *Journal of Palliative Care, 27*(4), 259–60.

Sinclair, S. & Chochinov, H. (2012). Communicating with patients about existential and spiritual issues: SACR-D work. *Progress in Palliative Care, 20*(2), 72–8.

Palliative Care Australia. (2018). *National Palliative Care Standards* (5th edn). Australian Government. Accessed March 2018 at <http://palliativecare.org.au/wp-content/uploads/dlm_uploads/2018/02/PalliativeCare-National-Standards-2018_web-3.pdf>.

Web resource

Spiritual Competency Resource Center

References

Abbas, S. & Panjwani, S. (2008). The necessity of spiritual care towards the end of life. *Ethics and Medicine, 24*(2), 113–18.

Amoah, C. (2011). The central importance of spirituality in palliative care. *International Journal of Palliative Care Nursing, 17*(7), 353–8.

Attard, J., Baldacchino, D. & Camilleri, L. (2014). Nurses and midwives acquisition of competency in spiritual care: A focus on education. *Nurse Education Today, 34*, 1460–6.

Australian Bureau of Statistics. (2012). *Cultural Diversity in Australia. Reflecting a Nation: Stories from the 2011 Census.* Accessed December 2012 at <http://www. abs.gov.au>.

Barton, K., Tate, T., Lau, N., Taliesin, K., Waldman, E. & Roseberg, A. (2018). I'm not a spiritual person. How hope might facilitate conversations about spirituality among teens and young adults with cancer. *Journal of Pain and Symptom Management*. doi: 10.1016/j.jpainsymman.2018.02.001

Brady, M., Peterman, A., Fitchett, G., Mo, M. & Cella, D. (1999). A case for including spirituality in quality of life measurement in oncology. *Psycho-oncology, 8*(5), 417–28.

Cacciatore, J. (2011). Psychosocial care. In C. Spong, *Stillbirth: Prediction, Prevention and Management* (pp. 203–28). USA: Wiley-Blackwell.

Casarez, R. & Engebretson, J. (2012). Ethical issues of incorporating spiritual care into clinical practice. *Journal of Clinical Nursing, 21*, 2099–107.

Chochinov, H., Hack, T., Hassard, T., Kristjanson, L., McClement, S. & Harlos, M. (2005). Dignity therapy: A novel psychotherapeutic intervention for patients near the end of life. *Journal of Clinical Oncology, 23*(24), 5520–5.

Cooper, K., Chang, E., Sheehan, A. & Johnson, A. (2012). The impact of spiritual care education upon preparing undergraduate nursing students to provide spiritual care. *Nurse Education Today*. In press: <http://www.ncbi.nlm.nih.gov/pubmed/22564926>

Edwards, A., Pang, N., Shiu, V. & Chan, C. (2010). The understanding of spirituality and the potential of spiritual care in end-of-life and palliative care: A meta study of qualitative research. *Palliative Medicine, 24*(8), 753–70.

Ford, D., Downey, L., Engelberg, R., Back, A. & Curtis, J. (2012). Discussing religion and spirituality is an advanced communication skill: An exploratory structural equation model of physician trainee self-ratings. *Journal of Palliative Medicine, 15*(1), 63–70.

Helming, M. (2009). Integrating spirituality into nurse practitioners' practice: The importance of finding the time. *Journal for Nurse Practitioners, 5*(8), 598–604.

Hodge, D. & Horvath, V. (2011). Spiritual needs in health care settings: A qualitative meta-synthesis of clients' perspectives. *Social Work, 56*(4), 306–16.

Levett-Jones, T., Dwyer, T., Reid-Searl, K., Heaton, L., Flenady, T., Applegarth, J., Guinea, S. & Andersen, P. (2017). *The Patient Safety Competency Framework (PSCF) for Nursing Students.* Sydney, NSW. Accessed January 2019 at <http://www.proftlj.com/wp-content/uploads/2017/07/UTS_PSCF_Brochure_2.pdf>.

Lovgren, M., Sveen, J., Steineck, G., Wallin, A., Eilertsen, M. & U, Kreicbergs. (2017). Spirituality and religious coping are related to cancer-bereaved siblings' long-term grief. *Palliative and Supportive Care*, 1–5.

Moore, T. (2010). *Care of the Soul in Medicine: Healing Guidance for Patients, Families, and the People Who Care for Them.* New York: Hay House.

Morrison, E. (2009). *Critical Issues for the 21st century* (2nd edn). Sudbury, MA: Jones & Bartlett.

Nelson, C., Rosenfield, B., Breitbard W. & Galietta, M. (2002). Spirituality, religion and depression in the terminally ill. *Psychosomatics, 43*(3), 213–20.

Noble, A. & Jones, J. (2010). Getting it right: Oncology nurses' understanding of spirituality. *International Journal of Palliative Care Nursing, 16*(11), 565–9.

Olson, M., Sandor, M., Sierpina, V., Vanderpool, H. & Dayao, P. (2006). Mind, body and spirit: Family physicians' beliefs, attitudes, and practices regarding the integration of patient spirituality into medical care. *Journal of Religion and Health, 45*, 234–47.

Phelps, A., Lauderdale, K., Alcorn, S., Dillinger, J., Balboni, M., Van Wert, M., . . . Balboni, T. (2012). Addressing spirituality within the care of patients at the end of life: Perspectives of patients with advanced cancer, oncologists and oncology nurses. *Journal of Clinical Oncology, 30*(20), 2538–44.

Puchalski, C. (2006). Spiritual assessment in clinical practice. *Psychiatric Annals, 36*(3), 150–5.

Puchalski, C., Ferrell, B., Virani, R., Otis-Green, S., Baird, P., Bull, J., . . . Sulmasy, D. (2009). Improving the quality of spiritual care as a dimension of palliative care: the report of the Consensus Conference. *Journal of Palliative Medicine, 12*(10), 885–904.

Reed, P. (1996). An emerging paradigm for the investigation of spirituality in nursing. *Research in Nursing & Health, 15*, 349–57.

Ronaldson, S. (2012). Spirituality in palliative care nursing. In M. O'Connor, S. Lee & S. Aranda, *Palliative Care Nursing: A Guide to Practice* (3rd edn) (pp. 52–75). Melbourne: Ausmed.

Ronaldson, S., Hayes, L., Aggar, C., Green, J. & Carey, M. (2012). Spirituality and spiritual caring: Nurses and practice in palliative acute care environments. *Journal of Clinical Nursing, 21*, 2126–35.

Ross, L. (2006). Spiritual care in nursing: An overview of the research to date. *Journal of Clinical Nursing, 15*(7), 852–62.

Sinclair, S. & Chochinov, H. (2012). Communicating with patients about existential and spiritual issues: SACR-D work. *Progress in Palliative Care, 20*(2), 72–8.

Smyth, T. & Allen, S. (2011). Nurses' experiences assessing the spirituality of terminally ill patients in acute clinical practice. *International Journal of Palliative Care Nursing, 17*(7), 337–43.

Stephenson, P. & Berry, D. (2015). Describing spirituality at the end of life. *Western Journal of Nursing Research, 37*(9), 1229–47.

Tang, V. (2002). Buddhist view on death and rebirth. Paper presented at 'Dying, Death and Grieving: A Cultural Perspective' conference. 11 March, Melbourne.

Tiew, L., Creedy, D. & Chan, M. (2013). Students nurses' perspectives of spirituality and spiritual care. *Nurse Education Today, 33*(6), 574–9. doi: 10.1016/j.nedt.2012.06.007

Vlasblom, J., van der Steen, J., Knol, D. & Jochemsen, H. (2011). Effects of a spiritual care training for nurses. *Nurse Education Today, 31*, 790–6.

van der Riet, P. (1999). Ethereal embodiment of cancer patients. *Australian Journal of Holistic Health, 6*(2), 20–7.

Vermandere, M., Warmenhoven, F., Severen, E., Lepeleire, J. & Aertgeerts. (2016). Spiritual history taking in palliative care: A cluster randomised controlled trial. *Palliative Care Medicine, 30*(4), 338–50.

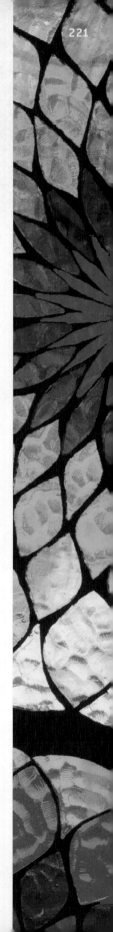

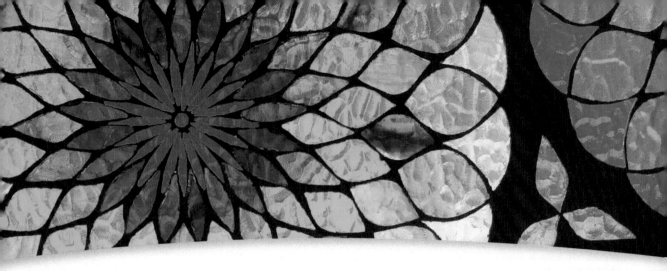

CHAPTER 19

COMMUNICATING WITH PEOPLE WHO ARE ANGRY OR AGGRESSIVE

Teresa Stone   Jeannette Walsh   Anna Treloar   Stephen Spencer

LEARNING OUTCOMES

Chapter 19 will enable you to:

- describe the context and causes of anger and aggression in healthcare
- discuss communication strategies that can prevent aggression and promote safe practice
- outline how to respond to people who are aggressive
- discuss the impact of psychological trauma on aggressive behaviours.

KEY CONCEPTS

aggression | anger | de-escalation | zero tolerance | misuse of power | cycle of aggression | trauma-informed care | respect

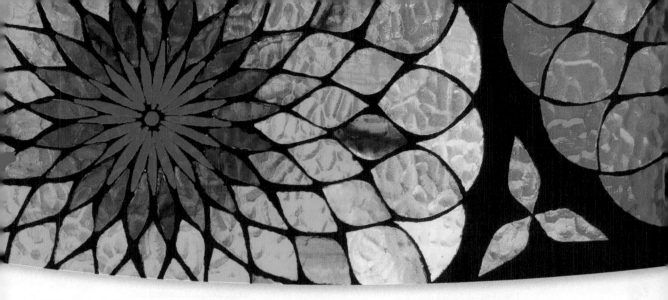

> The most basic of all human needs is the need
> to understand and be understood. The best way
> to understand people is to listen to them.
>
> (Nichols, 1980)

INTRODUCTION

Anger is an emotion that is experienced by virtually everyone (Hamby, 2017). Think of an occasion when you were needlessly kept waiting, becoming increasingly anxious and then perhaps annoyed; when loved ones were treated unfairly; when people were rude, abrupt or even quite aggressive. Did your anger make you aggressive?

Anger, aggression and violence are closely related: Aggression is the expression of anger in either actual or threatened violence. Violence is a sub-set of aggressive behaviour and is defined as 'the intentional use of physical force or power, threatened or actual, . . . that results in or has a high likelihood of resulting in injury, death, psychological maldevelopment or deprivation' (Krug et al., 2002). Workplace violence includes 'physical and psychological violence, abuse . . . bullying, racial harassment and sexual harassment and can include interactions between co-workers, supervisors, patients, families, visitors, and others' (McPhaul & Lipscomb, 2004). Given the complexities of providing healthcare to people who are experiencing distress, it is not surprising that healthcare staff experience work-related violence much more often than other workers (Hills et al., 2015).

To fully understand aggression, it is important to pay attention to the context within which it arises, otherwise healthcare professionals risk seeing aggression as coming just from within the patient. This is not in order to excuse the aggression, rather it is to help us understand and respond appropriately to the individual and to identify factors that may have precipitated the aggression or violence. Duxbury & Whittington (2005) identify these factors to be internal, external and interactional factors; these will be explored later in the chapter.

Talking with someone who is angry and aggressive can be challenging for healthcare professionals. Anyone can be pleasant to people who are grateful for the care they are receiving, but it takes self-control, integrity and self-awareness to connect positively with angry or aggressive people, especially those with stigmatising characteristics such as mental health or drug and alcohol problems, or who use swear words (Stone & McMillan, 2012).

This chapter describes aggression and anger and identifies some of the factors that exacerbate them. We then explore how to communicate with people who are angry or aggressive and set clear appropriate boundaries in our interactions with patients.

ONE SHIFT. THREE STORIES

My name is Caleb.

I've had this intense pain in my rectum for 2 weeks now. The doctor said I have haemorrhoids or a fistula.

I am supposed to have surgery, but the hospital has cancelled it twice now.

My doctor gave me painkillers but I ran out on Monday, and I haven't slept for the last 3 nights because of the pain.

I haven't been to work and I'm worried I'll get the sack.

I can't get in to see my doctor till next Monday and all the other doctors are booked out.

But I don't think I can stand this pain for another minute.

So I go back to the emergency department at the hospital.

I wait for ages, then the nurse at the front counter finally calls me in. I tell her how much agony I'm in and that I can't stand it.

She tells me that I will have to wait for a long time but that she will bring me some painkillers. She tells me to go and sit in the waiting area.

I say 'Don't you understand? . . . I can't sit down!!!'

Then she goes off and never comes back. Eventually I can't stand it anymore.

I get angry and yell for someone to bring me some painkillers.

The nurse comes back, and then this big male nurse comes over and tells me to be quiet.

I totally lose it.

Next thing I know they've called security and they push me outside. In front of everyone. My girlfriend sees it all. She is crying and screaming.

I can't stand the pain and nobody cares. What's wrong with these people?

Next thing the police arrive.

They stand around me, but I don't care anymore . . . the pain is so bad. They can shoot me for all I care.

Then another nurse comes over. She talks to me. She tells me she will get the doctor and give me some meds. Finally! I just start crying.

They put me in a wheelchair and wheel me over near the door outside. The police leave and the nurse and a doctor come out with my pain meds.

FINALLY!

My name is Karen.

It's a busy Friday evening and I'm working the triage desk. The department is full, and the waiting room crowded.

A 22-year-old male presents complaining of rectal pain. I know this guy—Caleb. He was here last week with the same presentation. He caused some trouble then and this time he has attitude from the moment we meet.

He was supposed to get surgical follow-up, but he is back.

I can see that he is in considerable pain. He says it's 10/10 and, unfortunately for all of us, he is going to have a long wait to be seen. I tell him I will get him some oxycodone to try to make him more comfortable.

At that moment, a critically unwell patient arrives by ambulance. The paramedics are preforming CPR and need some assistance to move the stretcher into resuscitation.

A couple of minutes later, as I walk back to the desk, I hear him yelling:

'Doesn't anyone here care how much pain I'm in? Can't someone do something? What type of hospital is this?'

He picks up a chair and throws it against the desk.

I'm scared; the clerical staff are scared.

One of our nurses, Michael, comes out to see what's up.

He is great in these sorts of situations. 'This behaviour is unacceptable my friend.'

Caleb steps up and pushes him hard. *'Don't get smart with me!'* he shouts.

Clerical call a code black, and then they call the police.

Two wardsmen and security arrive and pretty much manhandle him outside.

I'm still shaking when two police cars roll up a couple of minutes later.

I see one of our senior nurses, Jane, walk over to the group.

Next thing, the police are leaving . . . and the wardsmen sit Caleb in a wheelchair and wheel him over in front of the 'No Smoking' sign for a cigarette.

I was like . . . *what??*

Then Jane and a doctor go over and give him some painkillers, and a script. He leaves shortly afterwards with his girlfriend.

So much for zero tolerance. I mean . . . this guy was rewarded for this sort of behaviour. He assaulted a nurse and for that . . . he jumped the queue, and had a doctor and nurse attend to him outside while he had a cigarette!

Not happy.

My name is Jane.

I'm the team leader for this evening. It's super busy, and a cardiac arrest has just arrived when I hear trouble out at the Triage desk.

By the time I can get out there, security have moved this guy outside. I looked after him last week. He has had a pretty tough life. Just got out of jail and I remember him telling me he was scared that he might lose his new job if he took any more sick leave. He has three kids, and one of them has some sort of congenital heart disease—a poor prognosis.

Anyway, the police arrive, words are being exchanged and the whole thing is escalating. The whole group is now obstructing the main entrance to the department and I can see a few very upset people trying to get past. I think it must be the family of the man who had the cardiac arrest. The police have lost patience and are about to haul him off.

I feel kind of sorry for the guy. He is obviously in a great deal of pain . . . and has just lost the plot.

I think I can de-escalate this situation and bring some sort of resolution. I don't think he remembers me from last week but I walk in and sit down beside him. With all the police around, I'm not feeling threatened, and I spend some time talking to him.

He bursts into tears, sobbing loudly.

All he wants is enough painkillers to get him by till he can get in to see his doctor. If the police haul him off he is only going to come back later. It's the weekend and he won't get in to see anybody till next week.

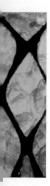

I think I can finish this quickly. I go and grab a doctor and explain the situation. The police are happy to leave once he calms down a little.

I feel good that I have managed to stop this situation becoming violent and ending up with Caleb being taken away from his family.

Within five minutes, he has had some painkillers, has a script, and leaves.

I notice the triage nurse give me a curt look as I walk by but I've got too much happening right now to talk to her. I hurry back to care for the family of the man who has just died in resuscitation.

Source: Adapted with the permission of Ian Miller, *theNursePath* blog.

The context and causes of aggression

Angry and aggressive patients are likely to be encountered in all settings, both clinical and non-clinical. A recent US study identified that nurses have a substantially higher risk of workplace violence than other occupations, and that injury from workplace violence has increased annually by 23 per cent (Groenewold et al., 2018). Internationally, violence towards healthcare staff is a growing concern with between 8 and 38 per cent of staff experiencing physical violence at some point in their careers; most at risk are nurses, paramedics and other staff directly involved in patient care (World Health Organization, 2017). Australian research indicates that as many as 88 per cent of emergency department nurses have experienced verbal aggression and over half had been physically assaulted in the last six months (Partridge & Affleck, 2017).

Healthcare professionals exposed to aggressive behaviours have higher rates of injury, absences from work, burnout and mental health problems than other groups. This inevitably affects patient safety and the quality of care they provide (Yassi & Hancock, 2005). However, understanding the factors that precipitate anger and aggression can help healthcare providers develop and utilise strategies aimed at preventing and de-escalation.

The internal, external and interactional causes of patient aggression

A number of factors have been identified as causes of aggression towards healthcare workers, including a lack of trust in health services, unrealistic expectations of what healthcare can provide, long waiting times to receive care, and poor communication (Zhang, Stone & Zhang, 2016). There are also internal, external and interactional causes of inpatient aggression that need to be understood.

Internal causes of aggression are the factors associated with the patient or client, commonly thought of as *risk factors*; they include:

- being male
- under 32 years of age
- cognitive state (e.g. psychosis, dementia)
- emotional state (e.g. scared, in pain, anxious, aroused, angry)
- substance misuse
- disinhibition
- past history of aggression
- brain injury, organic disease
- past history of trauma.

(Barlow, Grenyer & Ilkiw-Lavalle, 2000; Cutcliffe & Riahi, 2013a: Nijman et al., 2002; Worksafe, 2009)

External causes of aggression are those related to the environment and include:

- structure and layout of the healthcare setting
- patient mix, ward dynamics and milieu

- over-crowding
- inadequate staffing
- staff skill mixes
- organisational policies and procedures
- restrictive environment
- waiting times
- noise
- lack of natural light.

(Nijman et al., 2002; Worksafe, 2009)

Interactional causes of aggression include the attitudes, skills and behaviours of healthcare staff, such as:

- attitudes, knowledge and skill level
- communication skills
- limit-setting style
- willingness to help
- engagement styles
- ineffective staff–patient relationships.

(Duxbury & Whittington, 2005; Nijman et al., 2002)

Other causes of anger and aggression, which are not so easily controlled but should be recognised and factored into risk management planning, include:

- volatile emotional situations
- family disputes
- violence
- child protection issues.

(Worksafe, 2009)

'When someone is going through a storm, your silent presence is more powerful than a million, empty words' (Thelma Davis).

Situations when anger and aggression may be more common

- When a person is experiencing severe pain, or is very frightened or anxious, they may become angry or aggressive.
- If a person is intoxicated, disinhibition may occur and they may be irritable or oversensitive to perceived slights or insults.
- If a person brought to hospital is dependent on drugs, legal or illegal, they may be concerned about withdrawal symptoms and ensuring that their supply continues. Consequently, they may respond aggressively if challenged.
- If a patient is experiencing paranoid delusions or auditory hallucinations warning of great danger, they may lash out or do whatever seems necessary to gain protection from harm.
- Patients with delirium may have clouding of consciousness and inability to process information or new stimuli, and consequently become confused, frightened and aggressive.
- For people with dementia, the onset of night-time, or tiredness, thirst or hunger, may result in altered mood and aggressive outbursts.
- Patients with an intellectual disability or an acquired brain injury may be overwhelmed with unfamiliar settings, people and procedures, and respond with aggression.

Preventing aggression and promoting safe practice

Healthcare professionals can have a significant impact on the incidence and escalation of angry and aggressive episodes with patients. Providing person-centred care where each person feels respected and listened to is the foundation for positive engagement and safe patient care (Australian Commission on Safety and Quality in Health Care, 2017). The following communication strategies can help to promote safe and effective patient care and prevent anger and aggression:

Paying attention to relational aspects of healthcare: Positive engagement with patients is a key element of care (Doyle, Lennox & Bell, 2013). Negative engagement by healthcare professionals with patients leads to a climate of disrespect. It may occur because patients look strange to us; we may have been given prejudicial information about them; or their behaviour or sexual orientation may challenge our personal values. Sensing that we do not respect them, patients may perceive aggression and respond aggressively.

Managing how we exert power in our relationships with patients: Our role as healthcare professionals gives us power in the relationship and can cause patients to feel powerless. If we convey the message, 'I am in charge here and you need to do as I say', patients may attempt to assert themselves and regain power, withdraw or become aggressive. Further, if our expectations of appropriate patient behaviour are not met, we may also respond in an angry manner (Goodyear-Smith & Buetow, 2001).

Understanding patient's fear and distress: People can be very stressed and fearful when seeking healthcare in any setting. They often come to the health system distressed, in pain, and unsure of what is happening; they may be traumatised or afraid that a professional assessment will expose them to suspicion of violence against their child or partner. Such feelings can easily lead to aggressive behaviours.

Simple courtesies like greeting the person by name, explaining what will happen or that there will be delays and returning to provide updates, can often help minimise the frustration of waiting and worrying (Cohen et al., 2013).

Managing our own responses: It is helpful when you are faced with aggression to first 'check yourself' and to identify what you are feeling. If you are feeling fearful, angry or anxious, manage this response first. Reactive responses can escalate a situation. Considered, strategic responses that are empathic and appropriate to the situation can help to de-escalate aggression.

Systems approaches

All healthcare professionals and frontline staff should be educated about how to prevent, manage and report violence in the workplace (Bowers, Nijman et al., 2006; Spencer, Stone & McMillan, 2010). In addition, there needs to be risk assessments and the development of effective protocols to deal with workplace violence (Schindeler & Reynald, 2017). Looking after the wellbeing of staff is imperative and healthcare organisations have a responsibility to provide physical, emotional and social support to help staff feel safe; this in turn is likely to translate into patient safety (Yassi & Hancock, 2005). Education in violence prevention and reduction should be undertaken as part of undergraduate programs and should also form part of the induction program for all new staff (Victorian Taskforce on Violence in Nursing, 2005).

Aggression in the workplace can be emotionally distressing, both for staff who are directly involved and those who observe it. Individuals respond differently after such an incident and no response is necessarily right or wrong. While discussing an incident and debriefing with co-workers can be helpful for some people, professional counselling may also be beneficial.

Formal debriefing involves a step-by-step review of an incident by supervisors, without allocation of blame, so that learning from it may result in an improved response in the future. Seeking support and having a debriefing are positive steps towards taking care of one's self psychologically and promoting positive learning in the workplace. Remember, emotional wellbeing influences the quality of care health professionals can provide to the people they care for.

Healthcare organisations that have a zero tolerance policy towards violence demonstrate that any instances of aggression, threatened or actual, are unacceptable (NSW Health 2015a; Stone & Francis, 2010; Stone & McMillan, 2012). This is a worthy policy, but when routinely and inflexibly applied it can work against positive engagement with patients. Additionally, healthcare policies that mandate zero tolerance for swearing potentially discriminate against minority or traditionally disadvantaged groups. A rigid interpretation of the policy may also encourage intolerance in healthcare professionals (Duxbury & Whittington, 2005). Aggression and swearing should be met with a respectful request that the behaviour cease. If that is ineffective and patients are excluded from the service, an invitation should be issued to return for treatment when they have regained control of themselves.

Aggression should not be 'punished' by healthcare professionals (National Collaborating Centre for Mental Health, 2015). Decisions to exclude people from services in order to ensure patient and staff safety should be made at an appropriately senior level, in line with the duty of care, and should include suggestions of alternative access to care.

Effective communication and collaboration between healthcare professionals is essential as conflict within the treatment team can result in confusion and anxiety for patients, which may then surface as anger or aggression. Patients should also be involved in decision making so as to promote trust and mutual respect. In mental health settings, staff who positively value patients and regulate their fear and anger impact positively on rates of aggression, self-harm and absconding (Bowers, Eyres et al., 2006; Bowers, Simpson & Alexander, 2005).

Responding to people who are aggressive

Consistency, collaboration and consequences are the key to effective organisational management of aggression (Renker, Scribner & Huff, 2015). There are many reasons why a person may become aggressive and these potential reasons should be considered when planning how to manage or respond. However, if there is no identifiable clinical reason and if staff have done all they can to assist the person—given the constraints of triage, acuity, other patient priorities, staffing and time—then it is reasonable to remind them that it is not appropriate to speak to staff in such a manner. This is all that needs to be said; the aim is to maintain a constructive nurse–patient encounter (Falkenstrom, 2017). Demanding apologies, trying to engage in lengthy discussions or responding punitively will only exacerbate a volatile situation.

Where the person's behaviour and language are influenced by any of the factors listed previously, allowances will need to be made; and when the clinical issue has resolved, the person may, without prompting, choose to apologise later. Good relationships are still possible after strained beginnings (Lowry, 2016).

Avoiding aggression with empathic and appropriate communication is of course the ideal. However, it is important to have systems to safely manage aggressive and unpredictable behaviour when it occurs. It is also essential for staff to be aware of triggers such as long waiting times, and crowded or high-stimulus environments (Australian Commission on Safety and Quality in Health Care, 2017, p. 40). If things do go wrong, it is important that healthcare professionals apologise promptly, explain fully, and remain empathic when discussing the problem (National Patient Safety Agency, 2008). This alone may be sufficient to reduce anger and aggression.

When aggression does occur, de-escalation procedures may be required. De-escalation consists of a variety of psychosocial techniques designed to reduce aggressive behaviours (National Collaborating Centre for Mental Health, 2015). Competent de-escalation is a skill that requires much more than a theoretical understanding of aggression. The healthcare professional must undertake a developmental process, resulting in highly evolved self-awareness, so that the skills of de-escalation become almost instinctive (National Collaborating Centre for Mental Health, 2015) (See Figure 19.1). The communication strategies set out below are the basis for prevention and early intervention of aggression; the use of manual/mechanical restraint should only be used as a last resort (NSW Health, 2015b; SA Health, 2017).

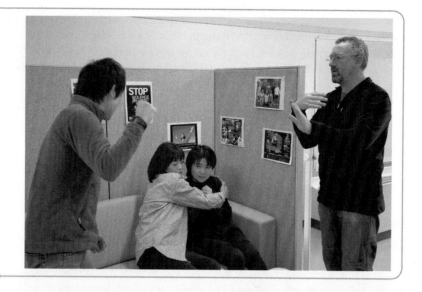

Skilled communication, non-confrontation, relationship-building and negotiation, as well as seeking to understand the reasons for the aggression, are the best ways to manage escalation and avoid harm (Harwood, 2017). The decision by a patient to use violence or aggression involves mental and emotional processes related to four simple issues: *justification*, *alternatives*, *consequences* and *ability* (de Becker, 2000). The focus of de-escalation is to convey willingness to understand the person's problem; to counter any perceived justification for violence; to produce alternative ways to resolve the situation; to modify expectations with an honest explanation of the consequences; and to remove the ability to commit an aggressive action by controlling the environment to ensure the safety of patients and staff.

Points to bear in mind when communicating with someone who is aggressive include:

- preserving the person's dignity
- being helpful
- staying calm
- offering alternatives.

Actions that can contribute to de-escalation include the following.

Non-verbal

- Remember your own safety.
- Monitor your body language and tone of voice; remember that 80 per cent of communication is non-verbal. Consciously notice where you are tense (such as shoulders and jaw) and try to relax your posture.
- Engagement should be in a place of safety for both parties, with a clear exit and where other staff can assist immediately.
- If possible, ask the person to sit down and sit down alongside them but at a safe distance.
- Place yourself at a 45-degree angle to the person, where you can maintain natural eye contact without appearing to stare.
- Angry and suspicious people need physical space around them to feel safe; do not encroach on it and avoid touching them.
- Separate people in conflict.
- Move dangerous objects out of reach/view.
- Remove people/objects that upset the person.

- Use people or objects that have a positive effect on the person.
- Move slowly and explain your actions.

Verbal

- Speak slowly and naturally and explain your actions.
- Keep your voice at a conversational level.
- One person should speak at a time.
- Allow the patient to tell their side of the story without interruption, to avoid a pattern of accusation–defence–reaccusation. Agree with what you can without telling an untruth: 'Yes, you have been waiting a long time. I can understand why you are angry about that and we are doing our best to have you seen as soon as possible.'
- Avoid confrontation and contradicting the person.
- If waiting causes a problem, 'underpromise and overdeliver': instead of 'the doctor will be here in just a minute', say it will probably be another 10 minutes (but only if you are confident that will happen).
- Reframe your language; instead of 'No, you can't have a drink', reframe it to something that you can assist with: 'I can give you some ice cubes to suck.'
- Following interactions, document all conversations and patient concerns according to your institution's policies.

Too often, without knowing, healthcare staff can make an angry person even angrier. These types of behaviour that undermine patient engagement, include:

- whispering or laughing, especially about the patient.
- touching—while therapeutic for some people when anxious or upset, it can trigger anxiety, fear and anger in others
- raising your voice and attempting to talk over the person
- lying—e.g. 'You can have a cigarette in the ward'
- direct eye contact—may be interpreted as a threat by some people
- giving multiple choices, especially in the one sentence: 'What are you angry about? What would you like, a cup of tea, or would you rather go and lie down, or see the doctor? Is there anyone I can call? Sugar with that?'
- taking a moral stance: 'You are not the only one waiting to see the doctor. Other people are far worse off than you. You should be grateful.'
- overreacting to language or gestures by commanding, ordering or threatening: 'Verbal aggression is against the zero tolerance policy. If you swear again I will call the police.'
- using analogies rather than being concrete: 'You know what they say about bending with the wind . . .'
- directly challenging delusions: 'Do you really think you . . .'

Managing aggressive phone calls

Angry telephone calls are often difficult to manage. In face-to-face conversations it is obvious you are listening and paying attention, but phone calls require verbal supportive and reflective comments. Sometimes you may need to set a limit to the expressed aggression: 'I am prepared to talk further, but at the moment I don't think it is useful. I am happy to call you or for you to call me when we can focus on a way forward.'

The cycle of aggression

Understanding the cyclic models of aggression can help healthcare professionals choose the most appropriate intervention for safe management of an incident, and to reduce the risk of injury to patients, staff and visitors. Background factors, which normally result from the internal, external and interactional causes of patient aggression, precede the five phases of the cycle discussed by Bowie (1996). Aggression typically starts with the triggering event; the subsequent escalation phase then lasts until the crisis point is reached, resulting in verbal or physical aggression. After that, comes the recovery phase, where appropriate behaviours are re-established. A post-crisis depression sometimes follows. A series of escalation/crisis/recovery phases without return to baseline may occur, particularly if there are multiple or continuing triggering events.

Psychological trauma and aggression

People who have experienced trauma as an adult—such as sexual assault or intimate partner violence—or stressful or traumatic events during their childhood—including abuse, neglect or exposure to other traumatic stressors (known as adverse childhood experiences)—may present with aggression and violence (Cutcliffe & Riahi, 2013b). This may be because they feel physically, socially or emotionally unsafe when receiving healthcare that results in anxiety and the possibility of the person feeling re-traumatised (Menschner & Maul, 2016). This may be interpreted by the healthcare professional as the patient being untrusting or aggressive. For example, a woman who was sexually abused as a child may fear receiving antenatal care, and something we might regard as harmless can trigger a powerful response because of her experience of past trauma.

This is best understood by considering the underlying physiology. In response to trauma and a heightened level of arousal, the amygdala can take over brain functioning and may activate the fight or flight response. The thinking part of the brain (pre-frontal cortex or cerebrum) is not involved, so the trigger will not be evaluated, and people cannot modulate their response. When waiting to see a healthcare professional, the person may become anxious, increasingly agitated and watchful, and then perhaps aggressive with staff and others. This example highlights the inseparability of the brain and the body, and the effect of trauma exposure, including neurological, biological and psychological responses (Menschner &Maul, 2016).

Recent research has indicated a high prevalence of trauma exposure in the general population, both as adults and as children (Baker et al., 2015; Cox, 2015; Fellitti et al., 1998; Cronholm et al., 2015). It is important, therefore, that healthcare professionals understand the meaning of trauma-informed approaches to care provision.

Trauma-informed approaches mean being alert to the possibility of trauma experiences for any person who receives healthcare. It is distinct from specific treatment for trauma. The principles of a trauma-informed approach lie in understanding the prevalence and nature of trauma from interpersonal violence and its impact on other areas of life and functioning, and creating cultures and practices that empower patients (Quadara, 2015; Kezelman & Stavropoulos, 2012; Bateman et al., 2013). This could include:

- engaging with patients collaboratively and treating them with respect: explaining what is going to happen and what you are going to do before you do it; not asserting power
- validating their experience: 'I'm sorry you have to wait. I know it can be frustrating.'
- asking whether the patient would like to call someone to wait with them
- ensuring that the environment is safe, both physically and emotionally, with responses that are consistent and predictable
- doing everything to be trustworthy, but not expecting the patient to trust you
- maintaining appropriate boundaries (this is always important, but is more so with survivors of trauma, because it provides a sense of psychological safety); not overstepping your role, and sensitively communicating its limits (e.g. if you see the person outside of the clinical setting be friendly but not friends)
- engaging patients in decision making and in the development of their care plan, rather than telling them what has been decided for them.

Conclusion

This chapter has examined some of the complexities associated with incidents of patient anger and aggression, and we have identified that simply implementing a zero tolerance policy is not enough. Hospitals and healthcare facilities are increasingly required to care for people who have chronic debilitating illness and multiple psychopathologies. Healthcare professionals see people when they are in pain, frightened, stressed, under the influence of drugs and alcohol, presenting with mental health difficulties, or they have experienced interpersonal violence. To practise safely and effectively we need to be aware of these factors. Such awareness will help us to communicate in ways that decrease the risk of aggression rather than escalating it, by adopting a positive, professional and proactive communication style.

Remember that accessing healthcare can be difficult for people who are marginalised or socially disadvantaged. Previous encounters with healthcare professionals may make them reluctant to return, and they may arrive expecting dismissive or abrupt responses from staff. Time spent communicating with courtesy and empathy can help to dissipate negative expectations and help build a foundation for partnership and cooperation.

Lastly, it is important to reflect on one's own state of wellbeing. Nurses are often exposed to stressful experiences and must manage complex situations in clinical environments that are often demanding and dynamic. If healthcare professionals are not provided with the necessary support, or do not deliberately engage in self-care strategies, compassion fatigue can result, and the sense of meaning and joy from helping others can be compromised. This can also have a flow-on effect to patients, with flawed decision making, frustration, irritability.

Critical thinking activities

A 15-year-old girl presented to the emergency department (ED) with persistent suicidal ideation and cuts to her forearm as a result of deliberate self-harm. It was a busy day in the ED and one of the nurses said to the child and adolescent social worker, 'We have two of your's here and can't move them along; so we have sick kids out there who can't get help.' The social worker took him to task about his attitude towards patients with mental illness and voices were raised. Unfortunately, this exchange was overheard by the young girl and her father, both of whom became visibly upset and teary. The social worker and nurse tried to explain to them that their needs were important, but during the discussion the father yelled that he would take his daughter somewhere 'where the staff would give a damn'. Hearing the yelling, the registrar poked his head around the curtains and told the father to tone it down, otherwise he would call the police: 'There are sick people around here and no call for this behaviour.' In the meantime the young girl had gone very quiet. She took out a razor blade that was hidden in the tongue section of her shoe and started slashing her legs and arms while her father struggled with her to get the blade. The nurse called for backup, and the social worker, the nurse, the registrar and a passing clinical psychologist tried to calm the situation by all talking at once.

1   How can a healthcare professional's attitudes, behaviours and beliefs influence patient aggression and safety?
2   Discuss the relationship between effective communication and aggression minimisation.
3   Discuss what specific communication techniques you could use to manage a similar situation more effectively.

Teaching and assessment activities

The story and questions below can be used as a stimulus for tutorial discussion.

Weak calls for 'nurse, nurse' come from behind a curtain but are not answered. Somebody begins to vomit. The swing doors crash open and a delivery from stores arrives. The trolley is left in the middle of the patient area. This area is already blocked by the dirty plates and cutlery from lunch, which are stacked on another trolley. An ambulance and a police van pull up. The patient in the ambulance seems to be handcuffed.

As police, paramedics and patient come through the ambulance door, a man who has been sitting on a chair in the corner of the ED near the toilet suddenly stands up and stamps into the clerk's office. 'Look!' he says, 'How much longer do I have to wait? I have a headache, I feel really sick, and I just want to get up into the ward and lie down. Seems to me you lot couldn't organise a booze-up in a brewery.' The clerk leaps to her feet, glares at the man, and says, 'There are other people here too you know. You are not the most important person here, don't you realise?' The man kicks the wall, knocks over the meal trolley, and pushes past the police and paramedics to get outside. He then runs off and disappears.

1   In small groups, students can be guided to discuss the following questions.
   a.   What were the internal, external and interactional causes of the aggression in this situation?
   b.   What do you think the patient was thinking and feeling in this situation?
   c.   How might the ward clerk have been feeling?
   d.   How could the environment have been modified to reduce triggers of aggression?
   e.   What communication techniques could been used in this situations?

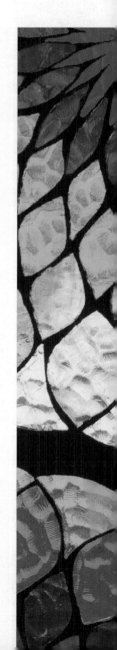

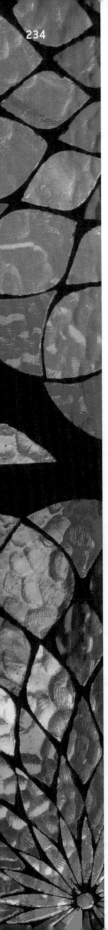

2   Provide the opportunity for students to reflect on and discuss the following.

a.   Think of a time when you felt yourself becoming angry: What were the triggers? What were your immediate thoughts and responses? What assisted you to calm down? How can you incorporate this learning into your clinical practice?

b.   Reflect on an occasion when you witnessed aggression in a work context. What were your immediate thoughts and responses? What are your thoughts now that you have read this chapter? What has changed/developed your thinking? How can you incorporate this learning into your clinical practice and your way of communicating?

Further reading

Brickell, T., Nicholls, T., Procyshyn, R., McLean, C., Dempster, R., Lavoie, J., . . . Wang, E. (2009). *Patient Safety in Mental Health*. Edmonton, Alberta: Canadian Patient Safety Institute and Ontario Hospital Association.

Muir-Cochrane, E. (2009). The person who appears aggressive or violent. In P. Barker (Ed.), *Psychiatric and Mental Health Nursing: The Craft of Caring* (pp. 230–6). London: Edward Arnold.

Web resources

NSW Ministry of Health. (2015). *Mental Health for Emergency Departments:* This reference guide is intended to assist emergency department staff and other clinicians in caring for people experiencing emergency mental health problems.
<https://www.health.nsw.gov.au/mentalhealth/resources/Publications/mental-health-ed-guide.pdf>

CDC: About Adverse Childhood Experiences (ACEs): Childhood experiences, both positive and negative, have a tremendous impact on future violence, victimisation and perpetration, and lifelong health and opportunity.
<https://www.cdc.gov/violenceprevention/acestudy/about_ace.html>

Trauma-informed care.
<https://www.chcs.org/resource/10-key-ingredients-trauma-informed-care/>

Safe Work Australia. Workplace violence: Definitions, resources and case studies.
<https://www.safeworkaustralia.gov.au/workplace-violence>

NSW Health: *Principles for Safe Management of Disturbed and/or Aggressive Behaviour and the Use of Restraint*
<http://www1.health.nsw.gov.au/pds/ActivePDSDocuments/PD2015_004.pdf>

SA Health: Restraint and seclusion in mental health: The current best available evidence on the prevention and elimination of restraint and seclusion, and eight fact sheets to assist with implementation.
<http://www.sahealth.sa.gov.au/wps/wcm/connect/public+content/sa+health+internet/clinical+resources/clinical+topics/mental+health/restraint+and+seclusion+in+mental+health>

References

Australian Commission on Safety and Quality in Health Care. (2017). *National Safety and Quality Health Service Standards* (2nd edn). Sydney, Australia: ACSQHC.

Baker, C. N., Brown, S. M., Wilcox, P. D., Overstreet, S. & Arora, P. (2015). Development and psychometric evaluation of the attitudes related to trauma-informed care (ARTIC) Scale. *School Mental Health, 8*(1), 61–76.

Barlow, K., Grenyer, B. & Ilkiw-Lavalle, O. (2000). Prevalence and precipitants of aggression in psychiatric inpatient units. *Australian and New Zealand Journal of Psychiatry, 34*, 967–74.

Bateman, J., Henderson, C. & Kezelman, C. (2013). Trauma informed care and practice: Towards a cultural shift in policy reform across mental health and human services in Australia, a national strategic direction. *Mental Health Coordinating Council.*

Bowers, L., Eyres, S., Grange, A., Hall, C., Nijman, H., Phillips, L. & Simpson, A. (2006). Serious untoward incidents and their aftermath in acute inpatient psychiatry: The Tompkins Acute Ward study. *International Journal of Mental Health Nursing, 15*, 226–34.

Bowers, L., Nijman, H., Allan, T., Simpson, A., Warren, J. & Turner, L. (2006). Prevention and management of aggression training and officially reported violent incidents. *Psychiatric Services, 57*, 1022–6.

Bowers, L., Simpson, A. & Alexander, J. (2005). Real world application of an intervention to reduce absconding. *Journal of Psychiatric and Mental Health Nursing, 12*, 589–602.

Bowie, V. (1996). *Coping with Violence: A Guide for the Human Services. London:* Whiting and Birch.

Cohen, E., Wilkin, H., Tannebaum, M., Plew, M. & Haley, L. (2013). When patients are impatient: The communication strategies utilized by emergency department employees to manage patients frustrated by wait times. *Health Communication, 28*, 275–85.

Cox, P. (2015). Violence against women: Additional analysis of the Australian Bureau of Statistics' Personal Safety Survey, 2012. *ANROWS Horizons,* (1).

Cronholm, P., Forke, C. R. Wade, R., Bair-Merritt, Davis, Harkins-Schwarz, M. . . . Fein, J. (2015). Adverse childhood experiences: Expanding the concept of adversity. *American Journal of Preventive Medicine, 49*(3), 354–61.

Cutcliffe, J. R. & Riahi, S. (2013a). Systemic perspective of violence and aggression in mental health care: Towards a more comprehensive understanding and conceptualization: Part 1. *International Journal of Mental Health Nursing, 22*(6), 558–67

Cutcliffe, J. R. & Riahi, S. (2013b). Systemic perspective of violence and aggression in mental health care: Towards a more comprehensive understanding and conceptualization: Part 2. *International Journal of Mental Health Nursing, 22*(6), 568–78.

de Becker, G. (2000). *The Gift of Fear.* New York: Bloomsbury Publishing PLC.

Doyle, C., Lennox, L. & Bell, D. (2013). A systematic review of evidence on the links between patient experience and clinical safety and effectiveness. *BMJ Open, 3*(1).

Duxbury, J. and Whittington, R. (2005). Causes and management of patient aggression and violence: Staff and patient perspectives. *Journal of Advanced Nursing, 50*(5), 469–78.

Falkenstrom, M. (2017). A qualitative study of difficult nurse-patient encounters in home health care. *Advances in Nursing Science, 40*(2), 168–83.

Fellitti, V. J., Anda, R. F., Nordenberg, D., Williamson, D. F., Spitz, A. M., Edwards, V., Koss, M. P. & Marks, J. S. (1998), Relationship of childhood abuse and household dysfunction to many of the leading cause of death in adults the adverse childhood experiences (ACE) Study. *American Journal of Preventive Medicine, 14*(4), 245–58.

Goodyear-Smith, F. & Buetow, S. (2001). Power issues in the doctor-patient relationship. *Health Care Analysis*, 9449–62.

Groenewold, M. R., Sarmiento, R. F., Vanoli, K., Raudabaugh, W., Nowlin, S., & Gomaa, A. (2018). Workplace violence injury in 106 US hospitals participating in the Occupational Health Safety Network (OHSN), 2012–2015. *American Journal of Industrial Medicine, 61*(2), 157–66.

Hamby, S. (2017). On defining violence, and why it matters. *Psychology of Violence, 7*(2), 167–80.

Harwood, R. H. (2017). How to deal with violent and aggressive patients in acute medical settings. *The Journal of the Royal College of Physicians of Edinburgh, 47*(2), 94–101.

Hills, D. J., Ross, H. M., Pich, J., Hill, A. T., Dalsbø, T. K., Riahi, S., . . . Martínez-Jarreta, B. (2015). Education and training for preventing and minimising workplace aggression directed toward healthcare workers. *Cochrane Database of Systematic Reviews*.

Kezelman, C. & Stavropoulos, P. (2012) *Practice Guidelines for Treatment of Complex Trauma and Trauma Informed Care and Service Delivery*. Adults Surviving Child Abuse.

Krug, E., Dahlberg, L., Mercy, J., Zwi, A. & Lozano, R. (Eds). (2002). *World Report on Violence and Health*. Geneva: World Health Organization.

Lowry, M. (2016). De-escalating anger: A new model for practice. *Nursing Times, 112*(4), 4–7.

McPhaul, K. & Lipscomb, J. (2004). Workplace violence in health care: Recognized but not regulated. *The Online Journal of Issues in Nursing, 9*(3).

Menschner, C. & Maul, A. (2016). *Key Ingredients for Successful Trauma-Informed Care Implementation*. Center for Health Care Strategies, Incorporated.

National Collaborating Centre for Mental Health. (2015). Violence and aggression: Short-term management in mental health, health and community settings. *NICE Guideline NG10* <https://www.nice.org.uk/guidance/ng10>, accessed 11 April 2018.

National Patient Safety Agency. (2008). *Seven Steps to Patient Safety in Mental Health*.

Nichols, R. (1980). The Struggle to be Human. Paper presented at the Convention of International Listening Association, Atlanta, Georgia.

Nijman, H., Merckelbach, H., Evers, C., Palmstierna, T. & a Campo, J. (2002). Prediction of aggression on a locked psychiatric admissions ward. *Acta Psychiatrica Scandinavica, 105*(5), 390–5.

NSW Health. (2015a). *Preventing and Managing Violence in the NSW Health Workplace: A Zero Tolerance Approach* (Document No. PD2015_001). Sydney, Australia: NSW Department of Health.

NSW Health. (2015b). *Principles for Safe Management of Disturbed and /or Aggressive Behaviour and the Use of Restraint* (Document No. PD2015_004). Sydney, Australia: NSW Department of Health.

Partridge, B. & Affleck, J. (2017). Verbal abuse and physical assault in the emergency department: Rates of violence, perceptions of safety, and attitudes towards security. *Australasian Emergency Nursing Journal, 20*(3), 139–45.

Quadara, A. (2015). Implementing trauma-informed systems of care in health settings: The WITH study. *ANROWS Landscapes State of Knowledge*.

Renker, P., Scribner, S. & Huff, P. (2015). Staff perspectives of violence in the emergency department: Appeals for consequences, collaboration, and consistency. *Work, 51*, 5–18.

SA Health. (2017). *Restraint and Seclusion in Mental Health*. Government of South Australia. Accessed January 2019 at <http://www.sahealth.sa.gov.au/wps/wcm/connect/public+content/sa+health+internet/clinical+resources/clinical+topics/mental+health/restraint+and+seclusion+in+mental+health>.

Schindeler, E. & Reynald, D. M. (2017). What is the evidence? Preventing psychological violence in the workplace. *Aggression and Violent Behavior, 36*, 25–33.

Spencer, S., Stone, T. & McMillan, M. (2010). Violence and aggression in mental health inpatient units: An evaluation of aggression minimisation programs. HNE Handover. *For Nurses and Midwives, 3*, 42–8.

Stone, T. & Francis, L. (2010). What's the bloody law on this? Nurses, swearing, and the law in New South Wales, Australia. *Contemporary Nurse, 34*(2), 248–57.

Stone, T. & McMillan, M. (2012). Warning—this job contains strong language and adult themes: Do nurses require thick skin and broad shoulders to deal with encounters involving swearing? In D. Holmes, T. Rudge & A. Perron (Eds), *(Re)thinking Violence in Health Care Settings: A Critical Approach*. Farnham: Ashgate Publishing.

Victorian Taskforce on Violence in Nursing (2005). *Victorian Taskforce on Violence in Nursing: Final Report*. Nurse Policy Branch, Victorian Government Department of Human Services, Melbourne.

Worksafe. (2009). *Prevention and Management of Aggression in Health Services: A Handbook for Workplaces*. Accessed January 2019 at <https://www.worksafe.qld.gov.au/_data/assets/pdf_file/0004/82822/Prevention_management_health_services.pdf>.

World Health Organization. (2017). *Violence Against Health Workers*. Accessed January 2019 at <http://www.who.int/violence_injury_prevention/violence/workplace/en/>.

Yassi, A. & Hancock, T. (2005). Patient safety–worker safety: Building a culture of safety to improve healthcare worker and patient well-being. *Healthcare Quarterly, 8*, 32–9.

Zhang, L., Stone, T. E. & Zhang, J. (2016). Understanding the rise of Yinao in China: A commentary on the little known phenomenon of healthcare violence. *Nursing and Health Sciences*. doi:10.1111/nhs.12311

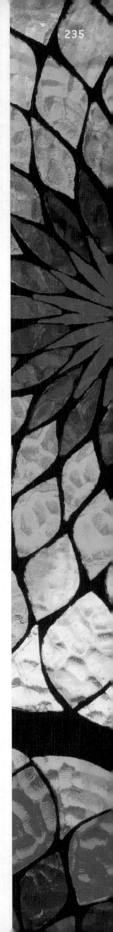

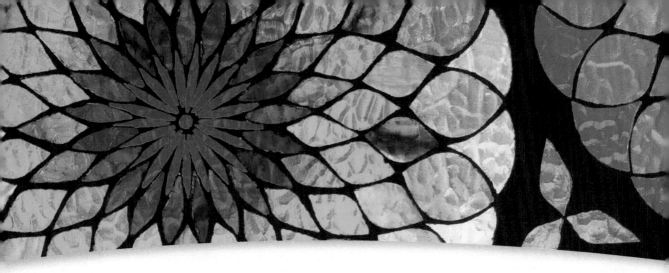

COMMUNICATING ABOUT END-OF-LIFE CARE AND DECISIONS

Lorinda Palmer   Graeme Horton

LEARNING OUTCOMES

Chapter 20 will enable you to:

- consider the range of contexts and situations in which end-of-life healthcare issues need to be discussed with patients, their families or carers and other health professionals

- consider the range of factors and barriers that may influence optimal communication about end-of-life decisions

- identify examples of best practice communication strategies for communicating about end-of-life care

- identify examples of communication behaviours that are likely to be unhelpful or may potentially be harmful when communicating about end-of-life care

- discuss the importance of advance care directives

- reflect on your values, beliefs, emotions and experiences to identify how they could affect your capacity to be professional and therapeutic in situations where end-of-life care options are being discussed and/or decisions are being made.

KEY CONCEPTS

end-of-life care | life-limiting illness | advance directives | advanced care planning | EOL decision making

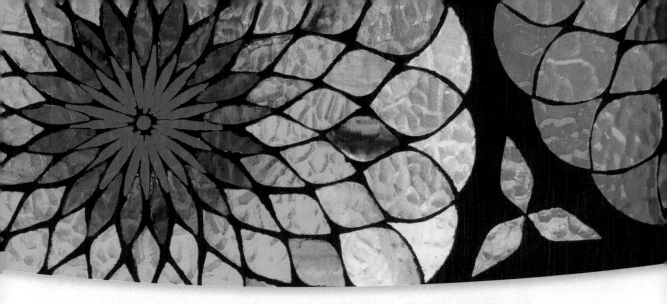

Conversations about uncertain prognosis, death and
dying require compassion, knowledge, experience,
sensitivity and skill on the part of clinicians.

(Australian Commission on Safety and Quality in Health Care, 2017, p. 10).

INTRODUCTION

Quality and safety are major concerns for everyone involved in delivering and receiving end-of-life (EOL) care. Patients and families are acutely vulnerable at such times and the potential for suffering is high. Unfortunately, adverse outcomes and experiences can occur in EOL care situations, particularly loss of dignity or personhood, a sense of abandonment, provision of unwanted or inappropriate treatments (Heyland, Barwich & Pechora, 2013), unmet needs or expectations, and unresolved or poorly resolved disagreements between patients, families and the healthcare team. In recent years, there has been considerable attention given to developing and disseminating models and standards of best practice for quality of EOL care (Shipman et al., 2008).

For some time now, lack of communication and inadequate communication have been identified as critical factors contributing to poor quality of EOL care (Clayton et al., 2007; Heyland et al., 2013). In an interview with *The New York Times*, oncologist, bioethicist and former presidential advisor Dr Ezekiel Emanuel (2013) suggested that the *number one thing* that could be done to improve the quality of EOL care was for *all* healthcare professionals to receive training in how to effectively talk about these issues with patients and families. When you think about it, that is a brutally honest thing for him to say. On the one hand it could be viewed as a sad commentary on the state of the health professions, but on the other hand it offers students a clear signal of one very important way to make a meaningful difference to the quality of people's lives when they are dying.

In Dr Emanuel's statement the word *'all'* is important and its significance should not be overlooked. This is because EOL care happens in a wide variety of contexts and circumstances, despite prevailing perceptions that it is limited to adult (or elderly) patients with diagnoses such as cancer, in locations like hospices. As the evidence shows (and despite their preference to the contrary), more people die in acute-care hospitals than in hospices or their own homes (Tabor et al., 2007). Therefore, capacity for good EOL communication skills are needed by all healthcare professionals in all areas of practice—particularly in areas not usually associated with specialist EOL care, such as acute hospitals, paediatrics and neonatal intensive care, surgical units, adult intensive care, residential aged care, and community care.

Furthermore, EOL care is not just about cancer care. There are many situations and conditions, diagnoses and age groups in which consideration of, and conversations about, life-limiting illnesses become necessary. No matter what your intended area of practice, it is inevitable that you will be involved in caring for patients and families in situations where life-limiting prognoses are involved, and EOL care communication and planning has to be done. Thus, you will need to skilfully engage in therapeutic conversations in order to provide care that it is truly person-centred.

SOMETHING TO THINK ABOUT	Fewer Australians are dying in their own homes than ever before and this trend is growing. 'Many of us have parents that are aging, and if we have the conversation with them about what they would like in the last phase of their life, most would say: "I want to be at home, surrounded by family and friends",' said the Productivity Commission social policy commissioner, Richard Spencer (The World Today, 2017, para. 4–5.). 'But that doesn't happen in Australia, it happens very rarely. Over 70 per cent would like that at the end of life, [but] less than 10 per cent experience that possibility.'

'If a patient is deeply distressed or panicked, we need to be able to acknowledge that. It should be an essential part of our skill set, but we haven't been trained in how to deal with emotions in interviews. If you can do that, you can do almost anything—break bad news, tell about recurrence, or make the transition to palliative care'

Robert Buckman, developer of the SPIKES protocol for breaking bad news (Baile et al., 2000).

Snapshots of critical conversations

The process of planning optimal EOL care must be person-centred and hence be done in genuine partnership with patients and those who most care about and for them. This requires the full range of therapeutic communication skills and attitudes (discussed in Chapter 11), aligned with a clear and deliberate purpose, to develop a deep understanding of the dying person's needs, wishes and values. This is especially crucial in EOL care, because people with a life-limiting illness do not have any time to waste in dealing with the deleterious effects of un-therapeutic interactions with healthcare professionals. The following snapshots provide an illustration of what such un-therapeutic communication might look like, as a basis for ongoing discussion. These snapshots, while by no means exhaustive in scope, give some indication of the potential quality and safety issues inherent in communicating about EOL care.

In Snapshot 1, the nurse conveys how she would deflect a patient's tentative but earnest attempt to start a conversation about their wishes for treatment: communicating, probably unintentionally but nonetheless effectively, the message that such conversations are not really welcome. Unfortunately, the likely outcome of this misguided attempt at humour is that, having once been rebuffed and made to feel as if they were crossing a forbidden line, the patient would be unlikely to attempt to broach the matter again, with anyone. This may also conceivably result in the patient receiving treatments or interventions that they do not want and would otherwise, if given the proper opportunity, have refused.

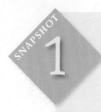

Nurse: I [often] have had patients say, 'Don't do any heroics on me.' They never say resuscitate. They say, 'I don't want any heroics.'

Interviewer: And how do you respond to that?

Nurse: I always say, 'We don't let people die here, because we've got too many forms to fill out.' Making it light.

Interviewer: In other words, telling them that you would resuscitate them?

Nurse: Yes. But I don't think they get the gist of what I say, really. They just say 'Oh, okay', whether they do understand or not.

Source: Schultz (1999), p. 112.

Snapshots 2 and 3 illustrate the deleterious effects caused by the use of certain forms of language, combined with the selection of highly inappropriate times and locations, for the communication of sensitive information. They also reveal a startling lack of awareness on the part of the healthcare professionals of the effect their disclosures were having on their listeners, and how much hurt and harm they were creating, despite their probable helpful intent. When it comes to effective communication, good intentions are clearly not enough.

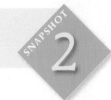

I was given a phone call . . . over the phone by the respiratory physiotherapist to tell me, 'By the way, thought you'd better know, 'cause you're going to get a copy of the letter . . . you're actually end stage now'.

Source: National Health Service (2011a), p. 8.

We had just settled my dad into his new room at the care home. He had motor neurone disease and was in a bad way. Walking down the corridor with my sister, the nurse turned to us and said, 'Of course, when your father dies, you can have a room to stay in here while he is dying.' Other people could hear this comment. This was the first time that anything had been said to us about my father dying. I felt dreadful and panic stricken.

Source: National Health Service (2011b), p. 5.

Snapshot 4 shows how the pain of a personal loss and grief can blindside even the best of communicators. Discussing issues around death and dying are never easy, but what should you do if you become overwhelmed with emotion relating to a personal loss in the midst of a patient-care situation? In this situation, the dietician involved was unprepared for both the patient's revealing disclosure and the effect that it had on her. All she was able to do was to conceal her distress from the patient as best she could, and somehow quickly bring the conversation to an end, presumably without responding to the patient's real and deep need for help, or without making sure that someone else did so.

I was having a bit of a dialogue with three of the four patients in the cubicle. The fourth patient I thought was sleeping . . . He was just lying there flat on his back. I hadn't heard anything from him and didn't know anything about him. He wasn't included in the conversation. Then he spoke. So I went over and chatted with him. Then the tea lady came in asking about morning teas and what not, and he said to me what I thought was 'I just want a cup of tea'. But what he actually said to me was 'I just want to die'. It came sort of not long after my dad's death, so I welled up . . . we had a bit of a brief chat and then I left. I just lost it completely.

Source: Schultz (1999), p. 152.

The final snapshot (Snapshot 5) illustrates how important it is to communicate effectively during the transition from curative to palliative care as, once options for cures are exhausted, healthcare professionals may feel uncomfortable and at a loss about what to offer patients next. They may even be embarrassed at what they perceive to be a tacit admission of failure. If not handled well (as was the case in this snapshot), it can come across to the patient as abandonment or as the clinician being uncaring, even when this was not what was intended. The physician's lack of situational awareness is also apparent here and this had a devastating effect on the patient. Possibly what is most striking about this snapshot is that it was not the actual bad news that was most devastating for the patient but rather the way in which it was delivered and what those implied messages of indifference conveyed to her about her worth as a human being.

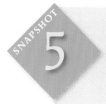

One woman with cancer explained how her doctor told her that she couldn't have the life-saving surgery she'd been hoping for. 'He just told me the news and then left me to go home,' she said. 'I felt devastated. He kept looking at his watch and shuffling in his seat, which made me feel I was an inconvenience to him and he needed to get on with some real work. I was given nothing and left with nothing. I left the hospital not even knowing what way to drive the car. Luckily my husband was with me and we knew we would find a way together.'

Source: National Health Service (2011b), p. 15.

These snapshots reveal just some of the costs for patients and families when healthcare professionals lack expertise in therapeutic communication skills. Studies demonstrate the impacts that both limited and poor communication can have (Thorne, Bultz & Baile, 2005; Heyland et al., 2013). These impacts are wide ranging and include:

- impairing the patient's ability to make the best decisions for their future
- directly increasing the overall costs of care (because patients were more likely to end up having treatments they would otherwise have refused, had they known that refusal was an option)
- psychological impacts such as increased fear and anxiety, feelings of hopelessness, reduced satisfaction with care, loss of trust and reduced quality of life.

Clinician stress and burnout can also be an outcome of poor communication in EOL care contexts. This is due to accumulated feelings of inadequacy arising from being aware of the inadequacy of one's communication skills but not having the opportunity to develop or improve them (Thorne et al., 2005). Read the skiing analogy (Box 20.1) and imagine what it would be like having to ski black diamond runs on a daily basis but without the requisite knowledge, ability or support to do so. While this review was conducted in relation to the costs of poor communication in cancer care, there is no reason to suppose that its findings would not apply to EOL care situations in general. Evidence shows that communication skills training for EOL contexts is both necessary and effective in improving clinicians' knowledge, confidence and skills in this critical area of practice (Brighton, et. al., 2017).

BOX 20.1   Communicating with patients who have life-threatening illnesses

Communicating with patients who have life-threatening illnesses is a critically important skill. Often, after watching an experienced clinician guide a patient through the transition from disease-modifying treatment to end-of-life care, students assume that this expertise comes naturally. Nothing could be further from the truth. In fact, end-of-life communication skills require deliberate intent, practice and reflective work—little of which can be detected by watching a master. An expert skier can make a black diamond run look easy; expert communicators can make difficult conversations look simple.

Source: Back & Arnold (2005), p. 582.

Barriers to critical conversations about end-of-life care

The communication snapshots in the previous section illustrate some of the barriers that can prevent good communication happening in EOL care. It is worth exploring them in some detail, since it is through awareness and understanding that such barriers can eventually be addressed and overcome. Some of the barriers arise from or are related to clinician-specific factors, some are patient or family related, and some are system or organisational level barriers (see Box 20.2). A number of systematic reviews (Hancock et al., 2007; Garland, Bruce & Stajduhar, 2013) have examined the reasons for health professionals' discomfort and avoidance in broaching discussions about EOL care. These have been identified as:

- a lack of specific, specialised training in communication skills
- the stressful nature and emotional impact of such encounters

---

BOX 20.2   Discussions about do-not-resuscitate orders

Over two decades ago, Tulsky, Chesney and Lo (1996) audio-taped 87 patient–physician discussions about do-not-resuscitate orders and advance directives. They found that these conversations were mostly left to the very junior, least-experienced doctors to undertake. On average, the conversations were less than 10 minutes in duration, and the doctors spent three-quarters of that time talking and only one-quarter of the time listening. They also very rarely explored deeper issues such as what was important to the patients, the patients' values, beliefs, fears and apprehensions, or the reasons for the choices the patients made.

The findings of this study stimulated a considerable debate about how to improve the quality of conversations about end-of-life care that is still ongoing today.

- fear of denying the patient hope or other negative effects on the patient
- the uncertainty of the dying trajectory, and how and when to explain that to the patient
- pressures of time or belief that they lacked the time to meet the patient's emotional needs
- requests from the family to refrain from disclosing bad news to the patient
- feelings of inadequacy in not having any further curative options to offer the patient.

It is not just at the clinician level that such barriers can be found. A study by Knauft and colleagues (2005) of COPD patients' perceptions of the barriers to effective EOL care communication found that the most often cited patient-related barrier was, 'I would rather concentrate on staying alive than talk about death'. This finding, albeit from one study, lends some credence to the perception that many healthcare professionals have that most patients have a deep-seated reluctance to talk about issues related to death and dying. Finding ways to broach this topic without causing additional stress to patients and families is clearly an essential element of therapeutic communication for EOL care. Garland et al. (2013) discusses, in the context of patients with heart failure, that there is much variation in the amount of information that patients wish to be given about prognosis and options for end-of-life care. Healthcare professionals must practice person-centred care in finding out how to meet the needs of their patients, which can change over time.

> 'It is possible that hope is derived not from prognostic disclosure itself but rather from the caring relationship in which it occurs' (Mack & Smith, 2012, p. 2716).

The two other most common patient-perceived barriers identified in Knauft et al.'s (2005) study were, 1. being unsure which doctor would be taking care of them if they became very sick; and 2. not knowing what kind of care they would want to receive if and when this happened. The former suggests a lack of clarity about what happens when transitions occur from acute or curative care to palliative care and is a barrier that needs to be systematically and carefully addressed. The latter reveals that there is likely to be a significant problem when patients have little or no knowledge about possible future treatment options and the risks and benefits associated with them. One aspect of end-of-life communication that is often identified as being a problem is the lack of disclosure of prognostic information to patients, and the prevailing myths about the effects that such disclosures may have on them; for example, the belief that truth will destroy hope (Mack & Smith, 2012).

This belief is fairly common and can give rise to situations where relatives are so fearful of a patient's reaction to the news of a poor prognosis that they seek to have this information withheld from the patient. While disclosure of prognostic information may be thought—incorrectly as the evidence shows (Mack & Smith, 2012)—to undermine hope and foster despair, concealment of the truth may also lead to aggressive and futile treatments being pursued and create ethical dilemmas for the healthcare professionals concerned. In those cases, it is important that opportunities are taken to explain the ethical and legal framework within which the professional works. An approach that balances respect for patient autonomy with the preservation of hope would focus on exploring with the patient what and how much information they want to know, based on the knowledge that truth, when carefully and sensitively conveyed, can foster hope and not destroy it (Pergert & Lutzen, 2012).

Misconstrued meanings can also be a barrier to good communication about EOL care and decisions. Sometimes this can be a lack of awareness of body language. This is illustrated in Snapshot 5, where the patient talks about how her doctor looking at his watch and shuffling in his seat affected her, and what she interpreted that to mean. He was probably acutely uncomfortable about conveying bad news and bracing himself for an expected emotional reaction from her—perhaps seeking to deflect what he did not know how to deal with—while she interpreted this as indifference and abandonment. EOL care situations can also be rife with jargon and terminology that is wide open to misinterpretation. Table 20.1 contains a few examples.

Feelings of abandonment, despair, confusion and failure are not what any healthcare professional would want to engender in their patients, so these kinds of stock phrases should not be used. Never say that there is 'no hope' (Workman, 2007). Hope has a spiritual dimension and comes in many guises. People can hope for all kinds of things: to live long enough to see their granddaughter graduate, to be comfortable and pain free, to be at peace, to see a loved one or friend that they have not seen for some time, to name but a few examples.

	Common phrase	Possible patient interpretation
TABLE 20.1 Commonly misconstrued phrases used in end-of-life discussions with patients	'There is nothing more we can do for you.' 'It's time to think about withdrawal of care.'	Abandonment/cessation of all care: 'My doctors/health carers don't want to help me any more' or 'I won't get any more care' or 'I am alone in this struggle'.
	'. . . Do you want us to do everything that we can to keep you alive?'	Confusion: 'If I don't have them do everything, I might not get the best medical care' or 'If I say I don't want everything, perhaps that means I will get nothing' or 'What do they mean by "everything"?'
	'You have failed the treatment (e.g. chemotherapy, radiation) . . .'	Personal failure: 'I'm a bad patient' or 'It's my fault the treatment didn't work.'
	'I think you should consider a hospice . . .'	Despair and hopelessness: 'I must be going to die very soon.'

Source: Adapted from Weiner & Roth (2006), Ngo-Metzger et al. (2008) and Blanclafor (2010).

Techniques and models for good end-of-life care communication

In order to address some of these barriers and to help clinicians to improve their communication skills in EOL situations, a number of different approaches have been developed. One of these is the six-step SPIKES protocol (Baile et al., 2000; de Sousa et al., 2017). While this is a model for breaking bad news, any of its elements could be adapted for use in a range of different contexts and situations. The six elements of this protocol are as follows:

1 **S = Setting up,** preparing for the interaction. This involves considering and planning carefully how you will approach the interaction, and ensuring that provision has been made for adequate time, privacy and having someone there to support the patient if that is what the patient wishes. This means that crucial information should never be blurted out over the phone or in public places like corridors, as happened in Snapshots 2 and 3.

2 **P = Patient's perceptions.** Assess these first. That is, use open-ended questions to assess the patient's and/or family's understanding of their current situation. Don't make assumptions about what and how much they know. If misunderstandings, misconceptions or lack of knowledge are apparent, these can be identified and addressed first.

3 **I = Invitation.** That is, seek and obtain the patient's permission to receive the bad news, and find out first how much of the truth they want to know. Don't make assumptions about what they do or do not want to know. This will also enable you to prepare to respond sensitively to the patient's emotional responses, rather than set up a barrier to deflect them, as happened in Snapshot 6.

4   **K = Knowledge and information.** This should be conveyed clearly and without jargon. It should be tailored to the patient and the situation, and unfolded gently, in stages, not rushed, pausing to give the patient and family time to take in the full import of what is being said to them. Elicit their responses and listen carefully to them. Some authors (Workman, 2007) say that key decision making and plans for future care should not be made at this time, but after the patient has had time to adapt to the situation. Phrases such as the ones in Table 20.1 should not be used, as they make the situation worse.

5   **E = Empathy.** Empathically respond to the patient's emotional responses. This is widely acknowledged to be the most difficult aspect of EOL communication. Know how to respond appropriately when patients express anger, shock or fear, or withdraw into silence. All of these are normal. Use comfort techniques such as touch (if appropriate) and express your sorrow, but be mindful that responding with 'I understand' can be a form of blocking with premature reassurance and is best avoided. Instead, use open-ended questions to explore these feelings rather than closing them off. That is, validate the patient's emotional responses rather than deflecting them or conveying the message that they should be suppressed.

6   **S = Summarise** and plan for the future. The patient and/or their family should not be left (as was the woman in Snapshot 5 and the family in Snapshot 3) feeling despair and as if there is nowhere to go and no hope for the future. This stage should involve clarifying the patient's understanding of the situation, ensuring that the patient is not left feeling distressed or abandoned, working with the patient to create a plan or strategy for the future, and listening for cues as to the patient's response to that strategy (Randen, 2012).

The SPIKES protocol is a way of preparing and engaging in a planned encounter, but sometimes these issues will arise unheralded and catch the healthcare professional unawares, as happened in Snapshots 1 and 4. In these kinds of situations it is a matter of developing a good situational awareness—particularly of one's own vulnerabilities and of 'expecting the unexpected'—and deliberate person-centred ways of responding. When patients raise issues they should not be deflected, made to feel as if they have done something wrong, or be left distressed, with their concerns and fears unattended to. It is up to all health professionals to ensure that they develop 'black diamond run' communication skills so that they can practise effectively in EOL care situations. For further suggestions and discussion on how to develop your EOL communication skills, review the 'Web resources' at the end of the chapter.

> 'It cannot be over emphasised how much trust is necessary for the patient or family to participate in shared decision-making with the clinical team, to participate in potentially noxious treatment, or to decide to withdraw life-extending care. Such trust needs to be earned by the clinician . . . [two ways to do this are to] 1. preserve the dignity of both patient and family 2. comprehensively elicit and treat suffering' [Maguire & Weiner, 2009, p. 165).

The use of interpreters during EOL discussions

The correct and timely use of interpreters is needed for EOL discussions with patients who have limited English proficiency (see also Chapter 17). The effect of not using professional interpreters has been reported as reduced understanding or diagnoses and prognoses during EOL discussions, and worse symptom management during EOL care. Many studies have suggested that it can be useful to use pre-meetings between clinicians and interpreters, to maximise familiarity of the interpreter with terminology to be used during the discussions (Silva et al., 2016).

Transitioning from curative to palliative care

For many patients there will come a point at which the focus moves from stabilisation and remission of illness to palliation and symptom control. This is widely recognised to be a difficult and emotion-laden step, yet in many instances its boundaries may not be clearly marked (Gardner et al., 2011). Factors that may initiate this transition include:

■   the patient's illness deteriorating (which can happen suddenly or unexpectedly) or not having responded to treatment as was anticipated

■   complications of the illness or of the treatment arising

■   the patient no longer being able to tolerate the treatment and its side effects

■   a shift in the patient's priorities and perspective.

'One goal of [end-of-life] conversations is to align patient and clinician views. This doesn't mean, "Get them to think about it our way"' (Centre for Palliative Care Education, n.d.).

This transition may also involve a handover of care from members of one team to that of another. For this reason, everyone involved needs to be sensitive to the patient's potential loss of personal contact with healthcare professionals with whom they have developed a rapport. This is a time when healthcare professionals must communicate with each other as seamlessly as possible, using the skills and practices outlined in the earlier chapters of this book. Some of the barriers to a smooth transition (apart from a lack of interprofessional communication) include uncertainty as to prognosis, as can occur in a relapsing chronic illness, or unrealistic expectations of the success of treatment. It is crucial that team members and/or patients and families are not at cross-purposes, and this will be facilitated by a shared understanding of the patient's condition and current needs.

Failure to recognise the role of family communication in decisions about EOL care can result in delays in accessing care and reduced quality of the experience (Wallace, 2015). Any member of the team can play a valuable role in patient advocacy by cueing the patient, family and other members to salient changes in the patient's symptoms that indicate a palliative approach needs consideration, and how agreement will be reached about how this will unfold (Thompson, McClement & Daenick, 2006). It is important that the perspectives of all involved are included as part of ongoing discussions, and it is crucial that the transition to palliative care be a shift in the focus of care and is not seen as a failure or abandoning of the patient. An ongoing person-centred focus, with exploration of and a response to the patient's needs as they evolve, will help to build the trust needed at this stage of care.

One of the most important reasons this needs to be done well is that, at this stage of illness, patients and families may have a very limited amount of precious time, perhaps only days or hours, in which to be with each other, to make peace and to say their goodbyes. More than anything they need what their healthcarers communicate and how they communicate to help them make these last days or hours the best they can be. This is crucially important, as the story of the final hours of Dr Gruzenski, described in Chapter 3, illustrates most effectively.

Advance care directives: the most critical of conversations

In the story below, John's wife and daughter are in a situation where they must make decisions about EOL care for John because he is no longer able to do so for himself. This is an increasingly common situation that families find themselves in. Sometimes there are warning signs that such a situation may be impending, but there may not be, such as in the case of acute illness or severe injury. Whether expected or unexpected, there is still profound shock. The person affected by the impaired consciousness or cognition may be a father, a mother, a daughter or a son, be young or old, chronically ill or previously well. The relatives must then decide what to do, to somehow come to know what is in the best interests of their loved one, to take account of what the loved one would have wanted and make decisions, all at an incredibly difficult time while overwhelmed (as were John's wife and daughter) by their own shock and grief. And in many cases the relatives have no clear idea as to what the patient's wishes would have been for such a situation, because they have never before discussed the possibility.

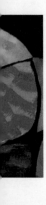

JOHN'S STORY

'"What on earth are we doing here?" I asked myself. It was 11 o'clock on a bleak winter Sunday morning in 2001. In the middle of my ward round as the intensive care specialist on duty at a large tertiary hospital, I was standing at the bedside of one of my patients, John, a 76-year-old man with advanced cancer. He had been admitted to the intensive care unit two nights earlier after becoming dangerously short of breath.

'One of my junior doctors had been called to see John at 3 am and had quickly established that he had pneumonia. It was clear John would die if we didn't do something to help him breathe. So the young doctor did what he was trained to do; he gave John some medication to drift off to sleep, carefully fed a breathing tube down his

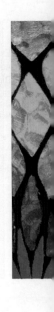

throat into his trachea and, with the help of the intensive care nurses, connected the tube to a mechanical ventilator to push oxygen into his sick lungs.

'Now, two days later, John was not getting better. In fact, he was slowly but surely getting worse: he needed more oxygen, the ventilator was working harder to push air into his lungs, his white cell count—crucial for fighting infection—was alarmingly low, and his blood circulation and kidneys were shutting down. His body, ravaged by the cancer that would certainly kill him, was also worn out by the chemotherapy he had been receiving.

'His oncologist was keen for "everything" to be done but the consensus among the ICU doctors and nurses was that John had no hope—he was going to die, despite our best efforts. So there I was, contemplating how we wound up in this situation, when I turned around to see John's wife and daughter standing in the doorway quietly watching me. "We're not winning the battle," I told them gently. It was like someone had finally given them permission to speak. Both women, with tears in their eyes, then told me that John would never have wanted any of this. But no one had bothered to ask.'

Source: William Silvester, 'A Good Death', The Age, 20 March 2011. This work has been licensed by Copyright Agency Limited (CAL). Except as permitted by the Copyright Act, you must not re-use this work without the permission of the copyright owner or CAL.

An Advance Care Directive (ACD) is a way to avoid this predicament. It is the means by which a person's EOL wishes are discussed and documented in case, at some time in the future, they are not able to participate in such a discussion. While this may be prompted by the development of a potentially life-threatening illness, or a change in circumstances such as moving to a residential aged-care facility, there is no need to wait for such events before an ACD is made. Patients and their families being clear on EOL wishes can make a very difficult situation easier for everyone (Mayer, 2011).

ACDs can take many forms, but there are a number of different templates available to provide guidance on what needs to be addressed. An excerpt of an ACD that is currently being used in New South Wales, Australia, is shown in Figure 20.1 It asks the patient to indicate the level of care they would prefer at a defined level of illness and/or impairment. ACD forms may also provide guidance for relatives on what the patient's wishes would be if death were imminent and the relative was out of the country. At least two persons responsible are asked to acknowledge and sign the ACD, which helps to ensure that issues that may be contentious, or actions that might be difficult for people to implement, can be discussed. In this way, support and appropriate advice can be obtained when there is likely to be time for it to be calmly and rationally considered.

There are limitations to this method of planning, including that patients find it difficult to make decisions in situations about which they have no experience or limited knowledge. They may struggle to decide based on not knowing how they would feel closer to the time. Other barriers include conflicting family dynamics and resistance to discussing EOL issues (Sampson et al., 2011). In some studies, ACDs have been shown to lead to greater satisfaction about EOL care and to reduce the amount of ineffective care that is delivered in the final days and hours of life (Mayer, 2011). One systematic review has found that written ACDs were related to an increased frequency of care outside of hospital that is focused on patient comfort rather than prolonging life, but there was no clear association with satisfaction of care or reduction in the symptom burden (Brinkman-Stoppelenburg, Rietjens & van der Heide, 2014). When advanced care planning included additional measures such as professional development of staff, and specifically trained facilitators to help patients and families reflect on their goals, there was greater compliance with patients' wishes and satisfaction with care.

The NSW Ambulance's Authorised Adult Palliative Care Plan is an example of good communication across different health professions that ensures a patient's wishes are respected in terms of location of care and where they wish to be transported after death, if this was to occur in an ambulance (https://www.slhd.nsw.gov.au/btf/pdfs/Amb/Adult_Palliative_Care_Plan.pdf).

'In terms of what makes a good death, the opportunity for life review, coming to a sense of peace and "taking care of unfinished business" is second only to pain relief and symptom management' (Steinhouser et al., 2000).

FIGURE 20.1
Excerpt from an
Advance Care
Directive

Source: NSW Health Ministry of Health. (2017).
*Making an Advance
Care Directive Package.*
Retrieved from <http://
www.health.nsw.gov.
au/patients/acp/Pages/
default.aspx>.

Section C: End-of-Life Treatment Instructions

In this section you are asked to give specific instructions for future healthcare and medical treatment decisions you do or don't want, if you are terminally ill.

Definitions of terms used in this section

- **Irreversible:** unable to be turned around—there is no possibility that the patient will recover.
- **Terminal phase of an irreversible illness:** the person is dying and the process is irreversible. Life expectancy is usually considered to be just a few days.
- **Permanent unconsciousness (coma):** when brain damage is so severe that there is little or no possibility that the patient will regain consciousness.
- **Persistent vegetative state:** severe and irreversible brain damage, but vital functions of the body continue (e.g. heart beat and breathing).
- **Palliative care:** compassionate care for people with a terminal illness, focused on prevention of suffering and relief from pain and other distressing symptoms.
- **Life-sustaining measures:** treatments (medical procedures) that replace or support an essential bodily function (e.g. cardiopulmonary resuscitation, artificial ventilation, artificial nutrition and hydration, dialysis).
- **Your treating medical practitioner:** this may not always be your usual doctor if you become extremely ill. It will be the medical practitioner (doctor) who is providing your treatment at the time your Directive will be used to inform your care and treatment.

5. **If in the opinion of my treating medical practitioner I am:**

   - in the terminal phase of an irreversible illness or condition; or
   - in a persistent vegetative state; or
   - permanently unconscious; or
   - so seriously ill or injured that I am unlikely to recover to the extent that I can survive without the continued use of life-sustaining measures

   Or I am in any of the following states that I consider to be an unacceptable quality of life, and the state is permanent *(tick all that apply):*

   - ❑ Not being able to recognise people important to me
   - ❑ Not being able to communicate
   - ❑ Not being able to eat by mouth
   - ❑ Not having control of my bladder and bowels
   - ❑ Other (please specify)

   Then, I request that everyone responsible for my care *(tick all that apply):*

   - ❑ Provide treatment for my comfort and dignity *only*, with particular emphasis on pain relief
   - ❑ Withhold or withdraw treatment that might obstruct my natural dying
   - ❑ Do not perform surgery on me, unless required for my comfort and dignity as part of my palliative care

6(a). **Do you have any other particular wishes about your healthcare or medical treatment that have not already been covered in this form?** *(for example, you may wish to write something like: 'I value life, but not under all conditions. I consider dignity and quality of life to be more important than mere existence' or 'I request that I be given sufficient medication to control my pain, even if this hastens my death'.)*

   - ❑ Yes—*complete 6(b)*
   - ❑ No

6(b). **Record your wishes here.**

Terminally ill patients, especially those experiencing intolerable pain or other symptoms, or fearing needless suffering at the end of their lives, may inquire about hastening their death. This might involve questions about withdrawing food and fluids and also about euthanasia or doctor-assisted suicide. The options that are open to patients and health professionals within a certain jurisdiction will depend on that jurisdiction's relevant laws; details of these are beyond the scope of this chapter.

Such an inquiry, however, must lead to an examination of the patient's mental health and decision-making capacity, and the adequacy of symptom management, employing whatever expertise is necessary. Healthcare professionals have a duty to honour the competent patient's request to cease treatment, but this must be in the context of having provided education about the options available, as well as support, empathy and appropriate reference to any ACD that the patient may have.

Healthcare professionals working in intensive care units and some other clinical areas may be involved in the care of patients identified as potential organ donors, or field questions from patients and their relatives about this possibility eventuating. A patient may be identified as a potential organ donor if they suffer 'brain death', defined as 'irreversible coma and irreversible loss of brain stem reflex responses and respiratory centre function', or 'cessation of cerebral perfusion' (Australian and New Zealand Intensive Care Society, 2010). Conversations about organ donation require specialised expertise and multidisciplinary input. A number of principles provide guidance and may help to ease the discomfort that many health practitioners feel in discussing this topic. Review the 'Further reading' list at the end of the chapter for more information about this topic.

A family's satisfaction with the process has been found to be higher when a grave prognosis and brain death are discussed before and separately from the offer of organ donation (Williams et al., 2003). The family should be given adequate time to contemplate the concept of brain death and this requires coordination between the different hospital teams. Despite there generally being a significant shortage of donors compared with those on transplant waiting lists, at no point must the patient or the relatives feel that the needs of the donor patient are being subordinated to the needs of any potential recipient. When this is handled appropriately, many families have found that having their relative become an organ donor has helped them to deal with the death and bereavement.

> **SOMETHING TO THINK ABOUT**

Conclusion

This chapter has explored some of the issues pertaining to EOL communication. There are many challenges to everyone involved in delivering and receiving EOL care. These include difficulty in predicting the prognosis of a patient's condition, healthcare professionals being unsure of how much information a patient is wanting, and patients themselves wanting varying amounts of information at different times, perhaps influenced by their understanding, their culture, and family and interpersonal dynamics.

The most important message is that good communication skills are essential to understanding the patient's perspective and providing person-centred care at the end of life. Person-centred care will help to ensure that patients and families receive the best quality care that is consistent with the patient's values and goals, and that patients are not subjected to preventable distress, pain or unwanted treatments in their final weeks, days and hours. This may enable them to use that time to attain peace and 'take care of unfinished business'. Both individual healthcare professionals and organisations need to work to improve EOL communication through the use of interpersonal techniques, such as the SPIKES protocol, and effective and appropriate use of ACDs.

> 'Advanced care planning can be seen as the larger process of communicating about end-of-life care—eliciting and understanding the patient's values and goals so as to ensure that they receive care that is congruent with those values' (Centre for Palliative Care Education, n.d.).

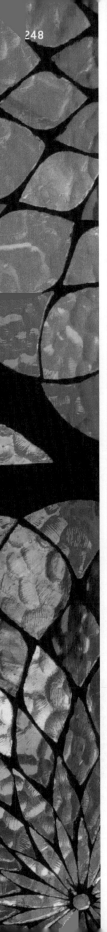

Critical thinking activities

1. Why do many people find discussing EOL issues difficult?
2. Do you think this reluctance varies between different cultures and generations, or is it a more universal phenomenon?
3. What would you personally find most difficult about discussing EOL care with patients and their families?
4. Refer back to Snapshot 1. If you overheard this conversation between a patient and a nurse, what would you do?
5. Refer back to the findings of Tulsky, Chesney & Lo (2006) (Box 20.2). In your clinical encounters, do you talk more than listen? What could you do about this?
6. How might a patient's intellectual disability or incapacity influence how you would communicate about EOL care?
7. What specific education strategies do you think you need in order to improve your communication skills when discussing EOL care issues with (a) patients and families and (b) other members of the healthcare team?

Teaching and assessment activities

1. Use the following questions as either the focus of a class debate or a discussion:
   a. With an ageing population dispersed across wide geographical areas in many developed countries, should more use be made of information and communication technologies in order for end-of-life care to be consistent with a patient's wishes?
   b. Could technologies such as mobile applications of video and web-based conferencing, personal electronic health records, and telemonitoring contribute to improved communication between patients and healthcare professionals, as well as better-informed patient decisions (Ostherr et al., 2016).
2. Use the six-step SPIKES protocol (see page 240) to structure classroom discussions about end-of-life care scenarios/ cases studies that you currently use in your teaching, or those illustrated in the videos found at these links:

   Example A
   <https://webconf.acu.edu.au/p28thuqaqua/>

   Example B
   <https://webconf.acu.edu.au/p5y3lv8u2yz/>

Further reading

American Society of Clinical Oncology (2008). Communication. What do patients want and need? *Journal of Oncology Practice*, 4(5), 249–53. doi: 10.1200/JOP.0856501

Back, A., Arnold, R. & Tulsky, J. (2009). *Mastering Communication with Seriously Ill Patients: Balancing Honesty with Empathy and Hope.* Cambridge, UK: Cambridge University Press.

Gaw, A., Doherty, S., Hungerford, P., May, J. (2012) When death is imminent: Documenting end-of-life decisions. *Australian Family Physician*, 41(80), 614–17.

Long, C. (2011). Ten best practices to enhance culturally competent communication in palliative care. *Journal of Pediatric Hematology/Oncology*, 33(Suppl 2), S136–S139.

Perrin, K. (2010). Communicating with seriously ill and dying patients, their families, and their health care providers. In M.L. Matzo & D.W. Sherman (Eds), *Palliative Care Nursing: Quality Care to the End of Life* (pp. 169–85). New York: Springer Publishing Company.

Web resources
Palliative care curriculum for undergraduates (PCC4U): This resource is a project by several leading Australian universities, funded by the Australian government Department of Health and Ageing. It contains a range of resources and learning modules designed to improve palliative care practice and is relevant for students and practitioners of all health disciplines. All the resources on the site are excellent, but *Module 2: Communicating with people with life-limiting illnesses* is particularly relevant to the material in this chapter.
<www.pcc4u.org/index.php/learning-modules/core-modules/2-communication>

Finding the words. National end-of-life care program: This resource is a workbook developed by the National Health Service (NHS) as part of a wider project to improve communication skills training for staff involved in the delivery of end-of-life care in the United Kingdom.
<http://endoflifecareambitions.org.uk/wp-content/uploads/2016/09/finding_the_words_workbook_web_1.pdf >

Communication at the end-of-life: This resource is a podcast on a site sponsored by Palliative Care Victoria. The podcast is by Associate Professor Brian Le who is a medical oncologist and palliative care specialist.
<www.pallcarevic.asn.au/library-media/communication-at-the-end-of-life/>

National Consensus Statement: Essential elements for safe and high-quality end-of-life care: This resource has been developed to help ensure that the end-of-life health care that people receive is appropriate and minimises the distress and grief associated with death and dying for both the individual, and their family, friends and carers. The principles that underpin systems and structures for delivering safe and high-quality end-of-life care are described.
<https://www.safetyandquality.gov.au/our-work/end-of-life-care-in-acute-hospitals/>

Let's talk about dying TED Talk: Dr Peter Saul is a Senior Intensive Care specialist in the adult and pediatric ICU at John Hunter Hospital, and Director of Intensive Care at Newcastle Private Hospital in Australia. Over the past 35 years Peter has been intimately involved in the dying process for over 4000 patients. He is passionate about improving the ways we die.
<https://www.ted.com/speakers/peter_saul>

References

Australian Commission on Safety and Quality in Health Care. (2017). *National Safety and Quality Health Service Standards* (2nd edn). Sydney, Australia: ACSQHC.

Australian and New Zealand Intensive Care Society. (2010). *The ANZICS Statement on Death and Organ Donation* (Edition 3.1). Melbourne: ANZICS.

Back, A. & Arnold, R. (2005). Dealing with conflict in caring for the seriously ill: 'It was just out of the question'. *Journal of the American Medical Association, 293*(11), 1374–81. doi:10.1001/jama.293.11.1374

Baile, W., Buckman, R., Lenzi, R., Glober, G., Beale, E. & Kedekla, A. (2000). SPIKES—A six-step protocol for delivering bad news: Application to the patient with cancer. *The Oncologist, 5*(4), 302–11.

Blanclafor, S. (2010). *Communication and End-of-life Decision-making: A Resource Guide for Physicians.* Accessed February 2013 at <www.ctendoflifecare.org/documents/CommunicationandEndofLifeDecisionMaking_000.pdf>.

Brighton, L. J., Selman, L. E., Gough, N., Nadicksbernd, J. J., Bristowe, K., Millington-Sanders, C. & Koffman, J. (2017). 'Difficult conversations': Evaluation of multiprofessional training. *BMJ Supportive and Palliative Care.* doi: 10.1136/bmjspcare-2017-001447

Brinkman-Stoppelenburg, A., Rietjens, J. A. & van der Heide, A. (2014). The effects of advance care planning on end-of-life care: A systematic review. *Palliative Medicine, 28*(8), 1000–25.

Centre for Palliative Care Education (n.d.). *Communicating with Patients and Families.* Accessed February 2013 at <depts.washington.edu/pallcare/training/curriculum_pdfs/CommunicationModule.pdf>.

Clayton, J., Hancock, K., Butow, P., Tattersall, M. & Currow, D. (2007). Clinical practice guidelines for communicating prognosis and end-of-life issues with adults in the advanced stages of a life-limiting illness, and their caregivers. *Medical Journal of Australia, 186*(12), S76–S108.

De Sousa, F. H., Valenti, V. E., Hamaji, M. P., de Sousa, C. A. P., Garner, D. M. & Sawada, N. O. (2017). The use of SPIKES protocol in cancer: An integrative review. *International Archives of Medicine, 10*(54). doi: 10.3823/2324

Emanuel, E. (2013). Better, if not cheaper care. *The New York Times.* Accessed at <https://opinionator.blogs.nytimes.com/2013/01/03/better-if-not-cheaper-care/>.

Gardner, C., Ingleton, C., Gott, M. & Ryan, T. (2011). Exploring the transition for curative care to palliative care: A systematic review of the literature. *BMJ Supportive and Palliative Care, 1*, 56–63. doi: 10.1136/bmjspcare-2010-000001

Garland, E. L., Bruce, A. & Stajduhar, K. (2013). Exposing barriers to end-of-life communication in heart failure: An integrative review. *Canadian Journal of Cardiovascular Nursing, 2*(1), 12–8.

Hancock, K., Clayton, J., Parker, S., der Wal, S., Butow, P., Carrick, S., . . . Tattersall, M. (2007). Truth-telling in discussing prognosis in advanced life-limiting illnesses: A systematic review. *Palliative Medicine, 21*(6), 507–17.

Heyland, D. K., Barwich, D. & Pichora, D. (2013). Failure to engage hospitalized elderly patients and their families in advance care planning. *JAMA Internal Medicine, 173*(9), 778–87. doi: 10.1001/jamainternmed.2013.180

Knauft, E., Nielsen, E., Engelberg, R., Patrick, D. & Curtis, J. (2005). Barriers and facilitators to end-of-life care communication for patients with COPD. *Chest, 127*(6), 2188–96.

Mack, J. & Smith, T. (2012). Reasons why physicians do not have discussions about poor prognosis, why it matters and what can be improved. *Journal of Clinical Oncology, 30*(22), 2715–17.

Maguire, P. & Weiner, J. (2009). Communication with terminally ill patients and their families. In H.M. Chochinov & W.S Breitbart (Eds). *Handbook of Psychiatry in Palliative Medicine* (2nd edn). London: Oxford University Press.

Mayer, D. (2011). Advanced care planning conversations. *Clinical Journal of Oncology Nursing, 15*(2), 117–18.

National Health Service. (2011a). *Finding the Words. National End of Life Care Programme.* Leicester: Crown Copyright. Accessed at <www.endoflifecare.nhs.uk/assets/downloads/ Finding_the_words_Workbook_web.pdf>.

National Health Service. (2011b). *Talking about End of Life Care: Right Conversations, Right People, Right Time. National End of Life Care Programme.* Leicester: Crown Copyright. Accessed at <https://www.bl.uk/collection-items/talking-about-end-of-life-care-right-conversations-right-people-right-time >.

Ngo-Metzger, Q., August, K., Srinivasan, M., Liao, S. & Meyskens, F. (2008). End-of-life care: Guidelines for patient-centred communication. *American Family Physician, 77*(2), 167–74.

Pergert, P. & Lutzen, K. (2012). Balancing truth-telling in the preservation of hope: A relational ethics approach. *Nursing Ethics, 19*(1), 21–9.

Ostherr, K., Killoran, P., Shegog, R. & Bruera, E. (2016). Death in the digital age: A systematic review of information and communication technologies in end-of-life care. *Journal of Palliative Medicine, 19*(4), 408–20. doi: 10.1089/jpm.2015.0341

Randen, H. (2012). *Best Practice for End-of-Life (EOL) Communication* [Presentation]. Accessed February 2013 at <www.stratishealth.org/documents/BestPrac_EOLComm_20120322.pdf>.

Sampson, E., Jones, L., Thune-Boyle. I., Kukkastenvehmas, R., King, M., Leurent, B., . . . Blanchard, M. R. (2011). Palliative assessment and advance care planning in severe dementia: An exploratory randomised controlled trial of a complex intervention. *Palliative Medicine, 25*, 197–209.

Schultz, L. (1999). Patterns of avoidance and involvement: Nurses' experiences of cardio-pulmonary resuscitation (CPR) decisions. Master's thesis, University of Newcastle, NSW.

Shipman, C., Gysels, M., White, P., Worth, A., Murray, S., Barclay, S., Forrest, S., Shepherd, J., Dale, J. & Dewar, S. et al. (2008). Improving generalised end of life care: National

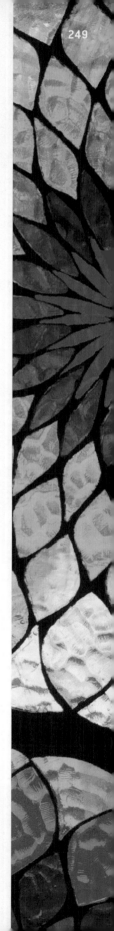

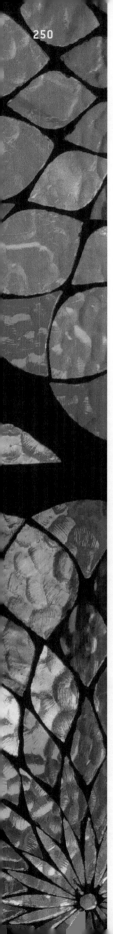

consultation with practitioners, commissioners, academics and service user groups. *British Medical Journal*, *337*, a1720. doi: 10.1136.bmj.a1720

Silva, M. D., Genoff, M., Zaballa, A., Jewell, S., Staber, S., Gany, F. M. & Diamond, L. C. (2016). Interpreting at the end of life: A systematic review of the impact of interpreters on the delivery of palliative care services to cancer patients with Limited English Proficiency. *Journal of Pain & Symptom Management*, *51*(3), 569–80.

Steinhouser, K. E., Christiakis, N. A., Clipp, E. C., McNeilly, M., McIntyre, L. & Tulsky, J. A. (2000). Factors considered important at the end of life by patients, family, physicians, and other care providers. *Journal of the American Medical Association*, *284*(19), 2476–82.

Tabor, B., Tracey, E., Glare, P. & Roder, D. (2007). *Place of Death of People with Cancer in NSW*. Sydney: Cancer Institute NSW.

The World Today (2017, 2 June). Where do you want to die? Most Australians say at home but end life in hospital. *ABC News*. Accessed January 2019 at <http://www.abc.net.au/news/2017-06-02/where-do-you-want-to-die-at-home-or-hospital/8584318>.

Thompson, G., McClement, S. & Daeninck, P. (2006). 'Changing lanes': Facilitating the transition from curative to palliative care. *Journal of Palliative Care, 22*(2), 91–8.

Thorne, S., Bultz, B. & Baile, W. (2005). Is there a cost to poor communication in cancer care? A critical review of the literature. *Psycho-oncology, 14*, 875–84.

Tulsky, J., Chesney, M. & Lo, B. (1996). See one, do one, teach one? House staff experience discussing do-not-resuscitate orders. *Archives of Internal Medicine, 156*(12), 1285–9.

Wallace, C.L. (2015). Family communication and decision making at the end of life: A literature review. *Palliative & Supportive Care, 13*(3), 815–25.

Weiner, J. & Roth, J. (2006). Avoiding iatrogenic harm to patient and family while discussing goal of care near the end-of-life. *Journal of Palliative Medicine, 9*(2), 451–63.

Williams, M., Lipsett, P., Rushton, C., Grochowski, E., Brekowitz, I., Mann, . . . Genel, M. (2003). The physician's role in discussing organ donation with families. *Critical Care Medicine, 31*(5), 1568–73.

Workman, S. (2007). A communication model for encouraging optimal care at the end of life for hospitalized patients. *Quarterly Journal of Medicine, 100*, 791–7.

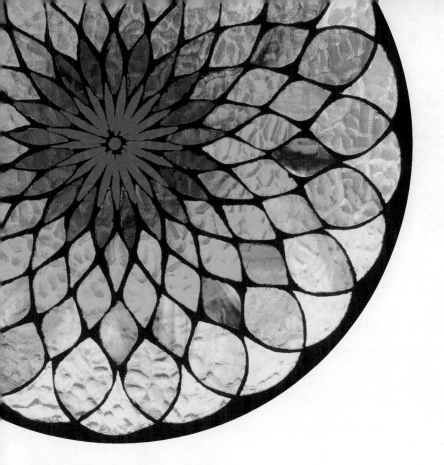

SECTION 4
Workforce issues and patient safety

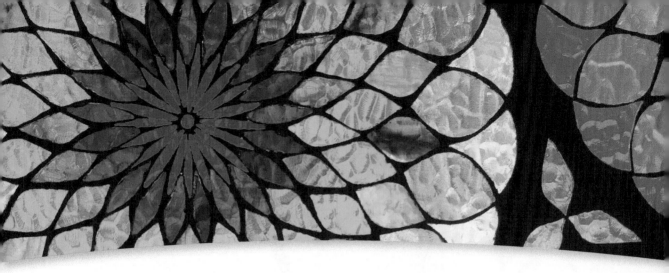

CHAPTER 21

WHEN WHISTLE-BLOWING SEEMS LIKE THE ONLY OPTION

Toni Hoffman AM   Kerry Reid-Searl

LEARNING OUTCOMES

Chapter 21 will enable you to:

- explain why whistle-blowing should be considered a 'last resort' for addressing healthcare concerns

- define the concept of moral distress, what causes it and how it can lead to whistle-blowing

- discuss the responsibilities of leaders in responding to errors and complaints

- explain the potential consequences of whistle-blowing for the individual, the organisation and for patients

- discuss how to proactively speak up to address errors and complaints in healthcare.

KEY CONCEPTS

moral distress | whistle-blowing | ethical leadership | proactive voice | patient advocacy

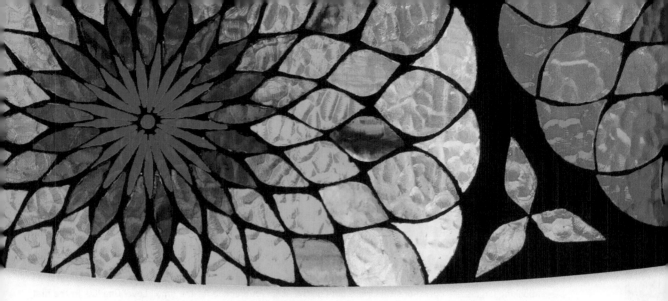

> All that is needed for evil to prosper is for
> people of good will to do nothing
>
> (Edmund Burke)

INTRODUCTION

One of the most important roles of healthcare professionals is patient advocacy. Speaking up for patients can be as simple as requesting an increase in analgesia or as difficult as advocating for end-of-life care. While being a healthcare professional is a privilege, at some stage you are likely to encounter morally distressing situations that challenge your personal and professional values, and where you will be called upon to respond assertively and empathically. This chapter has been written to help you negotiate these types of situations.

Have you ever been witness to a situation where a healthcare professionals' action or inaction resulted in permanent injury to a patient or even death? What if you decided to speak up about your concerns but no one listened or did anything? Or what if you were afraid to speak up but felt torn between your responsibility to your professional code of ethics ('to do no harm') and an organisational culture that seemed to not care?

This chapter will explore these types of situations and help you to understand the moral distress that healthcare professionals sometimes experience when confronted with poor practice. It will also provide examples of some of the challenges associated with speaking out, and outline strategies that can prevent the need for whistle-blowing. Importantly, this chapter will explain how to communicate effectively and use organisational structures to create leadership accountability and enhance the chance of being heard. Finally, this chapter will guide you on how to access the support you need when 'speaking out'.

At all levels of a healthcare organisation you hear people say that we need a better healthcare system. But what they sometimes fail to understand is that, in order to provide better healthcare for our patients, we first need to become better people.

TONI'S STORY

My name is Toni Hoffman and I would like to share my story of speaking up about patient safety and, ultimately, finding myself in a situation where my only option was to cross the line and blow the whistle.

In 2006, I was the recipient of a Local Hero Award in the Australian of the Year Honours list for showing courage and ethical conviction as a patient safety advocate at Bundaberg Base Hospital in Queensland; and in 2007, I was made a Member of the Order of Australia. However, these accolades came at significant professional, ethical and personal cost.

My story began in 2003. I was the nurse unit manager (NUM) of the intensive care unit (ICU) at Bundaberg Hospital. I found myself embroiled in a morally challenging situation following the appointment of a new surgeon—Jayant Patel—in April of that year.

Dr Patel was initially recruited as a general surgeon from the United States on a 457 visa. Within two weeks he was appointed to Director of Surgery. Early in his tenure, nurses and doctors expressed concerns when he started booking large-scale operations that were outside the scope of practice for the small Level One ICU. In the first eighteen months of his employment, Dr Patel completed seven oesophagectomies, and all but one patient died.

Concern about Dr Patel continued to grow. There were multiple cases of wound dehiscence, high infection rates, and in the renal unit a patient died after Dr Patel inserted a vascath. The renal unit consequently decided to outsource their vascath insertions to a private hospital to circumvent Dr Patel's surgery.

For two years I made complaints about the complications and deaths of ICU patients that Dr Patel had been responsible for and that were causing significant moral distress to myself and the other nurses. However, I felt powerless and intimidated because I was in a situation where my actions were being judged against those of Dr Patel—after all, he was the Director of Surgery. The Director of Nursing dismissed my concerns, stating that I had poor communication skills and that this was simply a personality clash. She gave me a book titled *How to Deal with Difficult People*. I approached the NUMs of the surgical ward and operating theatres to support me but, whilst acknowledging the issues, both declined to support my complaints.

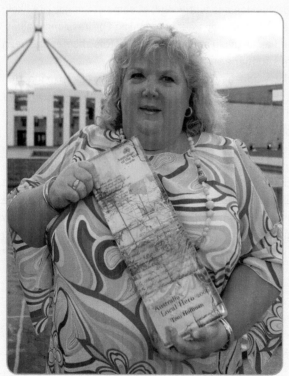

Source: © National Australia Day Council 2006.

Major incidents continued, including Dr Patel trying to perform a pericardiocentesis and abrading the patient's left ventricle. Finally, a major complaint was made to the District Manager and the Director of Nursing. However, other factors were at play. Bundaberg Base Hospital was 'on budget' for the first time in many years. Dr Patel had formed friendships and developed allegiances with a number of powerful people. He had also notified the local Jehovah's Witness Church that he was an expert in bloodless surgery and advised them to call for him if a member of their congregation was admitted to hospital. Dr Patel had stopped the normal reporting mechanisms of good clinical governance; he ran his own morbidity and mortality meetings, and no one challenged him. None of the deaths were reported to the coroner.

After doing an audit of ICU deaths and identifying that fourteen of Dr Patel's patients had died from preventable complications, I contacted the union. After they met with the Director of Nursing I was informed that the hospital planned to discredit me. I felt

For further information about my experience of being a patient advocate, access:

<http://cqu.kanopy.com/video/australian-story-deaths-door>

threatened, isolated, vulnerable and frightened. I could not believe that my colleagues and senior staff did not share my concerns and I didn't know what to do or where to turn.

Soon after, a young boy was admitted following a motorbike accident and Dr Patel operated on him. Dr Patel had told the mother she was lucky he was there, that he had been a trauma surgeon in the United States and the young boy was in safe hands. However, he tied off the wrong blood vessel and the boy lost his leg.

I was suffering terrible moral distress and I decided I had to escalate my concerns, so I called the coroner, the police and a journalist called Hedley Thomas. Eventually, after having contacted twelve different people, without result, I decided to 'cross the line' and 'blow the whistle'. I went to the local member of parliament and gave him a copy of the letter of complaint that I had previously given to the hospital executive. The letter was later tabled in parliament. The media then took up the cause and patients started to come forward, detailing their experiences with Dr Patel. The media called for a royal commission and pressured the government to have an investigation.

Dr Patel had been trying to negotiate a five-year contract at Bundaberg Hospital but, instead, decided to leave the country. When Hedley Thomas 'Googled' Dr Patel, he identified that Dr Patel had a long history (dating back to 1982) of deceitful behaviour and gross incompetence. He had even been forced to relinquish his licence to practice medicine in Oregon, USA. To avoid further prosecution for gross and repeated acts of incompetence, his licence had a notation on it saying 'see stipulated order' that neither the recruiters nor the Medical Board of Bundaberg Hospital admitted to having seen.

After this, there were two royal commissions, an extradition, two trials and two appeals. Dr Patel was initially convicted of three counts of manslaughter and one of grievous bodily harm. I spent two days in the witness box at the royal commission. I was afraid but I wanted to tell my story. The Queensland Nurses Union provided a lawyer to be with me and I was grateful for that support.

Dr Patel spent two years in jail and then his appeal was upheld on a technicality and a new trial was ordered. However, the DPP decided not to pursue him any further and he returned to the US.

For more than two years, I had consistently raised concerns about the patient safety record of Dr Patel. My ethical values would not allow me to turn my back on the problem. During this time, I was vilified and belittled; but I was eventually recognised for having 'placed my concern for patients and their families above my own well-being' (Commonwealth of Australia, 2006) and because my 'courage and persistence . . . in the face of inaction and even resistance, brought the scandalous conduct of Dr Patel to light' (Queensland Government, 2005, p. 1).

The message I would like to communicate to people working in healthcare is to maintain your objectivity, do not allow allegiances and friendships to cloud your thinking or interfere with robust clinical governance. An effective and ethical healthcare organisation does not need whistle-blowers. I, like many others before me, found whistle-blowing to be extremely damaging, both personally and professionally. However, healthcare professionals are charged with the moral responsibility for patient advocacy and . . . ***patient safety is everyone's business***.

My reflection . . .

As I reflect on how the above events have shaped my life, my hope is that other healthcare professionals will learn from my experiences and consider whistle-blowing only as a last resort. I hope my story helps others respond early and assertively when they identify clinical issues of concern, and that it helps them to be courageous and resilient when they have to negotiate complex ethical situations within healthcare organisations that are not always responsive. Integrity, transparency, accountability and responsibility are paramount as patient safety and peoples' lives depend upon a culture of safety that involves healthcare professionals and organisations working together to prevent patient harm, and learning from errors if they do occur.

Whistle-blowing: a last resort

Whistle-blowing occurs when an individual (or a group of employees) crosses organisational boundaries to take their concerns to the general public and/or regulatory bodies (Jackson et al., 2010b). The term originates from the United Kingdom whereby a whistle was blown to halt play and indicate an error or foul during a sports game (Bolsin et al., 2011). Therefore, a whistle-blower is someone who creates enough 'noise' to stop an organisation or person 'in their tracks' and force them to evaluate the situation.

There have been several high profile whistle-blowing incidents in Australian healthcare contexts where employees sought external support because internal attempts had failed or they believed management would not change its practices (McIlwraith & Madden, 2014). Whistle-blowing can be potentially damaging to healthcare organisations because it can highlight breaches to patient safety, leadership cover-ups, fraud (e.g. falsifying patient progress notes), or circumstances of bullying and harassment (Johnstone, 2016).

The ramifications of whistle-blowing are evident for many years afterwards and the associated professional and personal costs are significant. As well as damage to the reputation of the healthcare organisation, there may also be personal costs to the whistle-blower, such as career damage, loss of income and moral distress (Jackson et al., 2010b).

Robust and transparent clinical governance can reduce or even prevent the need for whistle-blowing. When there are clinical checks and balances, the issues associated with professional competence can be identified and addressed before they put patient safety at risk. Quality processes must include transparent morbidity and mortality meetings, the reporting of unexpected deaths to the coroner, meaningful unit-specific key performance indicators, and monitoring and reporting of infection rates, adverse patient outcomes and other relevant clinical data (Daly et al., 2014).

Following the recommendations from the Davies report in 2005, all healthcare-related deaths must be referred to the coroner who will decide whether an inquest is necessary (Dunbar, Reddy & May, 2011). Healthcare facilities must also have mechanisms to identify and address adverse outcomes. Healthcare professionals must be diligent in maintaining, protecting and observing these processes. Any attempt to change or discontinue these quality processes must be vigorously opposed. One of the reasons that Dr Patel was able to operate at Bundaberg Base Hospital for two years without detection was due to his own actions of interfering with the operating theatre reporting system, running his own morbidity and mortality meetings without robust examination of errors, and failure to report any of the 87 deaths that occurred during that period to the coroner (Queensland Government, 2005).

It is hoped that, by using the following information to gain insights into the dynamics that feed whistle-blowing, coupled with the strategies on how to best use your organisation's internal reporting processes, you will never need to 'blow the whistle'.

Dr Steve Bolsin's story (Box 21.1) highlights the ramifications of whistle-blowing for the whistle-blowers.

BOX 21.1   Dr Steve Bolsin's story

Dr Steve Bolsin was a consultant anaesthetist who worked at the Bristol Royal Infirmary in the UK in the early 1990s. During this time, he noticed several clinical anomalies in the post-operative care of paediatric patients by some of the cardiothoracic surgeons, with operations taking longer than usual and very high post-operative mortality rates. For six years, Dr Bolsin collected data and tried to improve service delivery. Although the mortality rate dropped from 30 per cent to less than 5 per cent, he faced ongoing confrontation and conflict with the surgeons. Dr Bolsin found it morally and ethically impossible to continue to anaesthetise children knowing that the post-operative mortality was so high. Because the hospital refused to investigate the two main surgeons, Dr Bolsin eventually decided to speak to the media. This action led to a wide-ranging government inquiry and a number of subsequent changes to the NHS in relation to cardiovascular services. However, Dr Bolsin's actions came at great personal and professional cost. Unable to find work in the United Kingdom following the whistle-blowing event, he had no choice but to relocate overseas with his family. He continues to work tirelessly to improve patient safety, transparency and clinical governance.

Source: Bolsin, S., Pal, R., Wilmshurst, P., & Pena, M. (2011). Whistleblowing and patient safety: the patient's or the profession's interests at stake? *Journal of the Royal Society of Medicine, 104*(7), 278–82. doi: 10.1258/jrsm.2011.110034

What creates moral distress?

Moral distress is the stress associated with the moral dimensions of practice (Varcoe et al., 2012) and can be due to inconsistency between one's values and one's actions (Cleary, 2014). It can occur when a healthcare professional is forced to act in a way that is destructive to the organisation and themselves. It can be heightened when what is happening is potentially destructive to patients and their families. Patients and families may have already suffered through an adverse outcome, complicated post-operative course or even worse, a death, only to find out that, in fact, malpractice has occurred, policies and procedures have been ignored and clinical governance has been compromised.

Both organisational constraints and personal insecurities can lead to an ethical dilemma, whereby the professional knows the right thing to do but is either prevented from acting or chooses not to act. Healthcare professionals may recognise the vulnerability of patients and care about their wellbeing, yet be reticent to speak up and fearful of conflict (Cleary, 2014). If, at the same time, they are committed to the values of their professional codes of ethics, this is likely to result in moral distress (Jackson et al., 2010a).

Signs of moral distress include fear, frustration, grief, anxiety, rage and powerlessness. Healthcare professionals may find that they are unable to sleep and worry continuously, thinking about a patient's situation and what they should have done but didn't do. They might feel anxious about going to work and become more isolated when at work. This poses a problem with patient care because distancing, avoiding or withdrawing from patients compromises their safety further and creates a vicious cycle (Wallis, 2015). See Box 21.2 for examples of morally distressing situations.

Qualitative research into moral distress (Jackson et al., 2010a), provides valuable insights into healthcare professionals' experiences—for example, doctors who describe themselves as 'powerless and resigned' and who state that 'my opinion means nothing', and nurses who complain that 'things are getting missed and we are spending less and less time with patients' (Varcoe et al., 2012, p. 492). Patient safety relies on 'healthcare professionals being able to speak up about matters of concern and adopting an advocacy stance for patients' (Harrison, 2003, p. 12). Healthy relationships and open dialogue between staff from all levels of the organisation are required, not just for better work satisfaction but to also foster patient safety (Malmeister, 2009).

BOX 21.2   Examples of morally distressing situations

- Witnessing unnecessary suffering due to cost cutting—for example, ambulance stations were running out of S8 drugs and patients suffering needless pain: '. . . the staff basically have to get patients to bite down on an old piece of leather or something' (NSW Parliament Legislative Council, 2008).

- Witnessing how the need for beds in a busy healthcare facility transcended concerns for patient safety—for example, a patient being disconnected from a ventilator before brain-death testing was completed because the doctor wanted a bed for a post-operative patient (Queensland Government, 2005).

- Witnessing inaccuracy in medical documentation—for example, the lack of veracity in documentation and verbal communication with patients and their relatives (Queensland Government, 2005).

- Negative judgments about patients and/or their families—for example, a newly employed social worker in a long-care unit for people with disabilities attempts to discuss resident abuse but is told by staff, 'You're new here, this is how we have to treat them otherwise they don't listen' (Greene & Latting, 2004, p. 219).

- Workload/overload—for example, a surgical nurse carrying a patient load of 10 patients: five post-op, two with epidurals and two on morphine needing observations every 15 minutes (Varcoe et al., 2012, p. 491).

REFLECTIVE THINKING QUESTIONS

- Have you experienced a situation in healthcare that caused you moral distress?
- What action, if any, did you take in the situation?
- What effect, if any, do you think your moral distress had on patient care?

Leadership responsibility

Speak your mind even if your voice shakes (Maggie Kuhn)

It is important for you as a healthcare professional to understand the environment in which you work, so that you can navigate and influence it for the better. The culture of a healthcare organisation is a reflection of all parts of the organisation and not just the leadership; it is also you and me. It is defined by shared assumptions, values, behaviours and frames of reference. A healthcare culture is especially complex due to the different educational and socialisation experiences of healthcare professionals and other staff, the different cultures that each healthcare profession stems from, and the fact that, historically, management has tended to focus primarily on the health of the organisation as opposed to individual patients (Leape et al., 2009). It is no wonder a conflict of values can occur.

Another important dimension to recognise is that healthcare systems and organisations are highly bureaucratic. They have hierarchical cultures (a ranking of seniority) and are rigid in structure and processes. This often limits flexibility, open-mindedness and creativity (Kassin, Fein & Markus, 2008). Decision-making flows downwards, while employees are expected to communicate upwards to those perceived as being better at making decisions, namely management (Scheeder, 2006). Unfortunately, this structure is not conducive to supporting a patient-safety culture and allowing healthcare professionals to deliver high-quality care. In such a structure, decision making can be slow and cumbersome, and those in positions of authority may lack the knowledge of those working at the patients' bedside and fail to engage healthcare professionals as part of effective change management. Competing priorities are often in conflict between management and clinicians, and sometimes the difference between right and wrong gets lost in the detail.

Ethical and empathic leadership is imperative. Studies highlight that employees' perception of the moral integrity of top management affects their own behaviour and performance (Daly, Speedy & Jackson, 2017). Senior management has greater authority to make decisions in four main areas: economic, legal, social responsibility and ethical. This means that senior managers have a significant responsibility to do the right thing morally and demonstrate the values and expected standards of patient care. When a healthcare system loses its conscience, bureaucratic structures, paternalistic control (abuse of power) and cover-ups can take precedence over transparency, accountability and dialogue (Ray, 2006). These increase the chance of there being a need for whistle-blowing.

The way an organisation's leadership responds to healthcare professionals who speak up provides valuable insights into how the organisation does business. Are the leaders of the organisation willing to meet with staff and take appropriate actions or do they ignore staff? Do managers actively listen to what staff say and act on it to promote quality improvement, or do they resist and deflect the concerns raised? (cited in Groves, Meisenbach & Scott-Cawiezell, 2011).

> A healthcare organisation that is not providing an adequate support system for staff to meet their professional responsibilities is not ethically responsive (Daly et al., 2017).

SOMETHING TO THINK ABOUT

Research conducted by Reid-Searl, Moxham, Walker and Happell (2010a) identified that more than 30 per cent of third-year nursing students admitted to having administered medications without supervision and had consequently made an error. Further, none of these students reported their errors for fear of retribution. This was described as 'Suck Up and Shut Up' behaviour (Reid-Searl et al., 2010). Healthcare professionals have an ethical responsibility to model behaviours that promote safety, and when an error occurs there is a need to speak up and take responsibility.

BOX 21.3　　　　Why do people conform?

Social psychology research has revealed a number of theories and explanations for conformity.

- **Informational influence**: People conform because they want to make correct judgments and assume that when others agree on something they must be right (Sherif et al., 1961).

- **Normative influence**: This leads people to conform because they fear the consequences of appearing deviant (Schacter [1951], cited in Kassin et al., 2008).

- **Primitive course of evolution**: Throughout history people have needed each other in order to flourish (MacDonald & Leary, 2005), so people conform when social pressure is intense as they may be insecure about how to behave.

Consequences of whistle-blowing

When a healthcare organisation has lost its moral conscience, it often views the actions of whistle-blowers as an act of disloyalty or a betrayal of trust. In these situations, leaders can fail to understand that the healthcare professional is indeed loyal—to their professional standards and patients (Johnstone, 2016). Further, the whistle-blower can be judged to lack the ability to work within a team, can be seen as a troublemaker, and their revelations may be viewed as vexatious. The source of the 'leak' is considered more threatening than the context of the accusations and can lead to negative consequences for the whistle-blower (Firtko & Jackson, 2005; Davis & Konishi, 2007). This difference in perception is often difficult to comprehend and shocking to the healthcare professional.

A study by Jackson et al. (2010a) revealed that whistle-blowing had a profound and overwhelming effect on working relationships. Participants spoke of colleagues excluding and bullying them or 'closing rank'; for example, doctors ignoring nursing input into patient care after nurses had blown the whistle about a medical colleague.

Acts of retribution and ostracism are often used to intimidate whistle-blowers, such as altering rosters to reduce employee income and make shiftwork difficult, refusing annual leave, and moving staff to hospital areas that are challenging to work in (Attree, 2007). Indeed, what began as a well-intended course of action can rapidly become extremely stressful. This is not unlike the moral distress that led to the act of whistle-blowing in the first place. In the end, the healthcare professional may be left with three options:

1　Leave the organisation.
2　Speak up.
3　Remain silent (see Box 21.4).

BOX 21.4　　　　A note on remaining silent

Remaining silent is not the easiest way out. It can be harder to live with the moral distress felt by remaining silent than actually facing the challenges of speaking up. However, healthcare professionals can sometimes rationalise their reticence to speak up. For example, in the Dr Patel case, nurses cited financial reasons (such as fear of being fired or demoted when they were the main breadwinner) and international doctors feared they may lose their visa and their position (because of the power wielded by Dr Patel) (Thomas, 2007).

Awareness is key

Recognising choice and making a change for the better first requires awareness. So far, this chapter has discussed external whistle-blowing, which is a last resort. The next part of the chapter will focus on ways that healthcare professionals can speak up about patient safety and be heard. The literature on whistle-blowing sometimes refers to this as internal whistle-blowing; however, we would like to reframe this as a 'concerned healthcare professional doing the right thing'.

A proactive voice

It takes courage to speak up, but it is necessary if change is to be enacted that, in turn, solves healthcare problems (Johnstone, 2016). Having a clear and persistent message, an awareness of organisational communication channels, and effective utilisation of resources are essential. Communicating your concerns can increase the safety and wellbeing of your patients, uphold your code of ethics, improve morale, maintain goodwill, and avoid legal and regulatory infringements (McIlwraith & Madden, 2014).

To help improve your chances of being heard, we have outlined a four-point cycle for the process of speaking up (see Figure 21.1). Such preparation and formality will not always be necessary; however, if your organisation bears some of the characteristics previously mentioned, then this process may help. The nature of your dilemma will also determine the initial route you take; for example, a clinical incident on shift would require completion of an incident report, while repeated staff shortages could require a letter to your immediate manager.

FIGURE 21.1
The process for having your voice heard

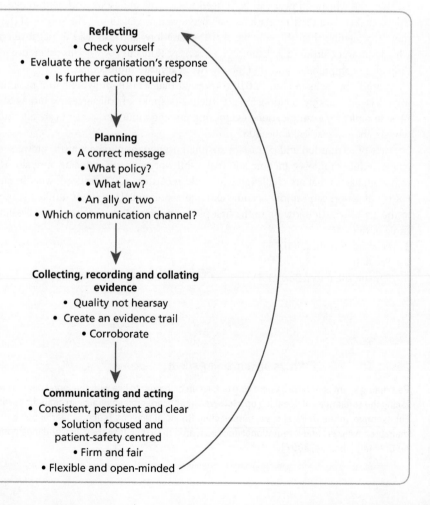

Reflecting
- Check yourself
- Evaluate the organisation's response
- Is further action required?

Planning
- A correct message
- What policy?
- What law?
- An ally or two
- Which communication channel?

Collecting, recording and collating evidence
- Quality not hearsay
- Create an evidence trail
- Corroborate

Communicating and acting
- Consistent, persistent and clear
- Solution focused and patient-safety centred
- Firm and fair
- Flexible and open-minded

© Kim Elkovich

1. Reflecting

Speaking up regarding concerns and influencing change requires careful consideration. The recipient of your well-meaning communication could respond favourably, or you could be embarking on an arduous journey, so make sure you are doing this for the right reasons. Ask yourself:

- What evidence do I have that patients or staff are at risk of harm? For example: Is the infection rate outside of the national average? Is the mortality rate for this particular surgery higher than average? Is there a stark increase in adverse patient outcomes, sentinel events or incident reports?

- Am I motivated by justified anger, based on the here-and-now situation that I am experiencing, or am I simply seeking revenge or being vexatious?

- Can I live with being silent?

- Will I be upholding the standards of my profession?

- Am I being true to myself? (adapted from Jensen, 1987; Martin, 1999)

2. Planning

- Define your concern(s) clearly. Your message needs to highlight the interaction between patient risk, your professional requirements and values, and the organisation's responsibility to deliver safe and effective patient care. Use words and phrases from policy, professional and workplace codes of ethics and resources. Be consistent and ensure you are presenting a correct and coherent position.

- Social psychology suggests that, for a minority group to have influence, the group needs to persistently express the same view (Carsten et al., 2008). Whether it is your first letter or your tenth meeting (now with the CEO), the fact that your concern has not altered shows that you have conviction and that there may be something in what you are saying (Siggall, Mucchi-Faina & Mosso, 2006). It also indicates that you are unlikely to yield when the majority may feel pressured to seek a compromise.

- Who do you approach first? If you are comfortable doing so, speak first to the person(s) directly involved; otherwise, your immediate manager is best. If the response isn't favourable or the problem is more systemic, the chain of command will need to be used. This means sequentially taking your concerns to the various levels of the hierarchy until you are heard (see your organisation's grievance policy). Following this process demonstrates professionalism, respect for the organisation, and a positive regard for each individual in the chain (Greene & Latting, 2004).

- Having one or more allies is beneficial. It is far more difficult to stand alone than to be part of a small minority (Kassin et al., 2008). Seek support laterally from your interprofessional team. If your concern pertains to patient safety and delivering quality outcomes, doctors, nurses and allied health professionals may be involved. Speak up and create solutions together.

- Using policy is a way you can introduce accountability. Before you act, identify the key policies and precedents relevant to your cause. If you lodge a grievance and the policy clearly outlines that the recipient must reply to you in writing within seven days, and this does not happen, document this breach. Then escalate your grievance to the next level of the process, outlining what has occurred. This forms a trail of evidence.

- Be aware of the law. In Australia, there is no federal legislation designed to specifically protect whistle-blowers; however, some states and territories do have a Whistle Blower Act. Check whether your employer has a whistle-blower or public disclosure policy. Does it protect you from any retaliatory actions after the lodgment of your complaint? Federal and state legislation can also offer protection for whistle-blowers.

  If you are finding that the response of your organisation is less than appreciative, it may be wise to meet with an industrial relations/employment solicitor. This person will listen to your story and read your policies, inform you of your rights, the evidence you need to highlight any breach, and legal avenues available to you.

If you are a member of a union, speak with someone from the union about your concerns and discuss what you are planning to do. It helps to be in contact with your representative early so that if the situation escalates, he or she is familiar with your case. However, in some cases health unions may limit their involvement because of a conflict of interest, as senior managers are often union members too (Skiveness & Trygstad, 2010).

3. Collecting, recording and collating evidence

■ Having quality evidence is imperative. Always ask yourself, 'Would this hold up in a court of law?' The notion of hearsay (that is, my word against yours) will not. Evidence includes witnesses (patients, visitors or staff) who have seen or heard first-hand what occurred and are willing to provide a statement if needed, and documentary evidence that provides a supportive account. Examples include letters, progress notes, minutes of meetings that contain conversations, emails, patient reports, audits, ward findings, or diarising shift requirements (to highlight overload, for example) (Martin, 1999). If you consider that veracity is an issue, photocopy documents to keep until after the investigation is over. You can de-identify the patients but remember to keep a copy of your documentation offsite as your access to your place of work may be limited.

■ As healthcare professionals, we are bound by confidentiality and privacy laws; however, for the purposes of whistle-blowing you may be protected for copying records. Why would we suggest this? Because it is not unusual during investigations for evidence and documents to go missing and/or be altered. At the bare minimum, prior to lodging any concerns (especially if you decide to lodge a complaint with external regulatory bodies) ensure that some of your trusted colleagues have sighted the documents. This is called 'corroborative observation' (NSW Health, 2011).

■ Keep a chronology of events and details as a record of evidence. It prevents confusion, allows you to see where your complaint or concern is at, and provides a trail and an index of evidence for future reference. For example:

> 16th April 2018. I spoke with the senior resident . . .
>
> 23rd May 2018. I forwarded a letter to the Nurse Unit Manager on ward 3 . . .
>
> 26th May 2018. I received a letter from HR. It stated . . .

■ Keep copies of emails in a diary so you have a chronological record of events. As the investigation of complaints can take months and sometimes years you cannot rely on memory to support your claims.

4. Communicating and acting

■ How you present yourself and articulate your message is everything. Take the time to draft a letter and have someone check it. Ensure that its purpose is primarily to protect the patient and that your reasoning is clear and rational. Be objective in your documentation and factual. If you are meeting a manager or others in person, prepare and rehearse what you would like to say (McIlwraith & Madden, 2014). Anticipate any objections the manager may have and prepare responses/solutions that address them. It is easy to fall into the trap of dichotomous thinking: expecting each party to choose one way over another as opposed to creating a solution together. The problem with this is that by the time a staff member has decided to take action they may have suffered a degree of moral distress and could be feeling very vulnerable. It is normal in these types of situations for the person to feel conflicted, unsure and to even doubt their own thoughts.

■ Active listening is an important skill to use. Try to understand the views of the other person or people. Hear what the others are saying and paraphrase or restate their words to validate them and ensure a common understanding (Birks, Davis & Chapman, 2015).

- Your attitude needs to be viewed as fair and positive. This is about a genuine desire to correct the problem. Explain to the other party that it is because you care about patients and the organisation that you are speaking up. Keep the emotion out of it and focus on the task you are there to perform.

- A balance is required for influence. On the one hand, you need to be even-tempered but strong, persistent and unwavering in support of your position. However, once you have been heard, stay flexible and open-minded to work on an agreed solution (Kassin et al., 2008).

- If your concerns are acknowledged and plans are made to resolve the situation, thank those involved for their professionalism and understanding.

Evaluating and reflecting

At this point, a response may or may not have been received. If it is a good outcome, you have fulfilled your professional and ethical obligations. If not, this is the time to once again reflect and decide on your next step. Remember to try and exhaust all internal channels before voicing your concerns outside of the organisation. Be mindful of talking to friends or any people outside of the organisation as they may not maintain confidentiality.

A healthy organisation

Healthcare organisations often have policies to support speaking up; however, effective communication channels are needed for dialogue, renewal and creating solutions. The characteristics of an effective leader include humility, empathy and a willingness to listen. Leaders believe they listen as much as they talk, but research has shown that they actually do 80 per cent of the talking when interacting with others (Birks et al., 2015). During meetings, leaders need to step back from taking a strong stand early in a group discussion and allow for open debate (Kassin et al., 2008).

Effective leadership encourages a culture of healthy criticism without fear of retribution. The 'no blame' culture of patient safety has promoted this. Effective leaders self-reflect and own their weaknesses (Stanley, 2011). They keep the focus on delivering safe and effective patient care as well as addressing conflicting organisational needs. They are accessible and the pathways to addressing issues are clearly communicated and understood by employees. Unfortunately, it is rarely within healthy organisations that clinical issues arise requiring whistle-blowing, rather it is in dysfunctional workplaces, where there is a multitude of complex contributing factors. Budgetary issues, alliances and co-dependencies as well as unethical behaviours create the conditions that may lead to whistle-blowing (Dunbar, Reddy & May, 2011).

There needs to be no compromise on organisational values and having an in-house ethics committee often assists. There needs to be a safe recourse for employees when they believe that the moral distress they are experiencing is irreconcilable, such as an internal ombudsman, a hotline or a trusted person in the organisation who has the autonomy to follow through on issues (Lachman, 2008). The option of remaining anonymous until organisational trust is regained must also be considered.

When internal efforts fail

When internal efforts fail, a number of external options are available, including hospital boards, regulatory agencies, complaints organisations (see Chapter 4), health advocacy groups, politicians and the media. The cycle of communication for external whistle-blowing is no different from internal mechanisms: reflection, careful planning, having quality evidence, and communicating clearly is important. Remember that communication should be objective, factual and consistent.

The option of remaining anonymous when lodging complaints depends on the individual agency. The NSW Health Care Complaints Commission suggests that healthcare professionals identify themselves as part of the investigation. Considerable evidence is needed to prove that your employment would be at stake before they allow anonymity. It is believed that the transparency adds credibility to the whistle-blower's case, but it does leave the individual exposed. However, the Aged Care Complaints

Scheme accepts anonymous complaints. Weighing up the options and risks is vital. We recommend phoning the appropriate agency to seek advice on this issue before proceeding.

Letters and email correspondence to government ministers, and visits to your local member of parliament (MP) can be beneficial. Although an advisor usually makes the initial response, it may be useful to your case to have a ministerial letter sent to a regulatory body investigating your complaint to let the body know that the minister is aware and watching.

Politicians are interested in serious matters that are important to public safety. Sometimes you have to seek the attention of government ministers for others to take notice or accept that the source is valid. That is where the media can play an important role. In an ethical society, public organisations should operate from a place of transparency. Healthcare organisations should not be afraid of this transparency. The public knows that mistakes occur and they recognise that healthcare organisations should operate from a basis of continual growth and quality improvement. This is one of the reasons open disclosure has been so effective (see Chapter 8). As long as the organisation is truthful with the public, the patients and their relatives will generally accept that errors do occur, and as long as they can see that procedures have been instigated to prevent reoccurrence they will be (mostly) satisfied (Johnstone, 2016).

The media can be a useful ally and a fairly safe option, as journalists will protect their sources. In the Bundaberg Hospital case of Dr Patel, both the local MP and a journalist became powerful allies for Toni Hoffman. Media attention can be damaging to the reputation of highly bureaucratic organisations, especially if the complaint involves professional negligence and cover-ups (Scheeder, 2006); this can provide a useful negotiating platform.

Conclusion

Speaking up and being a patient advocate is like stepping into the unknown. It takes courage, determination, commitment and an empathic stance. The unfortunate reality is that decisions and outcomes are reliant on the objectivity, professionalism and goodwill of others within healthcare systems that are often cumbersome, hierarchical and far from perfect. Many healthcare problems have existed for decades, so resolving issues may take considerable time. But remember, by speaking up you are planting a seed that, along with the courage and knowledge of others to come, may grow into a new cultural norm.

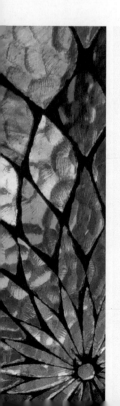

Critical thinking activities

Mr Brown was a 44-year-old man who returned from theatre following an oesophagectomy. He had chronic kidney disease as well as a number of other co-morbidities. Mr Brown had no recordable blood pressure for the last twenty minutes of his surgery and was maintained on adrenaline and dopamine. He was unresponsive to pain and his pupils were fixed and dilated. However, the surgeon documented that the patient was 'stable'. The nurses, who knew the family well from previous admissions, told them about the seriousness of Mr Brown's condition. The surgeon was furious with the nursing staff for telling the family the truth. Mr Brown died five days later having not regained consciousness (Queensland Government, 2005).

1   What is the ethical dilemma in this scenario?
2   What would your professional and ethical codes expect you to do in this situation?
3   In this type of situation, would you remain silent or speak up?
4   If you did decide to speak up, to whom would you take your concerns?
5   What would your message be and how would you frame it?

Teaching and assessment activities

1   The following activity can be presented as a classroom discussion or an assessment item:
    Imagine that you were one of the registered nurses working with Toni Hoffman at Bundaberg Base Hospital in 2003.
    a.   What advice would you have given Toni?
    b.   How would you have responded if Toni asked for your support in challenging and reporting the unsafe care being provided by Dr Patel?

c.   How would you have felt about 'crossing the line' and becoming a whistle blower?

d.   What could you have done to prevent the need for whistle-blowing?

e.   In what ways do you think the National Safety and Quality Health Service Standards (Australian Commission of Safety and Quality in Health Care [ACSQHC], 2017) could have been used by Toni to address the situation she encountered, and how might use of the Standards have changed the outcome?

f.   What have you learnt from Toni's story that will inform your own practice?

2   This activity can be used as a written assignment or for classroom discussion:

You have commenced your graduate year in a busy emergency ward. You have become increasingly aware of the poor communication skills of one of the senior nurses. For example, his clinical handovers to junior staff are very brief, his documentation is often unclear and inaccurate, and he sometime falsifies vital signs. However, the senior nurse has worked in the unit for more than 20 years and is very well regarded.

On one shift, when you make initial attempts to question the meaning of what the nurse has written in a patient chart, he responds aggressively, saying, '*Who the hell are you to question my practice? Come back when you have as much experience as I have.*' A week later you are called into the manager's office and told that a complaint has been lodged about your 'poor attitude' and 'lack of respect for senior nursing staff'. You feel isolated, unsupported and alone. You are concerned about what will be written in your clinical appraisal and whether it will impact your future employment at the hospital.

With reference to the a four-point cycle for speaking up (Figure 21.1) and the National Safety and Quality Health Service Standards (ACSQHC, 2017), describe how you would address this situation, both professionally and ethically.

Further reading

Ahern, K. & McDonald, S. (2002). The beliefs of nurses who were involved in a whistle blowing event. *Journal of Advanced Nursing, 38*(3), 303–9.

Goldie, J., Schwartz, L., McConnachie, A. & Morrison, J. (2003). Students' attitudes and potential behavior with regard to whistle blowing as they pass through a modern medical curriculum. *Medical Education, 37*, 368–75.

Philipsen, N. & Soeken, D. (2011). Preparing to blow the whistle: A survival guide for nurses. *The Journal for Nurse Practitioners, 7*(9), 740–746. Accessed January 2019 at: <http://whistleblowing.us/2011/10/preparing-to-blow-the-whistle-a-survival-guide-for-nurses/>

Web resources

AHPRA Public Interest Disclosure (Whistleblower) Policy
<https://www.ahpra.gov.au/about-ahpra/complaints/whistleblower-policy.aspx>

Australian Nursing and Midwifery Federation: Whistleblowing
<http://anmf.org.au/documents/policies/P_Whistleblowing.pdf>

Whistleblowers Australia

References

Attree, M. (2007). Factors influencing nurses' decisions to raise concerns about care quality. *Journal of Nursing Management, 15*, 392–402.

Birks, M., Davis, J. & Chapman, Y. B. (2015). *Professional and Therapeutic Communication*. Melbourne, Australia: Oxford University Press.

Bolsin, S., Pal, R., Wilmshurst, P. & Pena, M. (2011). Whistleblowing and patient safety: The patient's or the profession's interests at stake? *Journal of the Royal Society of Medicine, 104*(7), 278–82. doi: 10.1258/jrsm.2011.110034

Carsten, K., De Dreu, B., Nijstad, A., Baas, M. & Bechtoldt, M. (2008). The creating force of minority dissent: A motivated information processing perspective. *Social Influence, 3*(4), 267–85.

Cleary, S. (2014). *Nurse Whistleblowers in Australian Hospitals: A Critical Case Study*. Melbourne, Australia: Deakin University.

Commonwealth of Australia (2006). *Honour Roll*. Accessed January 2019 at <https://www.australianoftheyear.org.au/honour-roll/?view=landing&year=2006>.

Daly, J., Speedy, S. & Jackson, D. (2017). *Contexts of Nursing* (5th edn). Sydney, Australia: Elsevier.

Daly, J., Jackson, D., Mannix, J., Davidson, P. M. & Hutchinson, M. (2014). The importance of clinical leadership in the hospital setting. *Journal of Healthcare Leadership, 6*, 75–83.

Davies, G. (2005). *Report/Queensland Public Hospitals Commission of Inquiry*. Brisbane: Queensland Public Hospitals Commission of Inquiry.

Davis, A. & Konishi, E. (2007). Whistleblowing in Japan. *Nursing Ethics, 4*(2), 194–201.

Dunbar, J. Reddy, P. & May, S. (2011). *Deadly Healthcare*. Brisbane, Australia Australian Academic Press.

Firtko, A. & Jackson, D. (2005). Do the ends justify the means? Nursing and the dilemma of whistleblowing. *Australian Journal of Advanced Nursing, 23*(1), 51–6.

Greene, A. & Latting, J. (2004). Whistle-blowing as a form of advocacy: Guidelines for the practitioner and organization. *Social Work, 49*(2), 219.

Groves, P., Meisenbach, R. & Scott-Cawiezell, J. (2011). Keeping patients safe in healthcare organizations: A structuration theory of safety culture. *Journal of Advanced Nursing, 67*(8), 1846–55.

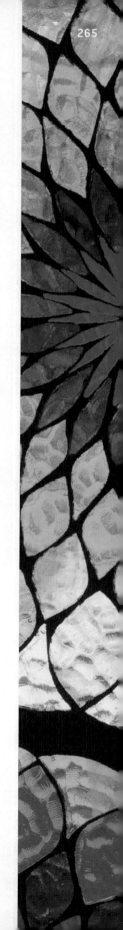

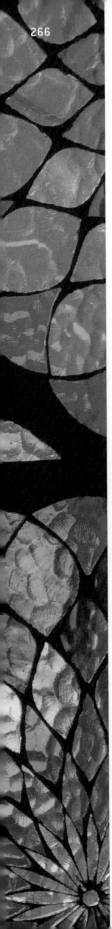

Harrison, S. (2003). Speak up . . . if you dare. *Nursing Standard, 17*(18), 12–13.

Jackson, D., Peters, K., Andrew, S., Edenborough, M., Halcomb, E., Luck, L. & Wilkes, L. (2010a). Trial and retribution: A qualitative study of whistleblowing and workplace relationships in nursing. *Contemporary Nurse, 36*(1-2), 34–44.

Jackson, D., Peters, K., Andrew, S., Edenborough, M., Halcomb, E., Luck, L., . . . Wilkes, L. (2010b). Understanding whistleblowing: Qualitative insights from nurse whistleblowers. *Journal of Advanced Nursing, 66*(10), 2194–201.

Jensen, J. (1987). Ethical tension points in whistleblowing. *Journal of Business Ethics, 6*, 321–8.

Johnstone, M. J. (2016). *Bioethics: A Nursing Perspective* (6th edn). Sydney, Australia: Elsevier.

Kassin, S., Fein, S. & Markus, H. (2008). *Social Psychology* (7th edn). Belmont, CA: Wadsworth/Cengage Learning.

Lachman, V. (2008). Whistleblowing: Role of organizational culture in prevention and management. *MEDSURG Nursing, 17*(4), 265–7.

Leape, L., Berwick, D., Clancy, C., Conway, J., Gluck, P., Guest, J. . . . Lucian Leape Institute at the National Patient Safety Foundation. (2009). Transforming healthcare: A safety imperative. *Qual Saf Health Care, 18*(6), 424–8.

MacDonald, G. & Leary, M. (2005). Why does social exclusion hurt? The relationship between social and physical pain. *Psychological Bulletin, 131*, 202–23.

Malmeister, L. (2009). Best practices in perinatal nursing. Promoting positive team interactions and behaviours. *Journal of Perinatal and Neonatal Nursing, 23*(1), 8.

Martin, B. (1999). *The Whistleblower's Handbook: How to Be an Effective Resister*. Sydney: Envirobook.

McIlwraith, J. & Madden, B. (2014). *Healthcare and the Law* (6th edn). Sydney, Australia: Thomson Reuters.

NSW Health (2011). Public Interest Disclosures [policy PD2011_061]. Ministry of Health, North Sydney.

NSW Parliament. Legislative Council, General Standing Committee No. 2. (2008). *The Management and Operations of the NSW Ambulance Service* [report 27]. NSW Parliament, Sydney.

Queensland Government. (2005). *Queensland Public Hospitals Commission of Inquiry* [Final Report]. Accessed January 2019 at <www.qphci.qld.gov.au/>.

Ray, S. (2006). Whistleblowing and organizational ethics. *Nursing Ethics, 13*(4), 438–45.

Reid-Searl, K., Moxham, L. & Happell, B. (2010). Enhancing patient safety: The importance of direct supervision for avoiding medication errors and near misses by undergraduate nursing students. *International Journal of Nursing Practice, 16*(3), 225–32.

Scheeder, F. (2006). Whistleblowers are not born that way—we create them through multiple system failures. *Journal of Healthcare Compliance*, July/August.

Sherif, M., Harvey, L., White, B., Hood, W. & Sherif, C. (1961) (reprinted in 1988). *The Robbers Cave Experiment: Intergroup Conflict and Cooperation*. Middletown, CT: University Press.

Siggall, H., Mucchi-Faina, A. & Mosso, C. (2006). Minority influence is facilitated when the communication employs linguistic abstractness. *Group Process & Intergroup Relations, 9*(3), 443–51.

Skiveness, M. & Trygstad, S. (2010). When whistle-blowing works: The Norwegian case. *Human Relations, 63*(7), 1071–97.

Stanley, D. (2011). *Clinical Leadership: Innovation into Action*. South Yarra, Victoria: Palgrave Macmillan.

Thomas, H. (2007). *Sick to Death: A Manipulative Surgeon and a Health System in Crisis—A Disaster Waiting to Happen*. Sydney, Australia: Allen & Unwin.

Varcoe, C., Pauly, B., Storch, J., Newton, L. & Makoroff, K. (2012). Nurses' perceptions of morally distressing situations. *Nursing Ethics, 19*(4), 488–500.

Wallis, L. (2015), Moral Distress in Nursing. *AJN The American Journal of Nursing, 115*(3), 19–20.

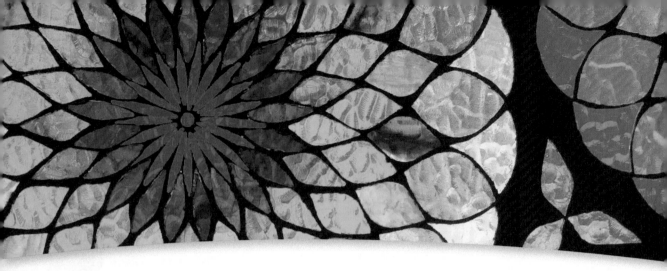

CHAPTER 22

CREATING SAFER
HEALTHCARE ORGANISATIONS

Joanne Travaglia   Deborah Debono

LEARNING OUTCOMES

Chapter 22 will enable you to:

- describe the goals and characteristics of safe, high-quality healthcare systems and healthcare organisations

- identify the organisational behaviours that foster safe high-quality healthcare

- discuss the levers that influence patient safety behaviours at different levels of the organisation

- discuss the importance of a population approach to patient safety, especially for people who are vulnerable to harm

- describe Safety-I and Safety-II approaches to patient safety, and how they relate to healthcare organisations.

KEY CONCEPTS

high-performing healthcare organisations | patient safety | quality care | culture | collegiality | communication | leadership | teamwork

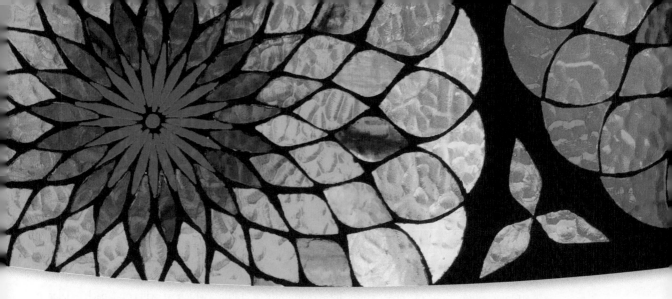

Improving the culture of safety within health care
is an essential component of preventing or reducing
errors and improving overall health care quality.

(AHRQ Patient Safety Network [PSNet], 2019)

INTRODUCTION

Health systems include people, actions and organisations with the common goal of improving, restoring or maintaining health (World Health Organization [WHO], 2007). This chapter focuses on one component of the health system—healthcare organisations—and in particular, what it takes for an organisation to function as a safe healthcare organisation.

What is a healthcare organisation?

Understanding how healthcare is organised is important when thinking about how healthcare can be made safer. Healthcare is organised in a series of concentric circles. Governments determine the funding for public healthcare, and also set regulatory requirements for organisations and professionals across both public and private healthcare. Accreditation and professional bodies determine and monitor standards. Public health systems operate within the frameworks established by government ministries and departments; private systems meet both public requirements and those of owners and/or shareholders. Services are delivered by individual organisations and/or networks of loosely or tightly linked providers. Formal and informal teams operate within and/or across disciplines, departments, units and/or locations. Lastly, individuals work with clients, patients, residents, families, carers, colleagues, supervisors and the public (including the media)—within the parameters of their individual and collective scope of practice and professional capabilities—directed by government, service and professional policies and guidelines.

Organisation is one of 'those' words, like community or culture (which we will come back to later in this chapter) that we all think we know the meaning of, but in reality, few people do. Davies (2003, p. 174) provides a succinct and useful definition for healthcare: 'Organisations are formally established goal-oriented structures with clear authority structures and boundaries.' Unpacking this definition provides us with more information about what organisations are, and helps us to understand the links to patient safety.

As *formally established* structures, organisations are more than just a group of people getting together (e.g. for the purpose of a train ride). Organisations are subject to rules and regulations, some internal and some external. They have purposes, practices, processes, life-spans, locations and histories. As *goal-oriented* structures, organisations have defined purposes that are (or should be) linked to defined and measurable outcomes. Having *clear authority structures* means that there are accountability and reporting pathways, and that these pathways flow upwards to an apex (be that to a minister of health or a chief executive officer, or both). Having *clear boundaries* means that specific organisations have specific remits—paediatric hospitals don't treat adults, laboratories don't do surgery, etc. Such boundaries are not immutable; they are a function of cultural and community expectations, and professional power and boundary negotiations.

It is common to limit the conceptualisation of organisations to the structural components. However, this approach fails to take into account what organisations *really* are, and what they do. As Grey (2017) argues, 'behind or beyond these abstractions are the lived experiences of people, not just working together, but joking, arguing, criticizing, fighting, deciding, lusting, despairing, creating, resisting, fearing, hoping or in short, organizing' (p. 2). In other words, organisations are also about communication, culture and collegiality (or more precisely, the relationships between colleagues) and can be understood in different ways. Mediating between what the structures are intended to achieve and what individuals actually do is the concept of culture, which seeks to describe the way in which organisational behaviour is shaped and motivated by communal expectations and sanctions (Braithwaite et al., 2017; Giorgi, Lockwood & Glynn, 2015).

Andy's story (see below) contrasts the approaches of two healthcare organisations in accommodating the specific needs of people with intellectual disability (ID) and/or autism spectrum disorder (ASD). It illustrates the importance of an organisational focus on, and implementation of, structures and processes that support the unique needs of different consumers for patient safety.

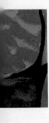

ANDY'S STORY

Andy is 17 years old and at the age of four was diagnosed with a moderate to severe ID and ASD. He also has a range of psychiatric and behavioural disorders. Andy's behaviour fluctuates with challenging, aggressive and violent outbursts. While he is non-verbal, it is possible to communicate with Andy using visuals such as hand signs and cards. Andy does not respond well to sensory over-stimulation. When the environment is noisy, chaotic, unpredictable or bright, it causes Andy pain, stress and confusion.

Andy lives in residential care in a group home, where he is cared for by a multidisciplinary specialist ID health team. This team coordinates and provides a range of community-based services that reduce the need for Andy to present to hospital. There is a strong relationship between these services and Andy's mother. All aspects of Andy's care follow a routine and are highly regulated—for example, Andy only takes his tablets with orange juice, and for lunch every day eats vegemite sandwiches with the crusts cut off.

Andy has episodes of suddenly-escalating, violent and self-injurious behaviour, which have required him to be taken to the emergency department (ED) at different hospitals. Mercy and Lakewood Hospitals are both large teaching hospitals that provide a wide variety of specialist healthcare services. Mercy Hospital has a hospital-centric administrative approach with limited networks to community services supporting people with ID. Lakewood Hospital is a disability community service-based hospital with strong links to multidisciplinary support services that specialise in the needs of people with ID. When people with ID need to be hospitalised, Lakewood Hospital enlists support from the healthcare team specialising in ID. This helps to provide person-centred care, build local capacity and implement processes and structures that cater for the unique needs of individuals with an ID.

Emergency departments are chaotic, bright, noisy and confusing, and make Andy distressed, anxious, panicky and agitated. Having to wait a long time in this over-stimulating and unfamiliar environment causes Andy's challenging behaviour to escalate and increases the chances of him lashing out. Andy's presentation at two different hospitals illustrates the impact of organisational approaches, structures and processes on patient safety.

Mercy Hospital: On Friday afternoon of a long weekend, Andy was taken to the ED at Mercy Hospital because his behaviour had become increasingly violent and the residential carers were unable to administer the medication he required. In the ED, with the bright halogen lights, noise and business, Andy began wailing, biting himself, spitting and lashing out. Security, nursing and medical staff worked to physically restrain Andy and administered different sedatives. Suddenly he stopped breathing; a cardiac arrest team was called; and Andy was intubated and transferred to intensive care unit where he remained overnight. When he woke up, Andy was transferred to a locked seclusion room in the psychiatric unit due to his challenging behaviour. During his admission, Andy's care deviated from his routine—he was served a variety of sandwiches for lunch and his medication was offered to him with apple juice. As a result, he refused to take his medications or eat, and continued to lash out. At the end of the long weekend, Andy's specialist ID team were contacted and recommended that he be discharged to his group home. His subsequent behaviours demonstrated that he had been highly traumatised by his experience.

Lakewood Hospital: Andy was taken to Lakewood ED some months later for the same reasons he had been taken to Mercy Hospital: increasingly violent behaviour and refusal to take medication. Unlike Mercy Hospital, this organisation had introduced improvements in the ED to manage presentations of people with ID and/or ASD in a person-centred way. For example, Lakewood Hospital had created a new field in the electronic medical record (EMR) that triggered an alternative triage process in ED and informed staff of Andy's particular needs. Rather than a noisy, bright, chaotic, over-stimulating ED triage room, Andy was taken to a quiet room to reduce sensory input and his stress. He was still agitated but did not need to be physically restrained. Andy was admitted to a quiet single room at the end of a ward. The location of the room meant that there was reduced stimulation for Andy and his mother was able to stay, comfort and interpret for him. From the point of admission, case conferences enabled Andy's caregivers—his mother, group home staff, hospital staff, and community and disability service staff—to discuss Andy's care and discharge planning. They recognised that Andy would respond negatively if he experienced delays when discharged so, rather than sit in a room waiting, as soon as it was advised that he would be discharged, transport was arranged to immediately return him to the group home. As a result of the processes outlined above, Andy settled back into his routine without the signs of trauma previously displayed when he was discharged from Mercy Hospital.

Source: Debono, D., Wille, J., Skalicky, D., Johnson, J., Leitner, R., & Chenoweth, B. (2015). Improving care for people with intellectual disability. In J. Johnson, H. Haskell, & P. Barach (Eds), *Case Studies in Patient Safety* (pp. 101–16). Burlington: Jones and Bartlett Learning.

The goals of safe, high-quality healthcare systems and organisations

The goal of health systems is to improve health and health equity in ways that are responsive, financially fair, and make the best, or most efficient, use of available resources (WHO, 2007, p. 2). Aligning with this, the main purpose of healthcare organisations is to provide high-quality, safe healthcare in a way that is responsive, fair and efficient. The Australian Safety and Quality Goals for Health Care (developed by the Australian Commission for Safety and Quality in Health Care [ACSQHC], 2018) are: safety of care, appropriateness of care, and partnering with consumers (see Table 22.1).

TABLE 22.1
The Australian Safety and Quality Goals for Healthcare in Australia

Goal	Goal described
Safety of care	People receive healthcare without experiencing preventable harm.
Appropriateness of care	People receive appropriate, evidence-based care.
Partnering with consumers	There are effective partnerships between consumers and healthcare providers and organisations at levels of healthcare provision, planning and evaluation.

Source: Australian Commission on Safety and Quality in Health Care. (2018). *Australian Safety and Quality Goals for Health Care.*

Along similar lines, the United States Committee on Quality of Health Care in America (Institute of Medicine, 2001) proposes six goals for healthcare systems, as summarised below and in Figure 22.1.

Safe healthcare organisations minimise adverse events (injuries, complications or deaths) arising from any aspect of care and make sure that quality of care is monitored and assured, all of the time. Systems for safety, such as double-checks and checklists, are in place; there are also systems for tracking adverse events and for disclosing them openly. All team members take responsibility for safety, and the organisation's communication systems maximise communication across units and professions.

Effective healthcare providers deliver appropriate care based on the best quality evidence available; there is a shared respect for science and evidence. As far as possible, the care of patients provides benefits to them, and avoids care that is not beneficial. Team members are committed to evidence-based and effective care, and their expertise is used to its maximum potential. Thus, staff members do not give treatment that is beyond their expertise or that could be better provided by another profession or person.

Person-centred organisations are respectful and responsive to each person's needs and preferences; the patient (and their family) is a partner and a key team member. Care is personalised, and there is full and appropriate communication with patients and between all members of the team, whatever their roles and wherever they are located. The expertise of all team members is valued as a part of optimal patient care.

Timely healthcare providers use systems to reduce waiting and delays in treatment as much as possible, so that patients are treated at the appropriate time. Furthermore, there is timely

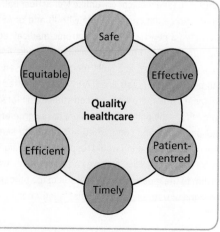

FIGURE 22.1 The six goals for healthcare systems in the United States

Source: Based on Institute of Medicine. (2001). *Crossing the Quality Chasm: A New Health System for the 21st Century.* Washington, DC: National Academy Press.

communication and information transfer to all members of the team, both inside and outside the organisation.

Efficient healthcare organisations avoid waste and duplication of care; essentially, they are cost-effective. The skills of all team members are used, with a good understanding of their expertise.

Equitable healthcare organisations provide care that is consistent in quality, regardless of patients' age, sex, location, socioeconomic status, ethnicity, and so forth. The organisation and its members show respect for all patients and healthcare professionals alike, and have systems to track any inequalities in care.

Characteristics of safe, high-quality healthcare systems and healthcare organisations

We have identified that organisations have defined goals, which differentiates them from a group of people who happen to be in the same place together but do not have a common goal. It is clear that patient safety is a primary goal of most healthcare systems and organisations. Structures within organisations are designed to achieve this goal and assess whether, and to what extent, it has been achieved by measuring performance on specific outcomes. Performance of healthcare organisations is assessed by adherence to evidence-based processes of care measures and risk-adjusted outcomes of care (Taylor et al., 2015, p. 2). While having appropriate structures in place is necessary to achieve defined goals, it is not enough. We know that factors such as culture and communication enable or undermine an organisation's ability to achieve its goals.

Characteristics of high-performing healthcare systems

According to the WHO (2007), in order to secure better health outcomes, health systems must be developed and strengthened. To this end, the WHO proposes six building blocks that are necessary for a healthcare system to perform well:

1   Good health services
2   A well-performing health workforce
3   A well-functioning health information system
4   Equitable access to cost-effective, good-quality, essential medical products, vaccines and technologies
5   Good health financing system
6   Good leadership and governance (WHO).

Good health services 'deliver effective, safe, quality, personal and non-personal health interventions to those that need them, when and where needed, with minimum waste of resources' (WHO, 2007, p. vi).

Characteristics of high performing healthcare organisations

The WHO's six building blocks help us to understand what is necessary for a healthcare system to perform well. What about healthcare organisations? What is necessary for a healthcare organisation to perform well and to provide safe care?

One way to determine this is to consider healthcare organisations that perform well (high-performing organisations) and to identify the characteristics that are common across them. High-performing healthcare organisations consistently achieve excellence in a range of measures across the organisation (Taylor et al., 2015) and these are sustained over time (Agins & Holden, 2007). Studies of high performing healthcare organisations have identified the following characteristics associated with sustained excellence: positive organisational culture; senior management support; effective performance monitoring; a proficient workforce; effective leaders across the organisation; expertise-driven practice; and interprofessional teamwork (Taylor et al., 2015). The interaction of these factors within a high-performing healthcare organisation is illustrated in Figure 22.2.

FIGURE 22.2
Characteristics
of a high-
performing
healthcare
organisation

Source: Taylor, N.,
Clay-Williams, R., Hog-
den, E., Braithwaite, J.
& Groene, O. (2015).
High performing hos-
pitals: a qualitative
systematic review of
associated factors
and practical strate-
gies for improvement.
*BMC health services
research, 15*(1), 244.

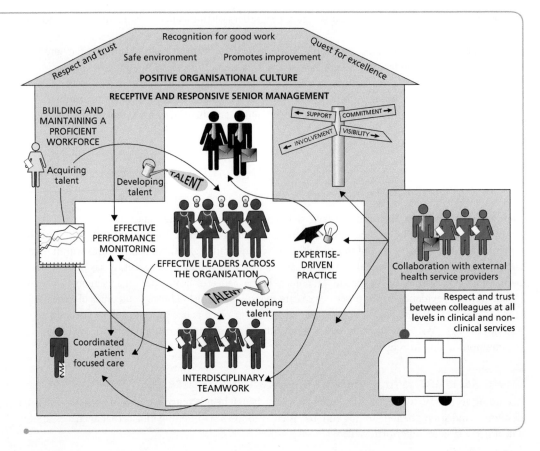

Organisational behaviours that foster safe high-quality healthcare

We will now consider four major elements in greater depth: culture, leadership, effective performance monitoring and interdisciplinary teamwork. One difference between a high-performing organisation and a group of people who are all interested in patient safety is that in high-performing organisations the behaviours across the organisation (i.e. individual behaviour, team behaviour, service behaviour and organisational behaviour) are all aligned.

Culture

There are many definitions of culture, but in general it can be defined as the espoused values and underlying assumptions that are learnt, passed on and shared within a group, which can be evidenced through the organisation's artefacts (including structures and processes) (Schein & Schein, 2017). Within an organisational culture are subcultures that may or may not align with each other and the overall culture of the organisation.

An expressed and specific focus on quality and safety has been identified as an integral characteristic of high-performing organisations. The positive culture of these organisations is demonstrated through: mutual respect and trust between clinical and non-clinical colleagues; a drive for excellence at every level; and vigilance across the organisation (Taylor et al., 2015). Recognition, rewards of good work and the freedom to innovate and 'speak up' also contribute to a positive culture (Taylor et al., 2015). Braithwaite et al. (2017, p. 1) found that, 'overall, positive organisational and workplace cultures were consistently associated with a wide range of patient outcomes such as reduced mortality rates, falls, hospital acquired infections and increased patient satisfaction'. However, subcultures within a healthcare organisation may differ in their attitudes and related practices about patient safety. These differences may individually and collectively undermine a positive organisational culture (Sirriyeh et al., 2012).

Leadership

Part of the positive culture in high-performing healthcare organisations is a responsive, receptive and supportive senior management and leadership. This is demonstrated by management's involvement and interaction with clinical and non-clinical staff across the organisation, and by their accessibility and visibility, along with an evident commitment to quality and safety (Taylor et al., 2015). Management teams play an important role in promoting and supporting a unified safety culture that is embedded across the organisation (Sirriyeh et al., 2012). According to Parand et al. (2014), senior management's activities that support patient safety and quality include: 'strategy, culture and data-centred activities, such as driving improvement culture and promotion of quality, strategy/goal setting and providing feedback. Significant positive associations with quality included compensation attached to quality, using quality improvement measures and having a . . . quality committee' (p. 1). Another important means of fostering a unified safety culture is with interprofessional training, in which teams work together to identify and solve patient safety problems (Sirriyeh et al., 2012).

Leadership does not simply equate with formal management roles and particularly not in the context of patient safety. The Francis Inquiry into Mid-Staffordshire Hospital found 'evidence of a large-scale failure of control and leadership at multiple levels' (Dixon-Woods et al., 2014, p. 2). As the Agency for Healthcare Research and Quality argues, 'although the concept of leadership has traditionally been used to refer to the top rungs of an organization, frontline workers and their immediate supervisors play a crucial leadership role in acting as change agents and promoting patient-centered care' (AHRQ PSNet, 2018).

Indeed in 2015, Peter Senge (who wrote one of the seminal books on learning organisations, *The Fifth Discipline*) announced the arrival of systems leadership, which he defined as arising from 'the deep changes necessary to accelerate progress against society's most intractable problems [that] require a unique type of leader—the system leader, a person who catalyses collective leadership' (Senge, Hamilton & Kania, 2015, p. 27). In other words, individual healthcare workers need to step up and practise in way that indicates that patient safety and quality improvement are every individual's responsibility. Further, every individual should expect that everyone they work with is equally accountable and active in ensuring that their organisation delivers safe, high-quality care.

Effective performance monitoring

Effective performance monitoring is associated with high-performing organisations. The characteristics of effective performance monitoring that have been identified as key include alignment of explicit goals to achieve good outcomes and collection of reliable data to allow for accurate measurement. According to Taylor et al. (2015) high-performing organisations value data systems that support monitoring and quality improvement. Importance lies in the active recognition of either poor or high staff performance, using individual and organisational outcome data, and data-informed feedback and continuous improvement (Taylor et al., 2015, pp. 15–22).

Interdisciplinary/interprofessional teamwork

Interdisciplinary (or interprofessional as it is more commonly known) teamwork has been the centre of many strategies to improve patient safety over the last decade (refer to Chapter 6). A single visit to a hospital requires many multidisciplinary teams to communicate effectively. The lack of interprofessional teamwork, and in particular effective interprofessional communication, has been implicated in large-scale patient safety inquiries, notably the Bristol Royal Infirmary Inquiry, that sparked the clinical governance movement in the UK and around the world (Hindle et al., 2006). Interprofessional collaboration and training help overcome the differences in disciplines' world views about patient safety (Travaglia et al., 2011). Effective interprofessional practice has been shown to improve patient safety, enhance the delivery of services, and improve health outcomes and treatment adherence for patients, particularly those with chronic diseases (Feldstain et al., 2018; Hall et al., 2011; WHO, 2009).

Levers that influence patient safety behaviours at different levels of the organisation

Since the US patient safety report 'To err is human' (Donaldson, Corrigan & Kohn, 2000) was published, most of the world's health systems have focused on quantifying and reducing medical errors, with mixed results. Although the error rates overall have not decreased, specific approaches have had success in reducing some types of errors (Mannion & Braithwaite, 2017). In a review of strategies to reduce medical errors, Singer and Vogus (2013, p. 375) identified groups of interventions that had been shown to improve safety culture and organisational behaviour. These include 'enabling' policies and practices that motivate the pursuit of safety, including *external actions* (e.g. accreditation and advocacy, surveys and rules around work hours) and *internal actions* (e.g. leadership behaviours, human resource practices and technology, such as electronic medical records). Singer and Vogus argue that these actions are translated into the organisation's *safety climate*—or the 'frontline interpretations of safety-related leader actions and organizational practices', which include: inter-personal processes such as effective teamwork; the ability to report and voice concerns; and the co-ordination of care at transitions (such as handovers) and across independent functions (through the use of checklists).

These types of activities are said to strengthen the safety culture; in other words, the values, attitudes, shared assumptions and patterns of behaviour that ideally become embedded in organisations as their 'way of doing things'. Safety culture is further strengthened by 'elaborating' or learning practices that reinforce safe behaviours, such as learning-oriented interventions, education (including simulation), operational improvements through case-based analysis and frontline systems improvement, and prospective, retrospective and concurrent systems monitoring (Singer & Vogus, 2013).

A population approach to patient safety

Because of the nature of medical errors, much of the focus of the patient safety movement has been on tertiary care, with more recent awareness of errors in primary and community healthcare systems. Attention largely focuses on errors of *commission* (or what goes wrong in an intervention). The latest field of patient safety goes even further. It considers the causes of ill health and the factors (economic, social, cultural and historical) that might prevent ill health in certain groups and communities, as well as preventing individuals and groups from accessing and utilising the care they require; in other words, there's a focus on the errors of *omission*.

This perspective, pioneered by health systems and services such as the Southcentral Foundation in Alaska (https://www.southcentralfoundation.com) and the Camden Coalition (https://www.camden-health.org) in New Jersey, have redesigned healthcare system delivery from the ground up and integrated service delivery, including social prescribing (which seeks to improve people's living conditions and prevent illness rather than focusing on curing once it has occurred). Southcentral provides services through interprofessional teams that work together in 'pods' providing constant interaction between team members. Co-location of these teams supports ongoing communication and reduces the risk of miscommunication about the people under their care.

Patient Safety-I and patient Safety-II approaches

The traditional approach to improving patient safety, *Safety-I*, defines safety as the absence of accidents or incidents (Raben et al., 2018). This view holds that identifiable problems (failures, errors, malfunctions)—including technology, procedures and humans working in the system—are the reason things go wrong. Safety, therefore, can be achieved by identifying and removing the causes of unacceptable risks in the system. This view assumes that the components of a system work together either correctly or incorrectly and does not account for the fact that healthcare organisations are complex and adaptive systems (Hollnagel, Wears & Braithwaite, 2015). Safety-I focuses on when human performance goes wrong rather than when it goes right. In contrast, *Safety-II*, a more recent view of safety which is informed by resilience engineering, defines safety as 'the ability to succeed under varying conditions, so that the number of intended and acceptable outcomes is as high as possible' (Hollnagel, 2018). This

Safety-II defines safety as 'the ability to succeed under varying conditions, so that the number of intended and acceptable outcomes is as high as possible' (Erik Hollnagel, 2018).

approach seeks to increase the number of things that go right (Hollnagel et al., 2015). Safety-II 'assumes that everyday performance variability provides the adaptations that are needed to respond to varying conditions, and hence is the reason why things go right' (Hollnagel et al., p. 4).

One of the implications for healthcare organisations of a Safety-II view is the necessity of understanding how care is actually delivered safely. Most of the time, interventions designed to improve patient safety are based on how organisations *imagine* their staff do their work (work-as-imagined) rather than how they *really* do their work (work-as-done). Safety-II holds that organisations need to understand how healthcare professionals adjust and adapt to accommodate constant changes. Given the complexity of healthcare systems, we need to balance the use of both Safety-I and Safety-II approaches to improve patient safety.

Conclusion

Safe healthcare organisations are characterised by processes and structures that support a positive culture that strives to deliver safe and excellent care. Effective leadership that fosters open communication between patients, carers, staff, teams and departments across the organisation is pivotal. Delivery of safe care requires communication within and between organisations. Boundaries between healthcare organisations must be traversed. This involves active communication between those who work within acute healthcare, community organisations, the person receiving care, and their carers. To provide safe and high-quality care, organisations must value what is important for patients/consumers and their carers from their perspectives. Communication must be provided in a way whereby the consumers and carers can understand it. To be effective, healthcare organisations must 'organise' in a way that supports communication and takes into account the needs of those communicating, including patients, carers and staff.

Critical thinking activities

Charles is a 46-year-old man who has an acquired brain injury resulting in an intellectual disability (ID). Charles experiences difficulties understanding instructions, is unable to read and write, and has difficulties retaining short-term memory. He does not like to be in a confined space. Charles has a dry sense of humour, enjoys meeting people, and likes to play sport and drive a car. He lives with his mother and father who understand what he is trying to communicate and act as interpreters for him. This includes checking that Charles has understood information given to him and has been understood by those with whom he is communicating. When he cannot make himself understood Charles gets frustrated, raises his voice and then withdraws.

At around lunchtime on a Wednesday in May, Charles was assaulted in the street near his home. He was pushed into the gutter and his leg jumped on, fracturing his tibia and fibula. Charles was taken by ambulance and admitted to Nightingale Hospital.

Charles has had several admissions to Nightingale Hospital and each time his mother and father have asked for it to be recorded in his notes that they hold power of attorney and are enduring guardians for him. They have also asked for it to be documented that his parents must be present during consultations with Charles so that they can support clear and effective communication by helping him to understand the information he is given, and ensuring the healthcare providers understand what Charles is communicating to them. That is, Charles' parents need to be involved in communication between Charles and the healthcare providers when information is being exchanged.

However, while his parents were not there, Charles was taken to the operating theatre where the fractures in his leg were stabilised. Charles' parents were not informed that he was going into surgery. After four hours in the operating theatre, Charles was moved to the ward. He woke after the operation to find his leg was plastered and he could not get out of bed. The next day, the physiotherapists put a 'moon boot' on Charles, and explained how to put it on and how to inflate the boot for comfort. Charles' parents were again not with him when this communication of information occurred.

When his parents arrived at the hospital, Charles was agitated and confused because he did not know what the moon boot was and why it was on his leg. He repeatedly tried to pull the boot off. Charles' parents could not explain nor pacify him because they did not know what the moon boot was for and they were confused about who they should talk to. They asked the nurse looking after Charles, and then the doctor, and then the dietician, and then any staff member who came to Charles' bedside, if they could speak to the person who had put on the moonboot. They wanted to understand so they could explain to Charles what was happening and why he needed to keep the boot on.

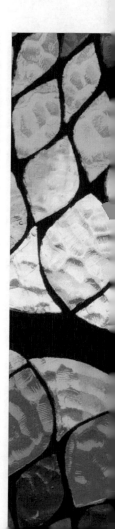

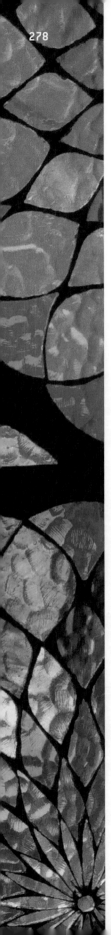

Three hours later, the physiotherapists brought crutches to Charles and tried to explain how to use them. He was told not to weight bear or get the moon boot or plaster wet. But because Charles was still agitated and confused about the moon boot, he found it difficult to concentrate on the instructions being provided by the physiotherapist about using the crutches. His parents were not included in the conversation despite repeatedly highlighting that they could assist with interpreting the information in a way that Charles could understand.

Charles was prescribed daily Clexane injections for ten days and a nurse explained how he should self-administer the injections at home. Again, Charles' parents were not included in the conversation and, until they read the discharge summary, had no idea that he would require injections or how to administer them. Charles was discharged three days after his admission and it was clear at this time that he did not know how to use the crutches correctly or how to self-administer his Clexane injections.

Because of his ID, Charles has trouble remembering instructions over a period of time. He was unable to self-administer the Clexane, his moon boot and plaster got wet in the shower and when he was allowed out of bed, Charles inconsistently and incorrectly ambulated with the crutches offering little support. Rather than using the crutches to bear his weight, Charles was semi-weight-bearing on his broken leg.

1   What are some potential implications of Charles not having understood the instructions and information communicated to him?
2   Who were the people involved in Charles' care, both during and following his admission to hospital?
3   How might the Nightingale Hospital have better supported effective communication between staff, patients and carers during the hospital stay?
4   How might communication with Charles and his parents have better prepared them for his discharge? (Consider whether the information about what to expect and do at home was explained.)
5   Charles' care in the hospital and community involved a multidisciplinary team. How might they have communicated better following Charles' discharge?

Teaching and assessment activity

In this activity, students should be instructed to work in teams of about five people. With reference to Andy's story (page 270) and Charles' story (above), teams should discuss strategies that might need to be implemented if their organisation was going to move to a Safety-II approach?

Students can compare the strategies of other teams, identifying who focused on knowing more about Andy and Charles (and their families) and who focused on learning more about the organisations' capabilities? Then, as a class, discuss the following questions:

1   What are the pluses and minuses of each approach?
2   Having heard from each team, which strategies or approaches would you prioritise?
3   Which strategies or approaches do you think would have the biggest impact on the services' culture?
4   What strategies or approaches do you think would have the biggest impact on the patients' quality and safety of care?
5   How important is it to see patients and their families as part of the 'team'?

Further reading

Braithwaite, J., Herkes, J., Ludlow, K., Testa, L. & Lamprell, G. (2017). Association between organisational and workplace cultures, and patient outcomes: systematic review. *BMJ Open*, 7(11), e017708.

Dellve, L., Strömgren, M., Williamsson, A., Holden, R. J. & Eriksson, A. (2018). Health care clinicians' engagement in organizational redesign of care processes: The importance of work and organizational conditions. *Applied ergonomics*, 68, 249–57.

Hollnagel, E., Braithwaite, J. & Wears, R. L. (Eds). (2018). *Delivering Resilient Health Care*. Routledge.

Hollnagel, E., Wears, R. L. & Braithwaite, J. (2015). *From Safety-I to Safety-II: A White Paper*. The resilient health care net: published simultaneously by the University of Southern Denmark, University of Florida, USA, and Macquarie University, Australia.

Johnson, J., Haskell, H. & Barach, P. (Eds). (2015). *Case Studies in Patient Safety*. Burlington, Jones and Bartlett Learning.

Web resources

Macquaire University: Practical-strategies: This resource provides an interactive demonstration of specific strategies that might be used to achieve the characteristics of a high-performing organisation.
<http://aihi.mq.edu.au/resource/practical-strategies>

US Department of Health and Human Services, Agency for Healthcare Research and Quality, PSNet: Highlights the latest patient safety literature, news and expert

commentary, including weekly updates, WebM&M and patient safety primers.
<https://psnet.ahrq.gov/>

Southcentral Foundation, Nuka System of Care
<https://www.southcentralfoundation.com/nuka-system-of-care/>

Safety and quality of health care: A website by the Australian Institute of Health and Welfare with useful links to safety and quality definitions, statistics, resources and international trends.
<https://www.aihw.gov.au/>

References

AHRQ Patient Safety Network (PSNet). (2019). *Culture of Safety*. Accessed January 2019 at <https://psnet.ahrq.gov/primers/primer/5>.

AHRQ Patient Safety Network (PSNet). (2018). *Leadership Role in Improving Patient Safety*. Accessed September 2018 at <https://psnet.ahrq.gov/primers/primer/32/leadership-role-in-improving-safety>.

Agins, B. D. & Holden, M. M. (2007). Defining a high performance healthcare organisation. *BMJ: British Medical Journal*, *335*(7629), 1055.

Australian Commission on Safety and Quality in Health Care. (2018). *Australian Safety and Quality Goals for Health Care*. Sydney, Australia: ACSQHC. Accessed January 2019 at <https://www.safetyandquality.gov.au/national-priorities/goals/>.

Braithwaite, J., Herkes, J., Ludlow, K., Testa, L. & Lamprell, G. (2017). Association between organisational and workplace cultures, and patient outcomes: systematic review. *BMJ Open*, *7*(11). doi:10.1136/bmjopen-2017-017708

Davies, C. (2003). Some of our concepts are missing: reflections on the absence of a sociology of organisations in Sociology of Health and Illness. *Sociology of Health & Illness*, *25*(3), 172–190.

Dixon-Woods, M., Baker, R., Charles, K., Dawson, J., Jerzembek, G., Martin, G., . . . West, M. (2014). Culture and behaviour in the English National Health Service: Overview of lessons from a large multimethod study. *BMJ Qual Saf*, *23*, 106–15. doi:10.1136/bmjqs-2013-001947

Donaldson, M. S., Corrigan, J. M. & Kohn, L. T. (2000). *To Err Is Human: Building a Safer Health System*. Washington, DC: National Academies Press (US).

Feldstain, A., Bultz, B. D., de Groot, J., Abdul-Razzak, A., Herx, L., Galloway, L., . . . Sinnarajah, A. (2018). Outcomes From a Patient-Centered, Interprofessional, Palliative Consult Team in Oncology. *Journal of the National Comprehensive Cancer Network*, *16*(6), 719–26.

Giorgi, S., Lockwood, C. & Glynn, M. A. (2015). The Many Faces of Culture: Making Sense of 30 Years of Research on Culture in Organization Studies. *The Academy of Management Annals*, *9*(1), 1–54. doi:10.1080/19416520.2015.1007645

Grey, C. (2017). *A Very Short Fairly Interesting and Reasonably Cheap Book about Studying Organizations*. London: Sage.

Hall, D., Buchanan, J., Helms, B., Eberts, M., Mark, S., Manolis, C., . . . Docimo, A. (2011). Health care expenditures and therapeutic outcomes of a pharmacist managed anticoagulation service versus usual medical care. *Pharmacotherapy: The Journal of Human Pharmacology and Drug Therapy*, *31*(7), 68694.

Hindle, D., Braithwaite, J., Travaglia, J. & Iedema, R. (2006). *Patient Safety: A Comparative Analysis of Eight Inquiries in Six Countries*. Sydney, Australia: Centre for Clinical Governance Research, Faculty of Medicine, University of NSW.

Hollnagel, E. (2018). *Safety-I and Safety-II: The Past and Future of Safety Management*. CRC Press.

Hollnagel, E., Wears, R. L. & Braithwaite, J. (2015). *From Safety-I to Safety-II: A White Paper*. The resilient health care net: published simultaneously by the University of Southern Denmark, University of Florida, USA, and Macquarie University, Australia.

Institute of Medicine. (2001). *Crossing the Quality Chasm: A New Health System for the 21st Century*. Washington, DC: National Academy Press.

Mannion, R. & Braithwaite, J. (2017). False dawns and new horizons in patient safety research and practice. *International Journal of Health Policy and Management*, *6*(12), 685.

Parand, A., Dopson, S., Renz, A. & Vincent, C. (2014). The role of hospital managers in quality and patient safety: a systematic review. *BMJ Open*, *4*(9), e005055.

Raben, D. C., Bogh, S. B., Viskum, B., Mikkelsen, K. L. & Hollnagel, E. (2018). Learn from what goes right: a demonstration of a new systematic method for identification of leading indicators in healthcare. *Reliability Engineering & System Safety*, *169*, 187–98.

Schein, E. & Schein, P. (2017). *Organisational Culture and Leadership* (5th edn). Hoboken, NJ: Wiley.

Senge, P., Hamilton, H. & Kania, J. (2015). The Dawn of System Leadership. *Stanford Social Innovation Review*, Winter, 26–33.

Singer, S. J. & Vogus, T. J. (2013). Reducing hospital errors: interventions that build safety culture. *Annual Review of Public Health*, *34*(1), 373–96.

Sirriyeh, R., Lawton, R., Armitage, G., Gardner, P. & Ferguson, S. (2012). Safety subcultures in health-care organizations and managing medical error. *Health Services Management Research*, *25*(1), 16–23.

Taylor, N., Clay-Williams, R., Hogden, E., Braithwaite, J. & Groene, O. (2015). High performing hospitals: a qualitative systematic review of associated factors and practical strategies for improvement. *BMC Health Services Research*, *15*(1), 244.

Travaglia, J. F., Nugus, P. I., Greenfield, D., Westbrook, J. I. & Braithwaite, J. (2011). Visualising differences in professionals' perspectives on quality and safety. *BMJ Quality & Safety*, *21*(9), 778–83.

World Health Organization. (2009). *Framework for Action on Interprofessional Education and Collaborative Practice*. Geneva, Switzerland: WHO.

World Health Organization. (2007). *Everybody's Business— Strengthening Health Systems to Improve Health Outcomes: WHO's Framework for Action*. Geneva, Switzerland: WHO.

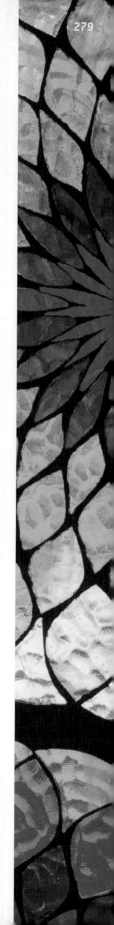

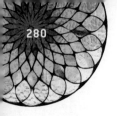

Glossary

Note: For many of these terms there are multiple definitions. The definitions here are those that are used and referenced throughout this book.

Aboriginal and Torres Strait Islander people People who are of Aboriginal or Torres Strait Islander descent, identify as such, and are accepted as such by their local community.

advanced care planning A process of communication and discussion about end-of-life care involving the person, those closest to them and their care providers, in which the person prepares for future scenarios and makes known their values concerning such issues as their quality of life, prognosis and wishes for future care.

advanced care directive A written, legally binding document (sometimes called a 'living will') in which a person consents to or refuses specific medical treatments or interventions, and that comes into effect at a future time when the person no longer has the capacity to make and communicate those decisions.

adverse drug reaction A response to a medication that is harmful and unintended, and occurs at normal doses.

ageism Prejudice or discrimination on the grounds of a person's age.

aggression The expression of anger in either actual or threatened violence.

augmentative and alternative communication (AAC) Strategies and systems that are used in combination with speech or in place of speech to enable a person to communicate.

Australian Open Disclosure Framework A nationally consistent approach for respectful communication following adverse events in all healthcare settings.

Balint group An experiential, small group educational activity in which healthcare professionals discuss cases from their practices with a focus on the clinician–patient relationship or health professional–client relationship.

caring Showing concern for or kindness to another person; the ability to create an emotional connection with patients.

clinical handover Transfer of professional responsibility and accountability for some or all aspects of care for a patient to another person or professional group on a temporary or permanent basis.

clinical reasoning A broad term denoting the thinking, judgments and decision making involved in clinical practice; the process by which clinicians collect cues, process the information, come to an understanding of a patient problem or situation, plan and implement interventions, evaluate outcomes, and reflect on and learn from the process.

collegiality Companionship and cooperation between colleagues who share responsibility for quality healthcare and patient outcomes.

communication A two-way interaction where information, meanings and feelings are shared both verbally and nonverbally, and when the message being conveyed is understood as intended.

communication impairment Difficulty in the use or understanding of speech and language that make it difficult for a person to communicate.

communication partner Anyone who talks or interacts with another person; this means we can all be communication partners.

co-morbidity The presence of one or more additional diseases or disorders co-occurring with a primary disease or disorder.

complex communication need (CCN) When a person has little or no speech and/or difficulty understanding the speech of others, and requires additional support in order to be able to participate in the process of communication.

conscious bias A particular tendency, trend or inclination, especially one that is preconceived or unreasonable.

critical conversations A verbal interaction that signals the need for immediate attention, addresses a situation that has caused (or could cause) patient (or staff) harm, or that focuses attention on practices or processes that call for improvement.

critical thinking A complex collection of cognitive skills and affective habits of the mind.

cultural awareness A recognition that people are not all alike; they have different values, different behaviours and different approaches to life; it includes knowledge and understanding of other people's cultures.

cultural competence A set of congruent behaviours, attitudes and policies that come together in a system, agency or professional group to enable that system, that agency or those professionals to work effectively in cross-cultural situations.

cultural diversity The existence of a variety of cultural or ethnic groups within a society.

cultural empathy The learnt ability to appreciate or imagine experiences through the unique lens of values, beliefs and perspectives of people from cultural backgrounds different to one's own.

cultural security Actively ensuring that cultural needs are met for all individuals, and in particular that cultural needs are included in policies and practices so that all people have access to safe and quality care in all contexts.

culturally and linguistically diverse (CALD) People from culturally and linguistically diverse backgrounds.

culture Ways of thinking and behaving that are socially accepted among a particular group or society.

culture of safety Safe performance in clinical care; the collective product of individual and group values and attitudes, competencies and patterns of behaviours in safety performance.

cycle of aggression Typically considered to start with a triggering event, then the subsequent escalation phase of verbal or physical aggression, and finally a recovery phase.

de-escalation A complex, interactive process in which a patient is directed towards a calmer 'personal space' through effective communication, identifying the patient's stressors, and providing functional alternatives to aggression.

delirium An acute confusional state that develops over a short period of time (usually hours to days) and tends to fluctuate during the course of the day.

diagnostic overshadowing A process where healthcare professionals wrongly presume that present physical symptoms are a consequence of their patient's mental illness; as a result, the patient with mental illness gets inadequate diagnosis or treatment.

effective leadership Leadership that is based on empowerment and change, challenging the status quo, creating a new vision and exciting the creative and emotional drives of individuals to strive beyond the ordinary to deliver the exceptional.

empathy The capacity for participating in and understanding the feelings or ideas of another; it involves cognitive, affective and behavioural elements.

end-of-life care A total and holistic approach to the care needs of people with a progressive, life-limiting prognosis.

end-of-life decision making A model of collaborative decision making by patients, families and physicians that focuses on the patient's interests, values and goals of care.

engagement The start of effective communication; when healthcare professionals engage effectively, patients feel a connection has been made with somebody trustworthy, that they are respected and valued as individuals, and that their needs are going to be met.

ethical leadership Leadership that is directed by respect for ethical beliefs and values and for the dignity and rights of others; it is related to concepts such as trust, honesty, consideration and fairness.

failure to rescue Mortality of patients who experience a hospital-acquired complication.

family-centred care A philosophy of a collaborative partnership between parents/carers and healthcare professionals; an approach that takes into account that each family is unique, and that the family is the constant in the child's life and the experts on his or her needs.

genuineness To be human or authentic.

Health Care Complaints Commission (HCCC) An independent body that deals with complaints about health professionals and healthcare services in New South Wales.

health literacy Health literacy refers to how people understand information about health and healthcare, and how they use that information to make decisions.

hierarchy A layered social structure that conceptualises superior and subordinate relationships in rank order; often depicted graphically; for example, in an organisational chart.

In healthcare, the 'clinical pecking order' is an example of an informal hierarchy.

holistic care A comprehensive model of caring that treats the whole person: mind, body and spirit.

interprofessional collaboration The intentional development of effective interprofessional working relationships with learners, practitioners, patients, their families and communities to enable optimal health outcomes.

interprofessional communication Occurs when healthcare professionals communicate with each other in an open, collaborative and respectful manner.

intrapersonal communication An internal process of communication (e.g. interpretation of messages from others, determining goals and tactics, self-assurance, self-discovery, and reflections on interactions with others).

leadership A collective cultural activity that is shared across all levels of an organisation.

life-limiting illness A term used to describe an incurable condition that will shorten a person's life, though they may continue to live active lives for many years.

linguistic diversity Differences in the language and linguistic traits—including grammar, syntax, vocabulary and verbal expression—of individuals and cultures.

medication incidents A mistake with medication, or a problem that could cause a mistake with medication.

mindful dialogue framework A model that allows healthcare professionals to reflect on their practice and the ways in which they empower patients/clients to co-construct an optimal quality of life.

mindfulness Focused attention and awareness; the awareness that emerges through paying attention on purpose, in the present moment, and non-judgmentally to the unfolding of experiences moment by moment.

moral distress The stress associated with the moral dimensions of practice due to inconsistency between one's values and one's actions.

non-verbal communication Behaviours and elements of speech that transmit meaning without the use of words; for example, pitch, speed, tone and volume of voice, gestures and facial expressions, body posture, and eye movements.

Noongar Aboriginal people whose traditional country is in the south-west corner of Western Australia.

open disclosure Health professional(s) communicating to the patient an explanation for what happened, an apology, a plan for the patient, and a practice improvement plan.

palliative care An approach that improves the quality of life for patients and families facing problems associated with life-threatening illness, through the prevention and relief of suffering by means of early identification, assessment and treatment of pain and other problems, physical, psychosocial and spiritual.

partnership Healthcare professionals working with patients to seek common goals and outcomes satisfactory

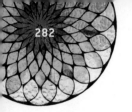

to all; partnership is an approach that seeks mutual understanding, consensus and an alignment, rather than a confrontational, authoritarian or paternalistic approach.

patient advocates Trained professionals who accompany patients to medical appointments in order to ask questions, explain disease concepts and treatment options, and provide patients with the confidence that someone is looking out for their health and wellbeing. Patient advocates are independent of any employer constraints and are typically medically savvy and health literate.

patient safety Actions undertaken by individuals and organisations to protect healthcare recipients from being harmed by their healthcare; an attribute of trustworthy healthcare systems that work to minimise the incidence and impact of, and maximise recovery from, adverse events.

patient-safe communication A goal-oriented activity focused on preventing adverse events and helping patients attain optimal health outcomes. It is a means by which health professionals gather and share information, clarify and verify accurate interpretations of information, and establish a process for working collaboratively with both patients and other healthcare professionals to achieve common goals of safe and high-quality patient care.

patient-safety incident Any unplanned or unintended event or circumstance which could have resulted or did result in harm to a patient; this includes harm from an outcome of an illness or its treatment that did not meet the patient's or the clinician's expectation for improvement or cure.

person-/patient-centred care A holistic approach to the planning, delivery and evaluation of healthcare that is grounded in mutually beneficial partnerships between healthcare professionals, patients and families. It is built on the understanding that patients bring their own experiences, skills and knowledge about their condition and illness; and that patients' perspectives (concerns, ideas and expectations) about their illness are as important as their physical examination and past medical history.

polypharmacy The concurrent use of multiple medications by a patient, especially for the treatment of a single disease.

professional identity A set of beliefs, attitudes and understandings about one's professional role and work activities.

reciprocity Mutuality of patient-care roles; it involves sharing of information with other healthcare professionals from different disciplines, and relies on goodwill towards others.

recovery (from the perspective of the individual with mental illness) Gaining and retaining hope, understanding of one's abilities and disabilities, engagement in an active life, personal autonomy, social identity, meaning and purpose in life, and a positive sense of self.

reflection A critical review of practice with a view to refinement, improvement or change; the process of looking back and the careful consideration of an experience; to explore the understanding of what one did and why, and the impact it has on one's self and others.

reflexivity Looking at *self* and changing in response to these reflections; it involves individuals reflecting on and monitoring their own actions.

religiosity A comprehensive sociological term used to refer to an organised system of beliefs and the numerous aspects of religious activity; it often includes certain rituals, retelling certain stories, prayer, worship, revering certain symbols, or accepting certain doctrines about deities and the afterlife.

respect A broad and complex term encompassing intentions, attitudes and behaviours towards people; it is related to people's differences as well as their inherent value as humans.

responsiveness Making situationally appropriate and contextually relevant adjustments; it involves the constant modifications that healthcare professionals make to their interactions as they deal with changes, unpredictabilities and uncertainties of practice.

self-awareness Being consciously aware of one's thoughts, feelings, beliefs, biases, assumptions, prejudices and values, and how they might influence and/or interfere with the ability to convey or hear a message as intended, or to interpret a situation or another person's perspective.

separation anxiety Children's experience of fear and anxiety in response to being parted from their family.

severe communication impairment (SCI) Situations where people have little or no intelligible speech.

social exclusion Exclusion from the prevailing social system and its rights and privileges, typically as a result of poverty or the fact of belonging to a minority social group.

socialisation of professional roles The process through which students and newcomers learn the roles, common values, problem-solving approaches and language of their profession.

spiritual care Healthcare that attends to spiritual and religious needs brought on by an illness or injury.

spiritual distress A disruption in a person's belief or value system and the impaired ability to experience and integrate meaning and purpose in life.

spirituality A core dimension of the human experience; an inner resource that helps people face illness and life-threatening events; often about a search for meaning or inner peace; it is an elusive, private and subjective term without a clear and consistent definition.

stigma A social process whereby an individual or a group is defined by society as deviant, other, different or dangerous.

team A group of people who do collective work and are mutually committed to a common purpose.

teamwork Working with a shared purpose, coordination of effort, exchange of resources and ability to adapt to change.

therapeutic communication Demonstrating care, genuine concern, empathy and interest in the patient as a unique individual by actively listening (hearing, understanding and believing the patient).

therapeutic presence The act of intentionally bringing one's whole self into the interaction with a patient; being fully

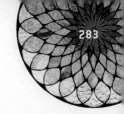

present and in a position to communicate in a way that is beneficial for the patient.

trauma-informed care A strengths-based framework grounded in an understanding of and responsiveness to the impact of trauma that emphasises physical, psychological and emotional safety for everyone, and that creates opportunities for survivors to rebuild a sense of control and empowerment.

unconscious bias Negative and positive stereotypes that exist in our subconscious and affect our decisions, behaviours and interactions with others.

validation Substantiating or confirming a person's position or feelings; it requires the healthcare professional to communicate to the person that their responses make sense and are understandable within their current situation.

verbal aggression Verbal abuse, threats and swearing.

verbal communication The use of words to convey an intended message and associated feelings.

violence The intentional use of physical force or power, threatened or actual, against one's self, another person, or a group or community, which results in or has a high likelihood of resulting in injury, death, psychological harm, maldevelopment or deprivation.

whistle-blowing When an individual or a group of employees cross organisational boundaries and take their concerns to the general public, media or regulatory bodies.

zero tolerance of violence The policy or practice of not tolerating violence, which ensures that in all violent incidents appropriate action is consistently taken to protect health service staff, patients and visitors, and health service property, from the effects of such behaviour.

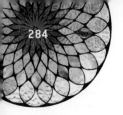

Index

Note: *Italicised* page numbers indicate figures, tables or boxes.

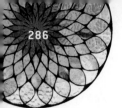

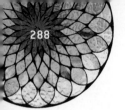